ALTERNATIVE MEDICINE

THE CHRISTIAN HANDBOOK

This book is designed to give information on various medical conditions, treatments, and procedures for your personal knowledge and to help you be a more informed consumer of medical and health services. It is not intended to be complete or exhaustive, nor is it a substitute for the advice of your physician. You should seek medical care promptly for any specific medical condition or problem your child may have. Under no circumstances should medication of any kind be administered to your child without first checking with your physician.

All efforts have been made to ensure the accuracy of the information contained in this book as of the date published. The authors and the publisher expressly disclaim responsibility for any adverse effects arising from the use or application of the information contained herein.

ALTERNATIVE MEDICINE

THE CHRISTIAN HANDBOOK

Dónal O'Mathúna, Ph.D., & Walt Larimore, M.D.

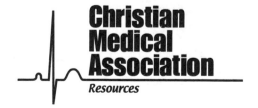

ZondervanPublishingHouse

Grand Rapids, Michigan

A Division of HarperCollinsPublishers

Alternative Medicine
Copyright © 2001 by Dónal O'Mathúna and Walter L. Larimore

Requests for information should be addressed to:

🏭ZondervanPublishingHouse
Grand Rapids, Michigan 49530

Library of Congress Cataloging-in-Publication Data
O'Mathúna, Dónal, 1961-.
    Alternative medicine : the Christian handbook / Dónal O'Mathúna, and Walt Larimore.
      p.   cm.
    Includes bibliographical references and index.
    ISBN: 0-310-23584-7
    1. Alternative medicine—Religious aspects—Christianity—Handbooks, manuals, etc. 2. Holistic medicine—
Religious aspects—Christianity—Handbooks, manuals, etc. I. Larimore, Walter L. II. Title.
R733.O48 2001
615.5-dc 21
                         2001017948
                              CIP

All Scripture quotations, unless otherwise indicated, are taken from the *Holy Bible: New International Version*®. NIV®. Copyright © 1973, 1978, 1984 by International Bible Society. Used by permission of Zondervan Publishing House. All rights reserved.

All rights reserved. No part of this publication may be reproduced, stored in a retrieval system, or transmitted in any form or by any means—electronic, mechanical, photocopy, recording, or any other—except for brief quotations in printed reviews, without the prior permission of the publisher.

Interior design by Todd Sprague

Printed in the United States of America

01 02 03 04 05 /❖ DC/ 10 9 8 7 6 5 4 3 2 1

To Dónal's parents

Mom, you exemplify true love in your unwavering care for Dad in his illness.

Dad, your strength and courage are a powerful example to us all.

CONTENTS

Chapter 13: Herbal Remedies, Vitamins, and Dietary Supplements 288

Chapter 14: Effectiveness of Therapies: Listed by Disease or Symptom 466

Foreword

DAVID STEVENS, M.D.

Have you ever noticed that the more we learn about health, the more complicated our lives become?

Scientific knowledge is increasing at a logarithmic rate. More knowledge means more options. Making choices—especially about something as important as our health—produces anxiety and stress.

Not only do we have to make a choice, we also have to evaluate the trustworthiness of each messenger and the validity of the message. What is the real motivation of the messenger? Is it to make money or a true altruistic motive? Have others verified the evidence?

Helping Christians Discern Truth and Make God-Honoring Decisions

Christians have yet another task. They must evaluate their choices in light of "What would Jesus do?"

With the explosion of health care knowledge has come a plethora of ethical and spiritual issues. Some are obvious ethical issues such as abortion, physician-assisted suicide, and human cloning.

Other issues facing Christians are not as obvious. How would Jesus have me deal with cancer or some other life-threatening illness? Should I select my treatment based solely on how well I think it might work, or do spiritual issues impact some of those decisions? Must I always pursue *some* treatment? What does it mean to die well? How should I prepare myself and my loved ones for my death?

You may feel there are more questions than answers. Most Christians do. As a physician who has cared for and counseled with tens of thousands of patients, I understand your confusion. You want and need a trusted expert to assist you.

That is why the Christian Medical Association has joined with Zondervan to produce a series of resources on health care issues. Resources you can trust. Each resource will be authored by one or more carefully chosen experts who are eminently qualified to give you guidance. They will provide solid scientific information in language you can understand.

Most importantly, our authors will present and evaluate your choices from a Christian world view. Then you can make God-honoring decisions.

What Is the Christian Medical Association?

The Christian Medical Association (CMA) is a *movement* of Christian doctors. The ministry was established in 1931 to help Christian health care professionals integrate their personal faith and professional practice.

Today, the Christian Medical Association helps thousands of members integrate faith and practice in hospitals and clinics, private practices, on the mission field, and in academic institutions. Presently, 93 percent of medical schools in the United States have a CMA student chapter that helps students from the first day of classes begin to integrate their faith and profession. Our goal is to help members become like the Great Physician, Jesus Christ.

The Christian Medical Association also holds conferences, produces resources, and develops positions on some of the tough ethical issues of our day. As the voice of Christian doctors, CMA provides testimony before Congress, submits amicus curiae briefs to the Supreme Court, provides public service announcements, and conducts national and local media interviews. We also want to fulfill an obligation to provide educational resources and other helpful information to the church.

Why This Book?

One of the most perplexing health care issues facing Christians today is how to evaluate alternative medicine in two areas:

- How can we evaluate therapies as effective, possibly helpful, or without merit?
- What alternative medicine systems contain non-Christian belief systems?

This book helps define what alternative medicine is, and provides a distinctly Christian framework to evaluate each modality. In encyclopedic format the authors evaluate dozens of alternative medicines and therapies, from reflexology to St. John's wort.

The book gives you the evidence for what is helpful. When the evidence is unclear, this book gives you the facts. When a method presents physical or spiritual dangers, this book sounds the alert.

This book has been created by experts in the area of alternative medicine. The manuscript has been reviewed by a committee made up of doctors with a variety of training and experience. The result is a resource that should make its way to every Christian's reference shelf.

May you use this book to learn the facts, weigh the evidence, and make sound, God-honoring decisions.

Acknowledgments

Many people have contributed to our writing of this book. We are deeply indebted to the Christian Medical Association (CMA) for their initiative in bringing us together to work on this project. Dave Stevens, M.D., and Gene Rudd, M.D., through their leadership roles in CMA, saw the need among Christian doctors and patients for a resource such as this and were actively involved in bringing this project to fruition. We are also grateful to William Carr Peel, Th.M., for the many hours he dealt with administrative issues related to the book and for his valuable theological insights on its content.

We are grateful to the Professional Review Committee organized by CMA, made up of primary-care physicians in private practice and in academic medicine who spent countless hours reviewing the manuscripts. This committee, ably directed by Andy Sanders, M.D. (Internal Medicine, Augusta, Ga.), included Ruth Bolton, M.D. (Family Medicine, Robbinsdale, Minn.), John Mulder, M.D. (Family Medicine, Nashville, Tenn.), and J. Scott Ries, M.D. (Family Medicine, Indianapolis, Ind.). These physicians volunteered their time to go through our book in great detail, evaluating its medical content. They offered invaluable suggestions as well as theological insights.

Our experience working with Zondervan has been superb. Cindy Hays has been our main contact, confidante, cheerleader, encourager, equipper, critic, and editor. We have been struck by her commitment to high-quality writing. Jane Haradine came on board to pull everything together and bring us down the home stretch. Her help was invaluable. Many others at Zondervan contributed to the final book. As first-time book authors, we feel we could not have been involved with a more superb publisher. We have been impressed with the pleasantness, professionalism, and efficiency of everyone we worked with at Zondervan.

Over the years there have been many others who have helped us become who we are. They, too, contributed to this book. Dónal's interest in scientifically evaluating herbal remedies was nurtured in pharmacy school at Trinity College, Dublin, Ireland. Desmond Corrigan, Ph.D., and A. I. "Sandy" Gray, Ph.D., gave him his first exposure to research, which was later developed at The Ohio State University under the direction of Raymond Doskotch, Ph.D.

Walt's interest in natural medicines began in the 1970s during his studies as a Queen's Fellow at Queen's Hospital in Nottingham, England. David Metcalf, M.D., and Derek Prentice, M.D., were both valued professors and mentors. This basic foundation in natural medicine expanded during residency in family medicine at Duke Medical Center under the direction of

Terry Kane, M.D., Woody Warburton, M.D., Christina Delatorre, M.D., and Ann Moore, M.D. Walt's first practical experience occurred in the early 1980s, in Bryson City, a small town in the Great Smoky Mountains of North Carolina, where the midwives and herbal therapists taught so much to the new doctor in town. Walt also acknowledges the more recent instruction in the use of natural medicines that he received from Andrew Weil, M.D.; Earl Mindell, R.Ph., Ph.D.; Joe Graedon; Teresa Graedon, Ph.D.; and especially Ellen Kahmi, R.N., Ph.D.

Dónal has learned much from the men and women who serve with him at Xenos Christian Fellowship in Columbus, Ohio. God has used many different churches and pastors in developing Walt's relationship with God, including Pastors Donald Tabb, Larry Miller, Mac Bare, Ken Hicks, and Nathan Blackwell. Doug Patch (for Dónal) and Bill Judge (for Walt) have fulfilled 2 Timothy 2:2 by demonstrating the lost art of mentoring. Their prayers and coaching have been priceless. Dónal learned much at Ashland Theological Seminary in Ashland, Ohio, especially from Luke L. Keefer, Jr., Ph.D., and David W. Baker, Ph.D. Walt acknowledges the teaching he received from R. C. Sproul, Ph.D., (of Knox Seminary) and the professors and staff at Reformed Theological Seminary in Orlando, Fla.

More recently, Dónal and Walt's involvement with the Center for Bioethics & Human Dignity in Bannockburn, Ill., has been an important source of encouragement and equipping, especially through its director, John Kilner, Ph.D. Many others could and should be acknowledged, but we limit ourselves to thanking Ann Schiele, Kip Sexton, Pat McKnight, and Cheryl Ney (all in Columbus), and John Littell, Jose Fernandez, Linda King, Amaryllis Sanchez, Leticia Romero, Vicki Roberson, Ned McLeod, and especially John and Cleta Hartman (all in Kissimmee).

We are both grateful to our fathers and mothers for giving us an abiding respect for God and for teaching us the importance of self-discipline. For Dónal, Marger Harman's prayers and encouragement have been a big factor in bringing this book to print.

We thank God daily for granting us the privilege of having our precious children—for Dónal, Catrina, Conor, and Peter, and for Walt, Kate, and Scott. We thank them for all the blessings they bring into our lives and for supporting us in so many ways through the labors required in this work.

We want to especially acknowledge the prayers, love, support, and encouragement of our wives, Cheri Lynn O'Mathúna and Barbara Shaw Larimore. We thank them for all the things they have done and sacrificed to make it possible for us to write.

Finally, we are most grateful to our Lord and Savior Jesus Christ, for choosing us to serve him through writing. Our deepest prayer is that this book will bring glory to God. To the extent that what we wrote is truthful and helpful, the praise and glory go to him. But if we have erred in anything, we accept sole responsibility.

Dónal O'Mathúna, Columbus, Ohio
Walt Larimore, Colorado Springs, Colorado
February 2001

Introduction

We have written this book together because we share two deeply held beliefs—one involving faith, the other science.

Growing up in different parts of the world has given us many different experiences. Our education and professional training give us different perspectives. But our lives have come to have a common purpose based on the relationship we each have with God. We seek to serve God and his people out of gratitude for the many blessings we have received from him. Our God is an awesome God, and we hope that others will come to know him and experience his love and grace as we have.

The second common belief that motivates us is the appreciation we have gained for science. This may seem like a contradiction to those who hear about arguments and antagonism between science and Christianity. We are aware of these debates and even participate in them. Science is a vital tool that helps us to not only understand God's creation but also to learn how to use the resources God has given us to improve people's health and lives. We disagree with those who misuse science in an attempt to deny God's existence or to validate some theory that is not only worthless but dangerous.

What led us to start asking questions about alternative medicine?

We saw patients taking herbal remedies and supplements about which very little information (good or bad) was known. We learned of people who were diagnosing and treating themselves with herbs and dietary supplements without first seeing a conventional doctor. We saw what such delays in seeking proper medical treatment could do—the unnecessary suffering, the risks, even death. We met students and patients who were being given "therapies" without being told of the religious roots or the spiritual implications of those therapies. We heard of churches embroiled in controversy over differences of opinion about alternative medicine.

Patients and even health care professionals didn't know where to get reliable information about alternative medicine. Although such information is becoming more available, we realized that none of the descriptions of the various therapies included theological evaluation to help Christians understand what spiritual risks may be involved.

We decided to put together a single resource that combines the latest and most accurate information on alternative medicine from these two important perspectives—science and Christianity. We look to science to provide valuable help in determining whether a therapy is effective and safe. We look to the Bible for answers on the spiritual questions.

Our goal in writing this book has been to examine the most popular alternative therapies, herbal remedies, vitamins, and dietary supplements. We combed the medical literature and published reports from the United States and many other countries. We discussed these therapies with conventional and alternative practitioners to find the best information on the effectiveness and safety of the most common alternative therapies. To compile this information in a practical and user-friendly manner, we developed categories of treatment, tools for ranking the research that's been done, and tools for ranking the effectiveness of the therapies and remedies. We organized all this information in such a way that you can quickly find information and our recommendations on a specific therapy or herb or dietary supplement.

We describe the research that has been done on each therapy or product and offer tips on understanding just what the results mean. We also describe the fundamental elements of research and clinical trials generally used to evaluate therapies to give you the tools you need to evaluate other therapies that will come along in the future.

Evaluating alternative medicine from a Christian perspective involves much more than just declaring which therapies are effective and which are not. We explain the spiritual issues that underlie some therapies, especially those contrary to Christian beliefs.

Christianity is much more than a list of do's and don'ts. Our reading and study of God's Word convinces us that God wants to influence how his people approach health and healing. We let you in on what we found during our study, giving you verse after verse to guide you in making your decisions and to help you answer those who would distort his Word for their own reasons. We offer guidelines for a Christian approach to health and healing, whether one pursues conventional medicine or alternative therapies.

We have done our best to be comprehensive and current. But we know that by the time this book is printed, new studies will be available on some of the therapies we evaluated. These new studies may contradict our conclusions. That is the nature of ongoing research, especially in such a controversial area. Yet in spite of this limitation, we believe our evaluations will, for the most part, give you reliable information that will be of value for many years.

We pray that this book will be a service to you, the reader. Pray with us that God will guide you as you make decisions about your health and the health of those in your care.

Dónal O'Mathúna, Columbus, Ohio
Walt Larimore, Colorado Springs, Colorado
February 2001

PART ONE

AN OVERVIEW OF ALTERNATIVE AND CONVENTIONAL MEDICINE

1

Alternative Medicine: The Issues

Physicians practicing conventional Western medicine at times see alternative medicine as unproven, worthless, perhaps even dangerous, steeped only in anecdotal case histories. Some view the alternative therapist as being naïve at best, a charlatan at worst.

A provider of alternative medicine may see conventional physicians as so focused on a disease or body part that they have no humanity, no compassion, and lack concern for the whole person. The conventional physician has been called a money-loving individual, in bed with pharmaceutical companies, who is out to take the life savings of the ill and infirm.

A truly accurate picture of both sides is a lot more complicated. But you need to understand the benefits and the dangers of alternative medicine before you make any serious mistakes.

What Is an Alternative Therapy?

The simplest definition of an alternative therapy is any therapy that is not accepted by the dominant medical establishment in a given culture. While the definition of alternative medicine can vary, there are some general characteristics and principles that most agree on.

- Alternative therapies are those approaches to healing that physicians and hospitals in the United States are unlikely to provide for their patients. The dominant medical establishment tends to look with disfavor (or disgust) on certain therapies and labels them "alternatives." Alternative medicine claims to have been pushed aside by practitioners of conventional medicine for reasons of political or financial gain.
- Practitioners of alternative medicine generally stress their holistic approach to health care—treating the body, the mind, and the spirit—relying on noninvasive "natural" methods of healing with an emphasis on prevention of disease. Although conventional medicine can be holistic as well, medical physicians frequently do not stress that fact.
- Some alternative therapies refer to the spirit in ways that are alien to Christianity. Unless you understand the roots of a particular therapy, you may find yourself

involved in a practice with a theology dangerously different from what Jesus taught
or what he would have us follow.

- Much in alternative medicine has little quality scientific evidence to support its
assertions of healing. However, as we shall show, some therapies have excellent
scientific support, yet are not utilized by many conventional Western physicians.
Other therapies, with proper testing, might gain proof of the value claimed. Without
such proof, no one, not even the experts in alternative medicine, knows for certain
whether the untested, unproven alternative therapies actually have healed anyone
or not. All we know is that patients relate how they were helped, or how they
entered long-term remission, or were cured after using some unproven alternative
therapy.

Before you embark on any path that takes you into the world of alternative medicine, even
if it's just to buy an herbal remedy that's being recommended by a friend, you need to investigate the realities of alternative medicine—the costs and the risks you might face as well as
the benefits.

Our purpose in this book is to point out the benefits, explain the risks, anticipate your
questions, and provide objective answers. We will show how conventional medicine has
evolved over the centuries, how what we commonly call "alternative therapies" have come to
exist, and the background for the various therapies and remedies. And we'll look at what the
use of alternative therapies could mean for a Christian.

In part 4 we discuss each of the most popular alternative therapies available today in
North America. This section lists not only what exists but also gives the origins, effectiveness,
and any reasons for caution and concern. We also give you detailed information on herbal
remedies, vitamins, and dietary supplements, since these are used as a form of self-help available without much direction in health food stores, most drugstores, many supermarkets, and
even on the Internet. Here, too, you'll be able to read our recommendations along with any
cautions and concerns.

Conventional Medicine Takes an Interest in Alternative Medicine

As more research is done, we believe that conventional medicine and alternative medicine will increasingly be used together. Some alternative therapy specialists recognize the
potential of a holistic approach in contemporary conventional medicine and work in tandem
with medical physicians to give high quality care. And many conventional medicine practitioners recognize that one or more alternative therapies might benefit their patients when used
in tandem with surgery and pharmaceuticals.

Increasing numbers of doctors, nurses, and other health care professionals are incorporating the best of both approaches into what is called "integrative medicine."[1] Professional
continuing medical education (CME) courses also are providing information on alternative
medicine. In fact, some of the most popular CME courses for doctors, nurses, and pharmacists

focus specifically on alternative medicine. Pharmacies are increasingly making alternative remedies available, although natural or health food stores, the Internet, and mail-order companies still account for most of these sales. According to a 1994 study, homeopathic preparations were being stocked by 69 percent of chain drugstores and by 3,000 independent pharmacies, accounting for annual sales at the time of about $100 million.[2]

Interest Grows Among Christians

Interest among Christians appears to mirror—and sometimes exceed—this general trend. Christian radio stations carry advertisements for herbal remedies and nutritional supplements even more commonly than the secular media. Specific "Christian" alternative therapies are promoted. One entrepreneur claimed to have figured out the recipe for manna and alleged it would protect people from all forms of illness, just as the original manna protected the Israelites in the wilderness. Another is the "Genesis 1:29 Diet" based on God's declaration that "I give you every seed-bearing plant on the face of the whole earth and every tree that has fruit with seed in it. They will be yours for food." Believers in this diet teach that people will be most healthy when eating a vegetarian diet.

Some Christians claim to have found particular ways to cure or alleviate cancer.[3] One prominent Christian author has written about the benefits he experienced from an alternative cancer therapy available only in Europe.[4] We frequently hear his case mentioned to encourage Christian involvement in alternative medicine. Research studies on prayer and religious faith have been published in mainstream medical journals. Although some of what is called "prayer" is very different from the prayer described in the Bible, some Christians now claim the power of prayer is supported by scientific research.

NIH Begins Evaluation of Alternative Medicine Treatments

In 1992, the National Institutes of Health began an evaluation of alternative medical treatments, establishing the Office of Alternative Medicine (since renamed The National Center for Complementary and Alternative Medicine). It has made grants available to a number of prominent universities and major medical centers to encourage both research and teaching of alternative medicine. In response, many medical schools and nursing schools have added courses in alternative therapies.

At least eight new journals devoted to alternative medicine were launched in the late 1990s, with their primary audience being physicians and other health care professionals. Well-established professional journals increasingly publish articles about alternative medicine. Some have even devoted entire issues to the topic, such as the November 1998 issue of the *Journal of the American Medical Association.*

Even medical insurance and managed-care companies have started to pay for some alternative therapies. In fact, by the end of 1998 an estimated 58 percent of major health maintenance organizations (HMOs) were covering some types of alternative medicine.[5]

Alternative Medicine Has Become Big Business

Despite the problems and concerns about alternative medicine, which you will learn about in this book, Americans are increasingly spending their money on alternative medicine. A frequently cited survey reported that in 1990 Americans spent between $9.4 billion and $13.2 billion on alternative therapies.[6] When this survey was repeated in 1997, expenditures had mushroomed to between $17.2 billion and $24.6 billion. Additionally, $5.1 billion was spent on herbal medicine, and $4.7 billion on therapy-specific books, classes, and equipment, bringing the total out-of-pocket expenses to somewhere between $27 billion and $34.4 billion.[7] Americans also spend about $12 billion annually on dietary supplements, with these sales growing each year by about 20 percent.[8] At this writing, the industry has become even stronger, much of the increase related to aging baby boomers and a younger population increasingly focused on wellness and looking for solutions outside mainstream medical practice.

The manufacturer of one herbal product alone, Metabolife 356®, a dieting product, was estimated in one review of the product to have sales in 1999 approaching $1 billion.[9] This review also noted that it was unable to locate any of the usual peer-reviewed, published research required of pharmaceutical companies to indicate that a product actually works and is safe.

Risks in Alternative Medicine Are Real and Sometimes Dangerous

In spite of all the interest in alternative medicine, the unquestioned reliance on unproven alternative therapies can have tragic results, especially for patients who try alternative therapies before seeking conventional help.

The harsh reality of delaying conventional treatment was obvious for a woman named Hazel (in this book, the cases are real; the names and some of the details, such as age or sex, may have been changed to protect the patient's confidentiality). She came to the office after nearly two years of trying a variety of alternative medicine treatments for a shoulder ailment. Her chronic bursitis was easily and quickly diagnosed using only a brief history, a physical exam, and an X-ray. An injection of a nonabsorbable steroid into the bursa—a common and proven conventional treatment—gave Hazel full use of her crippled shoulder within fifteen minutes. Hazel cried, realizing she had needlessly suffered chronic pain all those months while trying alternative therapies.

An even greater tragedy occurred with Brenda. I first became involved with Brenda's care after she was brought to the emergency room while having a seizure. The MRI (a diagnostic imaging test) showed cancer had spread to the brain and bones. Brenda told how for more than a year she had worried about a growing lump in one breast. She had thought it merely part of her fibrocystic breast condition, an annoying ailment though not dangerous.

Brenda had gone to her local health food store where the well-intentioned owner recommended a number of nutritional therapies and dietary supplements. Brenda also saw a local alternative medicine practitioner who, without even examining her, recommended other alternative therapies.

Days passed, then weeks. The lump continued to grow. By the time I saw Brenda, a young woman in her twenties, there would be no cure, no happy ending. I could only try to relieve her pain, her guilt and suffering, and comfort her as her family, the staff, and I helplessly watched her life fade away.

The outcome might have been the same with early conventional medical therapy. But medical literature is filled with well-documented proof that early detection and intervention in breast cancer frequently results in cure. Brenda probably died prematurely because she put her trust and faith in unproven alternative therapies suggested by those not trained in medical diagnosis. Although both of these patients were sincere in their beliefs about alternative medicine, they were sincerely wrong.

Unfortunately, these types of stories are not uncommon. A researcher for the Research Council for Complementary Medicine in London, England, visited twenty-nine health food stores in London asking advice for her numerous and severe headaches.[10] The symptoms were chosen so that a trained professional would easily recognize them as suggesting a brain tumor or other serious problem. The researcher was told by the health food store employees that her headaches were caused by the flu, low blood sugar, tension, the weather, or using her brain too much. Forty-two different therapies were recommended, with no consistency in the advice given. At fewer than one in four of the stores was the researcher advised to see a physician.

In another study in Hawaii, a researcher visited forty health food stores stating she was gathering information on herbal remedies for her mother, whose advanced breast cancer had spread throughout her body (metastasized).[11] In 90 percent of the stores, employees recommended various products to cure cancer, even though making such a claim is against the law. Shark cartilage was by far the most popular remedy, recommended at almost half the stores. Of great concern also is that almost one-fifth of the employees counseled against the use of conventional cancer therapy. We'll discuss the lack of evidence that shark cartilage cures cancer.

It is only fair to point out the many similar stories told by alternative medicine advocates, of how a large, noncaring, conventional medical system caused harm to patients. They cite pharmaceutical horror stories—thalidomide given to pregnant women to treat nausea that resulted in babies born with serious birth defects, including missing or shortened arms or legs. They relate how mass inoculation against the swine flu virus resulted in serious illness, even death. They tell of people who have become overly dependent on the latest tranquilizer or sedative. They note that wonder drugs, such as Viagra® to treat impotence, have been linked to heart attacks. They tell how people die every year from medication mistakes in hospitals and from prescription errors. And they are right. Conventional medicine is not perfect. It is a human enterprise where practitioners are always learning, where they sometimes make mistakes.

What the proponents of alternative medicine rarely, if ever, reveal to those seeking advice are the Brendas and Hazels from their past—those who suffered and even died needlessly.

With this book, we want you to become as wise as a serpent about the risks and benefits of conventional and alternative medicine. We don't want you to continue to merely ask the practitioners of conventional or alternative medicine, "What do you recommend?" or "What do you think is best?" We want you to learn how to ask, "What is the evidence that supports what you recommend?" We want you to wisely learn how to gather the information you need for the decisions you must make about your health. Jonathan Swift, the great eighteenth-century Irish satirist, summed up our concerns beautifully: "Falsehood flies and the truth comes limping after; so that when men come to be undeceived it is too late: the jest is over and the tale has had its effect."

Proof of Effectiveness Is Missing for Alternative Therapies

When the truth comes out, that most alternative therapies have little or no compelling clinical evidence to support their effectiveness or safety, most of the people we talk to are stunned. The evidence that does exist is often ambiguous or based on seriously flawed studies. In some cases the "proof" that a therapy is effective is based on controversial interpretations of scientific theories. For many therapies, the only evidence offered is a group of anecdotal reports—the testimony of users of the therapy.

Perhaps even worse is the way the popular media introduce alternative medicine concepts. As soon as a new therapy begins to show some positive results in some people, reports in the popular media promote it as though it has been proven. The fact that the idea may be wrong, that coincidence is more likely the reason for the positive result, is not mentioned. Instead, we see the touting of a cancer cure, a diabetes cure, or something similar based on very preliminary evidence and supposition.

Coenzyme Q_{10} is a good example of such a media blitz. Coenzyme Q_{10} at one time was one of the most popular of the newer dietary supplements. Physicians and researchers knew that Coenzyme Q_{10} is a critical factor in generating energy in all living organisms. They also knew that the aged and those with a number of different ailments have a reduction in levels of Coenzyme Q_{10}. Therefore, some alternative practitioners reasoned, if a person took Coenzyme Q_{10} as part of a regimen of daily nutritional supplements, it might slow or stop the aging process and the person would be assured of better health.

Soon they were touting this theory as fact. Coenzyme Q_{10} became a "must have" nutritional supplement. There was even talk that it could combat or reduce the severity of AIDS. Then long-term, carefully controlled studies began to be conducted. Now, at this writing, it has been noted in the University of California, Berkeley, *Wellness Letter* for April 2000 that there is no proof to support this theory. It's true that Coenzyme Q_{10} is critical for energy, and that it is lacking in the aged and many of the infirm. It may even provide a little benefit for those with heart problems. But the supplement is nothing like the "fountain of youth" it was originally advertised to be. Yet countless consumers, many Christians included, wasted millions of dollars because of premature claims made about Coenzyme Q_{10}.

Alternative Therapies Lack Adequate Regulation

Most European countries strictly regulate the manufacture and sale of herbal and other botanical products. In Germany, the Federal Health Agency set up what became known as

Commission E to evaluate the safety, efficacy, and quality of herbal products. Although the Federal Health Agency does not test herbal products, manufacturers are required to submit proof of a product's quality, safety, and effectiveness. Each product's license must be renewed every five years. Similar procedures must be followed for herbal and conventional drugs, although the type of evidence used to support an herb's safety and effectiveness is different from the requirements for a conventional drug.

Once established, Commission E functioned independently of the Federal Health Agency. From 1978 to 1994, Commission E reviewed all available literature on the safety and efficacy of 360 herbal remedies. These technical reports were published and are now available in English.[12] In countries with regulations like these, consumers are assured of the consistency and safety of what they purchase—and they have some confidence that the claims made about the substance are accurate.

Unfortunately, this is not true in the United States, as there are no such standards or regulations. The consumer not only has no guarantee of the safety or efficacy of what they purchase, in many cases they can't even be sure that the amount of the herb or other active ingredient indicated on the label is actually there.

- Some products don't contain the ingredients listed on the labels.[13]
- Others contain dangerous chemicals or pharmaceuticals not listed on the label.[14]
- Significant differences exist in the same product from different manufacturers (or even from the same manufacturer).[15]
- Different brands of some products contain dramatically different amounts of the active ingredients.[16]

For example, the *Los Angeles Times* commissioned a study to examine St. John's wort,[17] an herb known to be effective against some forms of mild to moderate general depression. *Times* reporters purchased the ten most common brands from several retail outlets, then had the pills tested by an independent laboratory.

The results were startling. Only one had between 90 and 110 percent of what the label indicated (an acceptable standard for over-the-counter products, based on the German standards). One manufacturer's pills had only 20 percent of the amount of active ingredient claimed on the label. Two others had a third *more* than the labels claimed.

Alternative Therapies Are Often Based on Ancient or Traditional Cultures

The ancient or traditional cultures with which many of these therapies are associated have been viewed through romantic lenses, their lifestyles seen as healthier than modern, fast-paced ones. The medicines, especially the herbs, used for centuries in these cultures would, it is claimed, never have gained acceptance if they were not effective. Thus, the therapies are declared by the proponents of alternative medicine to be valid. Some champions of a product will claim that their therapies were suppressed for years by Western imperialism and Christian missionary crusades. Only now, they say, are they being rediscovered and made available in the West.

Some of the more vigorous supporters of alternative medicine see many of the concerns about alternative medicine as the dying gasps of Western culture's two dominant institutions: science and Christianity. They claim that research on these therapies is lacking because of the biases of Western medical and pharmaceutical establishments. The claim has been made that the pharmaceutical industry will not research herbal remedies because it cannot patent the products and hence cannot make as much money from them. Conventional medicine, they claim, is only concerned with retaining power and market share.

Alternative medicine partisans advocate giving individuals the freedom to choose whatever form of health care they want. The argument is made that people's responsibility to care for their own health should be acknowledged and promoted by giving the individual greater freedom in matters of health care. They view those seeking to regulate alternative medicine, such as the Food and Drug Administration (FDA) and the Institute of Medicine (IOM), with suspicion.

Spiritual Part of Some Therapies Is a Problem for Christians

For Christians, there is another concern. Some alternative therapies are based on practices and rituals that have long been part of pagan traditions or other religious practices.

Spirituality is an important concept in alternative medicine. Unfortunately, the word *spirituality* may mean one thing to Christians and quite another to someone who practices therapies such as traditional Chinese medicine or India's Ayurvedic medicine. They both incorporate herbal remedies, meditation, and relaxation, with traditional Chinese medicine also using acupuncture and other therapies. Each system also has a very distinct world view based on the religious ideas commonly accepted in those cultures.

Some Christians have expressed the valid concern that some forms of alternative medicine may be vehicles for the promotion of a variety of religious perspectives, many of them opposed to Christianity, while other forms may actually involve occult practices. These concerns have been reinforced by *New Age Journal* editors who view the increased interest in alternative medicine as the most significant change contributing to the redefining of American culture.[18]

One of the central tenets believed by many in the New Age movement is that all spirituality is good, that no form is any better than another.[19] This is in opposition to the consistent message of the Bible that many problems people have originate, either directly or indirectly, in the conflict between the spiritual forces of good and evil. Paul wrote in Ephesians 6:12, "For our struggle is not against flesh and blood, but against the rulers, against the authorities, against the powers of this dark world and against the spiritual forces of evil in the heavenly realms."

Thus the "openness" advocated by many in the alternative medicine community could expose people to spiritual beings and practices whose primary concern is to harm people and lead them away from the loving Father of the Universe. Although some question the existence of evil spiritual forces, the Bible describes Satan as "a liar and the father of lies" (John 8:44) and warns Christians that "your enemy the devil prowls around like a roaring lion looking for someone to devour" (1 Peter 5:8).

Practitioners of alternative therapies frequently speak of the "spiritual" part of what they do. Some are devout Christians, while others believe in practices whose world view is radically different from biblically based beliefs. Both sides use some of the same terms, but the meanings are quite different.

For example, Therapeutic Touch (see page 275) seems, on the surface, to be related to the laying on of hands. The practitioners claim to be following in this tradition after removing the religious context from the practice. However, the nurse who helped develop the practice is a Buddhist and admits that the principles behind Therapeutic Touch are the three main principles of Buddhist teachings.[20]

Some alternative medicine practitioners believe they cannot help their patients without first introducing them to one or another of the ancient Eastern or New Age faith systems. This leads to potential conflict for Christians. They may hear anecdotal stories from friends about shamanism (see page 269) easing arthritis pain without drugs, Therapeutic Touch increasing the speed of healing after a severe burn, and Reiki (see page 266) easing a chronic health condition. The stories are positive. Nothing is said about the spiritual side of the treatments. But are they safe?

Some pastors might say that many of these therapies go against biblical teaching. They may even warn that some alternative therapies lead to involvement in the occult. But others teach that ultimately all healing comes from God. They emphasize that Jesus is called the "Great Physician." They point out that in his day, Jesus would have been considered an alternative healer. Both perspectives can't be right.

What to Do When Considering an Alternative Therapy

In the midst of this debate, most people, including physicians, are left confused and frustrated. People with health problems don't want philosophical or political debates; they want relief. They just want to know what they can and should do. Christians also want to please God in their actions, base their beliefs on his Word, the Bible, and reflect his character in the decisions they make.

We should all be concerned about our health. We should know why we are using whatever therapies or remedies we do use. We need to know that a particular remedy is not only effective but reasonably safe—that the label on the bottle is accurate and reliable. We need to know the costs, risks, and benefits of the choices available to us. Recommendations and experiences of certain people can be an important part of any evaluation; but these are not enough.

We should all investigate the claims made about the remedies we put into our bodies, the therapies we allow to be practiced on us, and the practitioners in whom we place our trust. "Do you not know that your body is a temple of the Holy Spirit, who is in you, whom you have received from God? You are not your own; you were bought at a price. Therefore honor God with your body" (1 Corinthians 6:19–20). Gather objective background information, weigh the options, and make as informed a decision as possible.

This investigation should be done whether we are pursuing conventional or alternative medicine. Yet with both forms of medical care, we see people trusting blindly in someone or something for no reason other than the chance happenings that led them to a certain practitioner.

We must also evaluate remedies from an investment, or stewardship, perspective. We are all limited in the amount of time and money available to us. We should not waste or squander our resources. Christians, especially, are called to be accountable stewards of these resources. Jesus asked, "So if you have not been trustworthy in handling worldly wealth, who will trust you with true riches? And if you have not been trustworthy with someone else's property, who will give you property of your own?" (Luke 16:11).

For us as Christians, then, we must evaluate whether our pursuit of alternative medicine is motivated by the values of our culture or by godly reasons. This book is intended to help you make these decisions.

Notes

1. Deborah A. Grandinetti, "'Integrated Medicine' Could Boost Your Income," *Medical Economics* 74, no. 18 (September 8, 1997): 73–99.

2. June H. McDermott, June E. Riedlinger, and Edward Chapman, "What Pharmacists Should Understand About Homeopathic Remedies," *American Journal of Health-System Pharmacy* 52 (November 1995): 2442–45.

3. Anne E. Frähm with David J. Frähm, *A Cancer Battle Plan: Six Strategies for Beating Cancer from a Recovered "Hopeless Case"* (Colorado Springs, Colo.: Piñon Press, 1992).

4. Larry Burkett with Michael E. Taylor, *Damaged But Not Broken: A Personal Testimony of How to Deal With the Impact of Cancer* (Chicago: Moody, 1996).

5. Michele Bitoun Blecher, "Gold in Goldenseal," *Hospitals & Health Networks* 71, no. 20 (October 20, 1997): 50–52.

6. David M. Eisenberg, Ronald C. Kessler, Cindy Foster, Frances E. Norlock, David R. Calkins, and Thomas L. Delbanco, "Unconventional Medicine in the United States: Prevalence, Costs, and Patterns of Use," *New England Journal of Medicine*, 328 (January 1993): 246–52.

7. David M. Eisenberg, Roger B. Davis, Susan L. Ettner, Scott Appel, Sonja Wilkey, Maria Van Rompay, and Ronald C. Kessler, "Trends in Alternative Medicine Use in the United States," *Journal of the American Medical Association* 280, no. 18 (November 11, 1998): 1569–75.

8. Joseph Weber and Sandra Dallas, "Cure? Well . . . Profit? Sure," *Business Week* (October 23, 1995), 58–59; Geoffrey Cowley, "Herbal Warning: Health-Food Stores Have Built a New Natural-Drug Culture. How Safe Are Their Wares?" *Newsweek* (May 6, 1996), 60–68.

9. E. P. Barrette, "Metabolife 356 for Weight Loss," *Alternative Medicine Alert* 3, no. 1 (January 2000): 1–6.

10. A. J. Vickers, R. W. Rees, and A. Robin, "Advice Given by Health Food Shops: Is It Clinically Safe?" *Journal of the Royal College of Physicians of London* 32, no. 5 (September/October 1998): 426–28.

11. Carolyn Cook Gotay and Daniella Dumitriu, "Health Food Store Recommendations for Breast Cancer Patients," *Archives of Family Medicine* 9, no. 8 (August 2000): 692–99.

12. Mark Blumenthal, ed., *The Complete German Commission E Monographs, Therapeutic Guide to Herbal Medicines* (Austin, Tex.: American Botanical Council, 1998).

13. J. Parasrampurra, K. Schwartz, and R. Petesch, "Quality Control of Dehydroepiandrosterone Dietary Supplement Products," *Journal of the American Medical Association* 280, no. 18 (November 11, 1998): 1565.

14. Marcia Angell and Jerome P. Kassirer, "Alternative Medicine—The Risks of Untested and Unregulated Remedies," *New England Journal of Medicine* 339, no. 12 (September 17, 1998): 839–41.

15. B. J. Gurley, P. Wang, and S. F. Gardner, "Ephedrine-type Alkaloid Content of Nutritional Supplements Containing *Ephedra sinica* (Ma-huang) as Determined by High Performance Liquid Chromatography," *Journal of Pharmaceutical Sciences* 87, no. 12 (December 1998): 1547–53.

16. "Herbal Roulette," *Consumer Reports* (November 1995): 698–705.

17. Terence Monmaney, "Remedy's U.S. Sales Zoom, But Quality Control Lags," *Los Angeles Times* (August 31, 1998), from Website.

18. Jonathan Adolph, "The New Age is Now: Twenty Ideas, Books, and Records That Have Redefined Our Culture," *New Age Journal* suppl. (1995), 27–40.

19. John P. Newport, *The New Age Movement and the Biblical Worldview: Conflict and Dialogue* (Grand Rapids: Eerdmans, 1998).

20. Robert Calvert, "Dolores Krieger, Ph.D. and her Therapeutic Touch," *Massage* 47 (January/February 1994): 56–60.

2

A Look Back
at Conventional
Medicine

Today, in the United States, we live in a society that expects most, if not all, of our infections and fractures, cancers and traumas, our aches and pains, to be fixed by modern medicine, and fixed quickly, thank you.

Our conventional medicine—Western medicine—has developed from the country doctor with little training who made house calls to today's specialists in sophisticated medical centers with amazing resources that can diagnose and treat a myriad of ailments and accidents. Our life expectancy has increased. Diseases that were certain killers fifty years ago are curable today. For others, there still is no cure, but advances in medicine have made it possible to effectively manage these diseases in order to extend the life span to near normal. In many ways, we take our modern medicine and its cures for granted.

To better understand where conventional medicine is today, how it got to where it is, and how it may have gone astray, we must look back at where it started and how it progressed. In many ways, it's a sad story, as the physicians of old struggled to cure the myriad of ills. It's a story of mistakes, bad theories, bad information, and errors in judgment, but it's also a story of brilliance and breakthroughs and successes.

Proponents of alternative medicine would have you believe that conventional medicine is ignoring therapies that have been in use for hundreds, even thousands, of years. Our brief trip through the history of medicine will reveal the rest of the story: how many of the ancient theories they rely on were once a part of conventional medicine, but were discarded years ago; how innumerable ancient remedies they praise and recommend as cures in the alternative medicine of today are useless.

While people have always yearned for cures, it is only in recent history that we could realistically expect medicine to have any *reliable* cures. For much of history, the only medical resources available were the comfort of a caring physician or healer and remedies made from local herbs. Some people recovered, their bodies healing naturally, regardless of the treatment (or lack of treatment) they received. Some patients could not be helped, and died in comfort from the loving ministrations of family and the "doctor" called in at the time of illness. That comfortable passage into death was a healing of sorts; in a way it was the forerunner of the hospice concept for the terminally ill. And some, their bodies ravaged by disease, got better after being treated with ministrations we now know are scientifically groundless. They believed the treatment would provide a cure, and they recovered.

The Many Benefits of the "Placebo Effect"

This type of recovery is called the "placebo effect." The placebo effect plays an important and often beneficial role in all forms of medical and surgical care. Some medical historians have even concluded that the history of medicine is mostly a history of the placebo effect. It helps to explain why, even today, people report that they feel better after receiving a particular treatment. So if a person feels better, have they actually been helped? Or is their "improvement" merely a temporary mind-over-matter impression that has nothing to do with curing their illness? It depends on the illness. And the treatment.

Placebos, and the placebo effect, have been defined in various ways. A placebo is any pill or injection or intervention, or part of any intervention, that results in some beneficial effect in a patient without the treatment itself having any known, specific effect on the body. Maybe the patient gets better because the physician instills hope. Or the patient believes the "pill" or "shot" offers a cure, even if it doesn't.

An early study demonstrating the impact of the placebo effect was published in 1801. A competent and respected New England physician, Elisha Perkins (1741–1799), claimed to relieve many painful ailments using metallic rods (called Perkins' tractors).[1] Perkins claimed his metal rods worked because of the magnetic properties of the metal. He would stroke the afflicted part of a person's body and reported great success. Perkins was so convinced of his tractors' effectiveness that he went to New York to cure people during a yellow fever epidemic, but contracted the disease and died. The reputation of the tractors lived on, with a Perkinean Institute being founded in England.

Another physician, John Haygarth, was skeptical of the successes Perkins had reported with his metal rods and devised an experiment—what we would now call a "placebo-controlled study." Haygarth made wooden tractors, painting them to look metallic—which made them the placebo, or "sham," treatment. He then treated five patients with rheumatism, using Perkins' metallic rods one day (what researchers today would call the "test intervention"), and his wooden rods the next (the placebo), alternating the treatments. The patients, who believed they were being rubbed with Perkins' rods, reported the same amount of relief with the wooden rods as they had with the metal rods.

Haygarth's experiment was a demonstration of the placebo effect. Patients improved, not because of being stroked by Perkins' tractors, but because of the complex dynamics that make up the placebo effect. "The curative factors...were the patient's and physician's imagination and faith. The physician's fame...was an additional factor that contributed to the patient's faith: that is, the more important the physician, the more likely it was that the treatment would be effective."[2] Haygarth's study is not only one of the earliest examples of a placebo-controlled study, it is also one of the earliest examples of what is now called the "single-blind study," where patients do not know which treatment they are receiving, but the physician or researcher does.

The positive placebo effect is much more prevalent, even today, than many health care professionals or the lay public are willing to admit. Placebo effects have been observed with drugs, herbs and other botanicals, surgery, medical procedures, inactive compounds, psychotherapy, and diagnostic tests. In 1938, a physician wrote, "The great lesson, then, of medical history is that the placebo has always been the norm of medical practice, that it was only occasionally and at great intervals that anything really serviceable, such as the cure of scurvy by fresh fruits, was introduced into medical practice."[3]

However, the term "placebo" often carries negative connotations. Many people think of placebos as useless fakes given to trick patients into thinking they are getting something helpful when the doctor can find no reason for their symptoms. Placebos are thought to be prescribed for people with psychosomatic illnesses (ailments that are "just in their heads"), as a pacifier. (The word *placebo* comes from the Latin verb that means "to please.") If the patient gets better with the placebo, then the placebo effect worked. The problem is solved. Or is it?

The Negative Effect of the 'Nocebo'

What usually is not mentioned outside scientific circles is the opposite situation, called the "nocebo effect," in which a patient has a negative, or bad, reaction to a placebo. We bring this up to help you understand how unpredictable a person's response to a treatment can be.

Here's how the nocebo works in research. Suppose a group of patients in a controlled study have the same illness and the same expectation of recovery. Half the group is given a new medication known to bring recovery faster. The other half is given a placebo pill. No one, not even the doctors, knows who gets what, but all participants are told they might recover faster if they receive the new medication.

What happens? The majority of participants who actually take the new medication get well noticeably faster than those who take only the placebo pill. Just what you would expect. A few receiving the placebo improve, maybe even as dramatically as those who received the new medication. They benefited from the "placebo effect." But a few who took the placebo get worse, a "nocebo effect." They have an adverse reaction to the placebo even though the inactive ingredients in the pill can produce no physical effect whatever. One review of more than 100 research studies found that almost one out of every five people given placebos had adverse, or nocebo, reactions.[4]

The placebo effect is real. It brings relief, at least temporarily. People think the pills they took helped because they feel better. Research can now tell the difference. Studies have now been designed to evaluate whether a therapy is effective in and of itself or merely appears to work as a result of the placebo effect. It's important to know the difference when you're considering any treatment.

Most Ancient Remedies Had Little Actual Effect

Physicians in ancient cultures developed a long list of drugs that were prepared and often available for use only with a prescription. There were at least 370 different drugs used by physicians in ancient Mesopotamia, the region east of ancient Israel. Ancient Greece had between 200 and 400 different drugs. Ancient Chinese writings describe the use of more than 2000 herbs, metals, and minerals in more than 16,000 different preparations. There were 600 used in ancient India, 1000 listed in the writings of the Roman physician Pliny, and 820 in the writings of a Greco-Roman physician, Galen, whose theories had a profound effect on the field of medicine.

Practically every known organic and inorganic substance has been used as a medicine at some point in history. Many strange substances have also been widely used in remedies. For example, unicorn horn was used for fevers, poisonings, and to restore strength. Believed for centuries to be from the legendary unicorn, the horn was actually the spiraled incisor tooth of the narwhal whale.[5]

In ancient Babylon, sores on people's heads were treated by shaving them until blood oozed out and then covering the exposed sore with boiled dung.[6] In ancient India, meditation, fasting, vomiting, purging, bloodletting, enemas, and about 600 herbal remedies were widely used.[7]

In Egypt, the Eber's Papyrus from 1500 B.C. recommends treating people with dirt; fly-specks off walls; blood of lizards, cats, and other animals; grated human skull; ram's hair; teeth of swine; and urine and feces from eighteen different creatures, including humans.[8] "Powdered Egyptian mummy" was another popular remedy viewed as effective for healing wounds and a wide variety of other ailments. If mummies were actually used, they would have been extremely toxic, since arsenic was a main ingredient in the Egyptian embalming process.[9] In addition, religious rituals and sacrifices were also incorporated into many ancient healing practices.

An authorized list of medicinal drugs, called a "pharmacopoeia," published in France in 1608, and reissued in 1637, described remedies made from centipedes, worms, lizards, ants, vipers, and scorpions. It included some surprising recommendations:

As to the parts of animals our physicians hold assuredly and truly that they are endowed with many and admirable virtues . . . the skull or the head of a man dead but not yet buried . . . the brain of antelopes . . . the intestines of the wolf . . . the genitalia of the deer . . . fat of man . . . human blood . . . the toe nails of the eland pearls . . . the scales of many fishes. Finally, since the excrements of the said animals have also their particular virtues, it is not unfitting for the pharmacist to keep them in his shop, especially the dung of the goat, hog, swan, peacock, pigeon, muskrat, civet. . . .[10]

Despite the large number of preparations that were used to treat a variety of ailments, modern research has been unable to prove that the vast majority of these therapies had any direct physiological effect. Any positive benefit (and there must have been benefits) probably was due to the placebo effect.

This conclusion is not just a recent finding. Celsus, a first-century Roman, said the hundreds of remedies offered by physicians were of no more benefit than "a sound body, or good luck."[11] He believed that the only reliable medical treatment available in his day was surgery. Pliny assembled 20,000 facts from the medical writings of the first century and concluded that people went to physicians because of "the seductive sweetness of wishful thinking."[12] According to him, physicians had nothing to offer but their caring presence. He believed that many physicians of his day used therapies that were really "experiments," thereby putting their patients in danger.

Galen's Bad Influence on Medicine Lasts 1500 Years

But the Greco-Roman physician Galen (circa A.D. 131–200) had the biggest influence on medicine. Little changed for centuries because of Galen. His writings dominated medical practice for 1500 years. Why Galen became so revered is unclear, but it was at least partly due to his confident assertions, such as: "I have continued my practice on until old age, and never as yet have I gone far astray whether in treatment or in prognosis, as have so many other doctors of great reputation. If any one wishes to gain fame through these, and not through clever talk, all that he needs is . . . to accept what I have been able to establish by zealous research."[13]

Galen taught that there were four "humors." The humors corresponded to the major fluids in the body: blood (from the liver), phlegm (from the lungs), yellow bile (from the gallbladder), and black bile (from the spleen).[14] A person was healthy when these fluids were in balance, ill when they were unbalanced. Belief in Galen's theory explains why the most common medical practices of that era were bloodletting and purging. These were supposed to restore "balance" between the humors. Purgatives, emetics, and enemas were used in the belief they were ridding the body of disease-causing humors.

Patients were also treated with remedies chosen for their influence on all or most of the humors. These remedies were usually mixtures of many different herbs, animal parts, and minerals, often concocted according to secret recipes. One of the most famous was theriac, originally called "mithridatum."[15] This concoction contained between thirty-three and a hundred ingredients, most important of which were the flesh of vipers, squill, wine, and opium. It took at least six months to mix and brew, and then was used for almost every known ailment. Galen was so convinced that it was the finest medicine available that he wrote an entire book about it, thus assuring that it would go unchallenged for centuries. In 1745 theriac finally was proven to be ineffective—other than as a source of opium, though in highly variable doses. Yet it was included in pharmacy textbooks as late as the 1870s and was still available for purchase in Austria in the 1940s.

The Harm Done By Early Conventional Medicine

Ancient cultures did use some herbs that conventional medicine has found to contain active therapeutic ingredients. But some were actually dangerous. Galen recommended pennyroyal to induce abortion, yet this herb can cause death.[16] Spreading feces over open wounds, another treatment, can cause infections, not promote healing.

Treatments frequently used throughout history also were dangerous. These include dehydration through spitting, enemas, vomiting, or bloodletting. We now recognize how dangerous dehydration is in any patient and do just the opposite, give IV fluids for hydration. Patients now survive problems that in the past, using treatments that resulted in dehydration, would have resulted in death.

Most of the ancient healers were doing the best they could with the limited knowledge of their times. After President Abraham Lincoln was shot by actor John Wilkes Booth, the treatment he received has led some to question whether the bullet or the physicians killed the president. As he lay unconscious, he was given brandy and water to drink. Then two physicians inserted their unsterile fingers as far as possible into the bullet hole at the back of the president's head, hoping to reach the bullet. Failing this, they inserted probes (also unsterilized) six to seven inches into the president's brain. These were methods commonly used at the time, before a scientific understanding of germs and infections existed.

In spite of how crude these methods appear to us, allegations that the physicians killed President Lincoln are unfounded. One authority concluded: "Lincoln could not possibly have survived this wound, even in modern times, and...it is remarkable that he survived for nine hours, as he did, after the shooting."[17]

In some cases, ineffective therapies were better for patients simply because they kept patients away from more harmful treatments. George Washington died in 1799 at the age of fifty-seven after developing a cold and quinsy (an abscess on the tonsils). The following report of his treatment exemplifies the worst of medical practice without concern for demonstrated effectiveness. "Within twelve hours, he was bled 2.5 to 2.8 quarts, followed by a moderate dose of American calomel, an injection, 5 grains of calomel, 5 to 6 grains of emetic tartar, frequent inhalations of vapors of vinegar water, blisters applied to the extremities, and a cataplasm of bran and vinegar applied to his throat, on which a blister had already been raised."[18] It is likely that this amount of bloodletting led to dehydration, and with the other remedies used, probably hastened President Washington's death.

Late in the nineteenth century, the widely respected physician Oliver Wendell Holmes declared "that if the whole materia medica [a list of remedies, their properties, and their preparation], *as now used*, could be sunk to the bottom of the sea, it would be all the better for mankind,—and all the worse for the fishes."[19]

Looking back at these treatments, we wonder how people could have believed they would actually help them. They did what we do—depended on the word of "experts." Official conferences were convened to discuss the preparation and merits of particular remedies. Concerns about the adulteration and counterfeiting of preparations were sometimes addressed. Seventeenth-century merchants in Copenhagen, Denmark, brought in the best zoologists of the time to identify what they were selling as unicorn's horn. It turned out to be teeth with a spiral shape that are found in certain species of whales.[20]

When Franz Mesmer moved to Paris to practice his form of hypnotism and magnetic healing, the French Royal Academy of Medicine appointed a committee to evaluate the claims. This committee, which included Benjamin Franklin, issued its report in 1784, concluding that the effects of Mesmer's therapy were all due to what today would be called the placebo effect. The report found that the observed effects were explained better "by the touches of the operator [i.e., therapist], the excited imagination of the patient, and by the involuntary instinct of imitation."[21] The tests conducted by the committee used women who reported they could feel when the magnetic energy was sent from the mesmerist. However, when the women were blindfolded, they were unable to correctly judge when the mesmerist was sending magnetic energy or to which part of their body it was directed. These studies formed the beginnings of what would later be called the single-blind and double-blind methods in clinical research.[22]

Conventional medicine has relied on basic medical research and clinical trials and experience—demanding proof that a treatment works—in its move from those simple days of the country doctor to the sophisticated medical centers of today that can replace a damaged heart, cure a life-threatening infection, and repair broken and diseased bodies.

Conventional medicine also recognizes its limitations. There remain those diseases for which there is no cure, symptoms for which there is no relief. Medicine cannot fix everything.

All physicians, if they practice long enough, will also encounter the unexplainable: the patient who is too healthy to die, yet dies at an early age; the man who's been given only a few weeks to live, but years later is still doing well. Some people will do everything right as we understand healthy living and still die young. Some will do everything wrong and live to a grand old age. We don't know why.

As you can tell from this quick review, conventional medicine is not an exact science. It's been a long road of trial and error, of theory and testing—and change—to get where we are today.

Notes

1. Jacques M. Quen, "Elisha Perkins, Physician, Nostrum-Vendor, or Charlatan?" *Bulletin of the History of Medicine* 37 (1963): 159–66.

2. Arthur K. Shapiro and Elaine Shapiro, *The Powerful Placebo: From Ancient Priest to Modern Physician* (Baltimore and London: Johns Hopkins University Press, 1997), 127.

3. W. R. Houston, "Doctor Himself as Therapeutic Agent," *Annals of Internal Medicine* 11 (1938): 1416–25.

4. Judith A. Turner, Richard A. Deyo, John D. Loeser, Michael Von Korff, and Wilbert E. Fordyce, "The Importance of Placebo Effects in Pain Treatment and Research," *Journal of the American Medical Association* 271 (May 1994): 1611.

5. Odell Shepherd, *The Lore of the Unicorn* (Boston: Houghton-Mifflin, 1930).

6. Shapiro and Shapiro, *Powerful Placebo*, 3.

7. Ibid., 9.

8. Ibid., 4.

9. Arthur K. Shapiro and Elaine Shapiro, "The Placebo: Is It Much Ado about Nothing?" in *The Placebo Effect: An Interdisciplinary Exploration* (Cambridge, Mass.: Harvard University Press, 1997), 15.

10. Quoted in Francis R. Packard, "Gui Patin and the Medical Profession in Paris in the Seventeenth Century," *Annals of Medical History* 4, no. 3 (1932): 232.

11. Celsus, quoted in Guido Majno, *The Healing Hand: Man and Wound in the Ancient World* (Cambridge, Mass.: Harvard University Press, 1975), 355.

12. Pliny, quoted in Majno, *The Healing Hand*, 348.

13. Galen, quoted in Henry E. Sigerist, *The Great Doctors: A Biographical History of Medicine* (Freeport, N.Y.: Books for Libraries, 1933), 76.

14. Shapiro and Shapiro, *Powerful Placebo*, 6–7.

15. Bernadine Z. Paulshock, "William Heberden, M.D., and the End of Theriac," *New York State Journal of Medicine* 82, no. 11 (October 1982): 1612–14.

16. Ilene E. Anderson, Walter H. Mullen, James E. Meeker, Siamak C. Khojasteh, Shimako Oishi, Sidney D. Nelson, and Paul D. Blanc, "Pennyroyal Toxicity: Measurement of Toxic Metabolite Levels in Two Cases and Review of the Literature," *Annals of Internal Medicine* 124 (April 1996): 726–34.

17. John K. Lattimer, *Kennedy and Lincoln: Medical and Ballistic Comparisons of Their Assassinations* (New York: Harcourt Brace Jovanovich, 1980), 47.

18. Shapiro and Shapiro, *Powerful Placebo*, 25.

19. Oliver Wendell Holmes, *Medical Essays, 1842–1882* (Boston: Houghton Mifflin, 1891), 203.

20. Shepherd, *Lore of the Unicorn*, 261.

21. Quoted in Frank Podmore, *From Mesmer to Christian Science: A Short History of Mental Healing* (New Hyde Park, N.Y.: University Books, 1963), 59.

22. Ted J. Kaptchuk, "Intentional Ignorance: A History of Blind Assessment and Placebo Controls in Medicine," *Bulletin of the History of Medicine* 72, no. 3 (Fall 1998): 389–433.

PART TWO

GOD, HEALTH, HEALING, AND THE CHRISTIAN

3

The Christian
Principles of Health

Good health is everything."

"The most important thing in life is your health."

When someone goes through a bad time or an economic downturn, we may say, "Well, at least you have your health."

Slogans about good health abound. Many people think of physical wellness when they think about health, but the trend today is of a much broader view, a "holistic" view of health that acknowledges the many different influences on our health and healing—the physical, mental, emotional, relational, and spiritual factors, both prevention and treatment. We now know that many nonphysical factors play an important role in the development of certain illnesses and in keeping us healthy.

An Expanded View of What It Means to Be Healthy

How do we define health? One definition of health was included in the Constitution of the then newly formed World Health Organization back in 1948.

> Health is a state of complete physical, mental and social well-being and not merely the absence of disease or infirmity. The enjoyment of the highest attainable standard of health is one of the fundamental rights of every human being without distinction of race, religion, political belief, economic or social condition.[1]

Thirty-six years later, in 1984, the World Health Organization added "spirituality" to its list of factors involved in health.[2]

Admitting that health involves social, emotional, and spiritual factors allows us to include many different values in our definition of health. This has many advantages, not the least of which is that it is more realistic for good health.

But it also creates problems. For example, if a person is designated as relationally unhealthy, who defines what this means? Parents might say that it is not healthy for their children to hang around certain neighborhood kids. As adults, we may wish to define "relationally healthy" by the number of friends someone has, or by a certain track record in marriage, or by the extent of a person's involvement in social organizations. But which, if any, of these criteria is valid?

Things get more murky when we move to spiritual issues. What form of spirituality is needed to be healthy? Should you go to church once a week? Twice a week? Several times a week? Should you pray daily? Read the Bible? Take a walk in the woods and delight in God's creation? Or on that walk, does it count if you give all the credit to nature? Or what if you give credit for your health to spirits you believe inhabit trees and animals?

This expanded view of health impacts many aspects of health care. Hospitals now offer courses in marriage and parenting. The amazing popularity of Viagra® represents, in part, a broadening of health to include sexual satisfaction. Products to reduce wrinkles, overcome baldness, and enhance sports performance are also said to make us healthier.

These also take us into the gray area of aging and natural ability. Are we healthier if our skin makes us look younger than our years? Or are we unhealthy if we need to appear younger than we actually are?

Clearly, how we define health has profound spiritual, psychological, and social—even financial—consequences that go far beyond the issue of biological wellness. One philosopher of medicine put it this way:

> If health and disease are nothing more than socially determined, culturally mediated and individually subjective concepts, then there will be little if any possibility of either placing medicine on a firm scientific footing or of finding consensus among experts and patients as to the proper limits of medical concerns.[3]

This broader view of health does not mean that physical health should be neglected. It is important and good. It can and should be enjoyed and appreciated. The teaching of the Bible, and the miracles of Jesus, show that God cares for people's physical health. One of the best-known exemplars of biblical love is the Good Samaritan (Luke 10:30–37). He cared for the injured man holistically, including his relational and financial needs. But first the Samaritan bandaged the man's wounds, poured oil and wine on them, and took the man to where he could rest and recover physically.

What Does the Bible Say About Health?

The word "health" is rarely found in English translations. The Old Testament uses a number of Hebrew terms to reflect a broad concept of "health as wholeness." Obedience to God and humility before him are frequently associated with promises of health and blessing: "Do not be wise in your own eyes; fear the LORD and shun evil. This will bring health to your body and nourishment to your bones" (Proverbs 3:7–8; see also Deuteronomy 30:15–16).

Some of the Old Testament laws reflect God's concern for the health of his people and how he expected them to use natural means to promote health. Obeying some of these laws would have promoted health in the same way that public health regulations do today. For example, the Israelites were forbidden to eat meat that we now know was more likely to carry diseases. They were to quarantine people with possible signs of infectious diseases, just as we use certain "isolation techniques" today to prevent spread of infection (Leviticus 11; 13; 14).

The clear teaching of the Old Testament is that good health depends on living one's life according to God's will. This produces *tsedeq*, which means righteousness, or being in a right relationship with God, which leads to a long and healthy life.

This multi-dimensional description of health is carried into the New Testament, which shows us different aspects of health in various contexts. An underlying principle is that humans are more than simply physical beings; we are complicated persons with physical as well as emotional, relational, moral, and spiritual dimensions. The following are some of the passages where this principle is described throughout the Bible.

- Emotions are linked to health, as in Proverbs 17:22: "A cheerful heart is good medicine, but a crushed spirit dries up the bones."
- The morality of our actions influences our health. "For anyone who eats and drinks without recognizing the body of the Lord eats and drinks judgment on himself. That is why many among you are weak and sick, and a number of you have fallen asleep" (1 Corinthians 11:29–30).
- Our spiritual vitality is linked to our health. "Dear friend, I pray that you may enjoy good health and that all may go well with you, even as your soul is getting along well" (3 John 2).

The biblical view of health can also be expressed as blessedness, which was a theme in the Old Testament, and is most clearly described in the Sermon on the Mount (Matthew 5:3–12; Luke 6:20–26). The poor, the meek, the downtrodden, and the underprivileged are blessed, not rejected, by God. This aspect of health takes into account the role of values and beliefs in our view of health.

People can be blessed, and therefore healthy, despite undesirable circumstances. A quadriplegic can be blessed and right with God and "healthy" in the biblical understanding of health. The beatitudes describe the overall well-being of people who are poor, in mourning, or persecuted. In many ways, according to the Bible, our health depends on our inner life, which God wants to nourish and promote.

However, we sometimes need to prioritize the different aspects of our health. The Bible describes situations in which even physical health must be sacrificed for the promotion of spiritual health. Jesus tells us, "If your right eye causes you to sin, gouge it out and throw it away. It is better for you to lose one part of your body than for your whole body to be thrown into hell. And if your right hand causes you to sin, cut it off and throw it away. It is better for you to lose one part of your body than for your whole body to go into hell" (Matthew 5:29–30). The point of this passage is to show us how to order our priorities, not to take it literally. We are not saying that Christians should neglect their physical health. In most situations promoting physical health is completely compatible with promoting spiritual health. But sometimes a choice has to be made.

There will be times when, for the sake of our spiritual health, we will have to make a difficult choice not to pursue some aspect of health. Jesus sums up this principle: "What good will it be for a man if he gains the whole world, yet forfeits his soul? Or what can a man give in exchange for his soul?" (Matthew 16:26).

Central to all of these ideas is the declaration that Jesus Christ came to offer ultimate health to people in the form of a life on earth that would be full and satisfying and meaningful, coupled with the promise of a disease-free, sin-free, tear-free eternal life. "I have come that they may have life, and have it to the full" (John 10:10).

Good Health Should Not Be Our God or Our Ultimate Goal

If someone minimizes the importance of the spiritual, or does not believe in an afterlife, then this life is all there is, and maintaining physical life and health can become the most important focus.

Many of the more recent, controversial developments in conventional medicine (cloning, assisted suicide, test-tube babies) have arisen because some believe that the purpose of life is to promote life itself—and not just *any* life, but life that is judged by human standards to be valuable or of good enough quality.

For many, the focus of their lives is maintaining a certain quality of physical life for as long as possible. Thus, some people hold that cosmetic surgery, the impotence pill Viagra, and medical "treatments" for baldness and wrinkles are important for maintaining a certain quality of life, or "health." Each of these may have a legitimate use in specific cases, but their popularity is a natural outgrowth of the idea that the purpose of life is to promote life itself.

Those who focus only on health also pursue whatever spiritual, relational, emotional, or physical factors will contribute to their goals in life. If religion and spirituality are said to help people live longer, healthier lives, they are willing to try them. Whether the beliefs are based on truth doesn't matter to someone with such a mindset. To such individuals, the purpose of life remains rooted in the here and now, the period from birth to a painless, free-of-suffering physical death.

For many within the New Age movement, this attitude toward life is taken one step further. Health involves self-actualization. "The self-actualized individual is happier, healthier, and more creative."[4] Methods that allow self-actualization to occur involve ways of getting in touch with one's intuitive side, the inner self. Various forms of meditation therefore take on an important role. One's own health in this life becomes of central importance.

> One is responsible only to one's own feelings. Only you can judge your values, [Carl] Rogers said. . . . Within the parameters of the experiential, anything that could conceivably contribute to human growth, whether scientifically verified or not, was admissible—and was admitted.[5]

This type of thinking underlies the openness within New Age thought to alternative therapies. With health defined as broadly as well-being—and the most important test being how people feel after a therapy—almost anything could be included as "therapy."

While the alternative therapies used might be different from the drugs and technology sought by others, the underlying drive is the same. The ultimate purpose in life is good health. Therefore, according to this view, the individual ought to pursue anything that might improve health.

This belief actually makes it more difficult to accept illness, limitations, aging, and death. When the most important thing in life is to be physically healthy, a lack of health can be devastating—and even lead people to belittle their own value, worth, and purpose. People's very identity can be shaken by illness if that illness appears to prevent them from having what they view as most important in life—good health. This may partially explain why people spend huge amounts of resources keeping their bodies "healthy," then demand assistance in suicide when they deem their lives to be of no further value.

The Problem of Living in a World That Deifies Physical Health

Problems arise when we blindly accept our culture's view of health. Christians should be especially concerned about spending their time and money on things with artificial value rather than things of real value.

- Plastic surgery and breast implants for purely cosmetic reasons are based on changing views about physical attractiveness.
- Giving healthy children of below-average height powerful hormones to help them grow taller is based on the artificial value society places on tallness.
- Performance-enhancing drugs in sports are based solely on the questionable value of winning competitions while minimizing the true benefits of sports.

Winning has become everything. More than twenty years ago surveys revealed that some athletes were willing to do anything to win a gold medal. In 1997, *Sports Illustrated* asked almost 200 current or aspiring U.S. Olympic athletes if they would take a drug that would make it possible for them to be world champions for five years even though the drug would then kill them.[6] More than half said they'd take it!

Medicine is being used to promote a form of "health" that is based on personal choices and questionable cultural values. Yet we can't ignore the fact that people who are not sports stars, who are less beautiful, or are shorter than average do suffer for not having traits that society values. Their pain is real, but the problem is prejudice. The answer is not to encourage them to undergo medical "treatment." The answer is in understanding that their suffering is caused by an artificial value, and then rejecting that value, just as God rejects other forms of discrimination: "There is neither Jew nor Greek, slave nor free, male nor female, for you are all one in Christ Jesus" (Galatians 3:28).[7]

What Value Should We Place on Our Health?

Health is good for the reasons God said it is good. We should maximize our physical, emotional, relational, and spiritual health, but they are not ends in and of themselves. The pursuit of physical health must be balanced against other values. Good health is a means by which we can glorify God and serve others. We saw this in Jesus' greatest commandments (Matthew 22:36–40), but it is also expressed by Paul when he says to Christians, "You were bought at a price. Therefore honor God with your body" (1 Corinthians 6:20).

In God's system, there are sometimes good reasons to sacrifice our health and even our lives. Jesus touched the lepers and other "untouchables" of his day for the greater value of their spiritual health. Doctors, nurses, and others still imitate Jesus when they take care of those with infectious diseases. Those who go on the mission field to countries where little health care is available make these same choices for themselves and their families. They are to be admired. They know that there is more to life than just physical health.

Devout Faith Helps But Does Not Guarantee Good Health

Does religious commitment help you live a healthier life? Beneath this question lies an assumption that "good people" shouldn't have to undergo bad things. That "good people," if they are living for God and doing things his way, should reap some benefits of a longer, healthier life here in this world.

God in his Word gives us general guidance for a healthy lifestyle. Those who follow his advice will tend to reap the health benefits, just like following the guidelines in your car manual will generally keep your car running better.

But all the attention in the world to these guidelines won't protect us from others' mistakes or malice—leading to smashed cars, broken bodies, and twisted relationships. Nor can we isolate ourselves from events, like falling trees and hurricanes and genetic illness.

Although we wish it were otherwise, God never promised us perfect health. The church should not act as though he did, promising his healing at a certain time on Sunday. But the church also should not ignore how God does work through natural mechanisms to bring healing.

Some religions, including some that are actively involved in alternative medicine, claim to offer complete health to their adherents. Evaluating the health of believers in those religions would provide important evidence about the truth or falsity of those religions (as has been done for the First Church of Christ, Scientist, or Christian Scientists).[8] For this reason, it is important to examine in detail what the Bible says about healing, and whether God promises to heal Christians.

Scientific studies seem to support the idea that religion is an important factor for health. Numerous studies show a positive correlation between involvement in religious practices and people's health. One researcher said it this way: "A large proportion of published empirical data suggest that religious commitment may play a beneficial role in preventing mental and physical illness, improving how people cope with mental and physical illness, and facilitating recovery from illness."[9]

A national adult sample in 1991 found that the frequency with which people both prayed and attended religious services significantly impacted their health status, regardless of their age.[10] The more involved people were with religion, the better they scored on various measures of health outcomes. This benefit is greatest when the individual is not just actively involved with services and programs in a religious community but when religious faith is an important part of who that person is. A strong faith not only influences a person's understanding of the meaning of life but also serves as a guide for living.[11]

The benefit of faith is not so dramatic for the faithful who worship in isolation, such as those whose involvement in religious services is by radio or television.[12] Other people use religion for self-justification and for sociability, as a means of obtaining status or personal security, thus making religion more utilitarian and self-oriented.[13]

Studies of the impact of religion on health have not been uniformly positive. And a small number of researchers found no correlation between faith and health, and in some cases, they found a negative effect.

From a scientific perspective, many of these studies have significant limitations.[14] Some of the studies were poorly designed, often because of the obvious complexity of religion and health. Most used simple questions like "Do you attend church?" to measure people's religiosity.

In spite of these limitations, the studies seem to indicate that those who rarely attend religious services, or have little personal faith, are at higher risk for disease and illness.

Prayer also has been found to have a beneficial effect in healing by medical researchers.[15] The Bible records numerous instances where God, in answer to prayer, directly intervened to cause healing. Two examples are King Hezekiah (2 Kings 20:5) and the centurion who asked Jesus to heal his servant (Matthew 8:5–13).

These general health benefits of faith are important—and the deeper and more internalized the faith, the greater the benefits. Scientific research has demonstrated that much even if it hasn't (and probably can't) prove *why* people benefit from religious faith. That also is a matter of faith.

Christians Are Told to Expect Suffering

Although faith can improve our health, we should not assume that our lives can, or will, be trouble-free. In fact, the Bible tells Christians both to expect suffering and to not be surprised by suffering. "For it has been granted to you on behalf of Christ not only to believe on him, but also to suffer for him" (Philippians 1:29; see also 1 Thessalonians 3:4; 1 Peter 4:12).

We are to comfort one another and encourage one another with the knowledge that our destiny is secure in the arms of the Lord, even in the face of suffering and death (1 Thessalonians 4:13–5:11).

Some claim illness and suffering reflect weakness in an individual's faith, but this is not borne out by the biblical record. The New Testament mentions by name a number of early church leaders, people we can assume had strong faith, who got sick. All of them died. Every faith healer in recorded history has gotten sick and died—some at a young age.

The faith that moves mountains is not "big faith," but small amounts of faith, faith the size of a mustard seed, one of the smallest seeds known (Matthew 17:20). In fact, Jesus dramatically healed those who stated they had faith even when it was very weak faith. The man with a demon-possessed son did not appear to have much faith when he asked Jesus:

"But if you can do anything, take pity on us and help us."
"'If you can'?" said Jesus. "Everything is possible for him who believes."
Immediately the boy's father exclaimed, "I do believe; help me overcome my unbelief!"

Mark 9:22–24

Their depth of faith was not as important as what they put their faith in—Jesus. This is in direct contrast with the current popular view that it doesn't matter what your faith is in, just that you have faith.

Notes

1. World Health Organization, *Constitution*, available at http://ecco.bsee.swin.edu.au/studes/ethics/WHO-constitution.html (accessed March 23, 2001).

2. Duncan Vere and John Wilkinson, "What Is Health? Towards a Christian Understanding," in Ernest Lucas, ed., *Christian Healing: What Can We Believe?* (London: Lynx, 1997), 59–84.

3. Arthur L. Caplan, "The Concepts of Health and Disease," in *Medical Ethics*, ed. Robert M. Veatch, (Boston: Jones and Bartlett, 1989), 60–61.

4. John P. Newport, *The New Age Movement and the Biblical Worldview: Conflict and Dialogue* (Grand Rapids: Eerdmans, 1998), 118.

5. Ibid., 119.

6. Michael Bamberger and Don Yaeger, "Over the Edge," *Sports Illustrated* 86, no. 15 (April 14, 1997): 60–70.

7. Dónal P. O'Mathúna, "The Case of Human Growth Hormone," in *Genetics and Ethics: Do the Ends Justify the Genes?*, ed. John F. Kilner, Rebecca D. Pentz, and Frank E. Young (Grand Rapids: Eerdmans, 1997), 203–17.

8. William Franklin Simpson, "Comparative Longevity in a College Cohort of Christian Scientists," *Journal of the American Medical Association* 262, no. 12 (September 1989): 1657–58; Andrew Skolnick, "Christian Scientists Claim Healing Efficacy Equal If Not Superior to That of Medicine," *Journal of the American Medical Association* 264, no. 11 (September 1990): 1379–81.

9. Dale A. Matthews, Michael E. McCullough, David B. Larson, Harold G. Koenig, James P. Swyers, and Mary G. Milano, "Religious Commitment and Health Status: A Review of the Research and Implications for Family Medicine," *Archives of Family Medicine* 7, no. 2 (March-April 1998): 118–24.

10. Kenneth F. Ferraro and Cynthia M. Albrecht-Jensen, "Does Religion Influence Adult Health?" *Journal for the Scientific Study of Religion* 30, no. 2 (1991): 193–202.

11. J. LeBron McBride, Gary Arthur, Robin Brooks, and Lloyd Pilkington, "The Relationship Between a Patient's Spirituality and Health Experiences," *Family Medicine* 30, no. 2 (February 1998): 122–26.

12. Mike Mitka, "Getting Religion Seen as Help in Being Well," *Journal of the American Medical Association* 280, no. 20 (December 1998): 1896–97.

13. Gordon W. Allport and J. Michael Ross, "Personal Religious Orientation and Prejudice," *Journal of Personality and Social Psychology* 5, no. 4 (April 1967): 432–43.

14. Jeffrey S. Levin and Harold Y. Vanderpool, "Is Frequent Religious Attendance *Really* Conducive to Better Health?: Toward an Epidemiology of Religion," *Social Science & Medicine* 24, no. 7 (1987): 589–600.

15. Mitka, "Getting Religion," 1896–97.

4

The Christian Explanations for Illness and Suffering

Sincerely religious individuals, active in their faith, can be and are struck down by fatal illnesses while young. This is why people often wonder, "Why do bad things happen to 'good people'?"

Their basic question is: Why? Or, why me, God?

Some Illness Is Caused By Sin

We can say, in one sense, that all sickness has its ultimate origin in sin because human suffering stems from the Fall and the sin of Adam and Eve (Genesis 2:15–17; Romans 1:28–32). But that's not the way most people think of sin causing sickness. The connection between sin and sickness is not a simple cause-and-effect relationship. The Bible doesn't claim that sin always leads to illness. But where sin and sickness are explicitly connected, God is said to either "cause" or "allow" the specific illness.

The Bible teaches that disobedience to God can lead to sickness that ultimately is of supernatural origin. "If you do not obey the LORD your God and do not carefully follow all his commands and decrees I am giving you today, . . . The LORD will plague you with diseases until he has destroyed you from the land you are entering to possess. The LORD will strike you with wasting disease, with fever and inflammation, with scorching heat and drought, with blight and mildew, which will plague you until you perish" (Deuteronomy 28:15, 21–22).

In various cases described in the Bible, the illness could be said to represent a specific judgment for specific sins.

- If the Israelites did not obey God, he promised, "I will bring upon you sudden terror, wasting diseases and fever that will destroy your sight and drain away your life" (Leviticus 26:16).

- After Miriam and Aaron questioned Moses' authority, God afflicted Miriam with leprosy (Numbers 12:9–10).
- The sins of Jehoram, king of Judah, led God to pass judgment on him: "So now the LORD is about to strike your people, your sons, your wives and everything that is yours, with a heavy blow. You yourself will be very ill with a lingering disease of the bowels, until the disease causes your bowels to come out" (2 Chronicles 21:14–15).

Jesus himself made a strong connection between sin and sickness when he healed the man at the pool in Bethesda (John 5:1–15). He basically equated forgiveness with healing, although his emphasis was on the fact that only God brings about either. As Jesus bid farewell to this healed man, he made the clearest connection between sin and sickness, warning: "See, you are well again. Stop sinning or something worse may happen to you" (John 5:14). The clear implication is that if the man sins again (possibly in some specific way well known to the man) something worse than thirty-eight years of crippling illness would befall him.

This incident may have left the disciples (and readers of John's gospel) wondering if every illness is the result of sin. Some people held to this belief at that time, and others have promoted it down through history.

John warns that sin can even lead to a person's death: "If anyone sees his brother commit a sin that does not lead to death, he should pray and God will give him life. I refer to those whose sin does not lead to death. There is a sin that leads to death. I am not saying that he should pray about that" (1 John 5:16). Two believers, Ananias and Sapphira, were struck dead because of a specific sin (Acts 5:1–11). Some Corinthian believers got ill and died because of their sin (1 Corinthians 11:27–34).

Today when someone gets seriously ill, has a tragic accident, or is told their disease will be fatal, it is common to ask, "Why? What have I done wrong?"

Actually, there is no simple one-to-one cause-and-effect relationship between sin and illness. God related to the ancient nation of Israel in significantly different ways than he relates to people today. Israel entered into an agreement with God, where they knew they would be blessed by God if they obeyed him—and swiftly punished by him for disobedience. God told them, "See, I set before you today life and prosperity, death and destruction" (Deuteronomy 30:15).

The Christian church today does not have such an agreement with God. We know from experience that God does not cause people to be ill every time they sin. We also know that God not only has the ability but also the right to punish sin by inflicting illness or death—even today.

But sickness can be related to sin in another, less direct fashion. The guilt most people experience after sin can be a debilitating state, leading to ill health. Most religions emphasize the importance of confession and forgiveness, and offer means by which these can be obtained. The burden of guilt can be very heavy, only matched by the relief of God's forgiveness. King David recounts his experience in Psalm 32:3–5:

When I kept silent,
my bones wasted away
through my groaning all day long.
For day and night
your hand was heavy upon me;
my strength was sapped
as in the heat of summer.
Then I acknowledged my sin to you
and did not cover up my iniquity.
I said, "I will confess
my transgressions to the LORD"—
and you forgave
the guilt of my sin.

Part of the general healing available through Jesus Christ is the total and complete forgiveness of sin, which provides a person relief from both the penalty of sin and the guilt of sin. This forgiveness cannot be earned by keeping rules or performing rituals. Forgiveness, and its healing benefits, is available as a free gift from God. "For it is by grace you have been saved, through faith—and this not from yourselves, it is the gift of God—not by works, so that no one can boast" (Ephesians 2:8–9). We believe this is an important aspect of the connection between healing and confession in James 5:14–16 (see Prayer for Healing, page 252).

Some Illness Is Caused By Demons

Paul's thorn in the flesh is a reminder of another source of illness (2 Corinthians 12:7–10). Paul states that the thorn was a messenger of Satan.[1] It is especially clear from the gospels of Matthew and Luke that illness can have a demonic source.

In these cases, prayer can lead to exorcism of the demons, or the effects of the demons, and result in complete healing. Jesus was asked why he, and not his disciples, could cast out a demon from a boy who was deaf and mute and bring healing. His reply: "This kind can come out only by prayer" (Mark 9:29).

Some Christians claim that all illness has a demonic origin, and that, therefore, all illnesses can be healed through prayer. They hold that since illness is from Satan, and healing is from God, prayer expressed in faith always leads to healing. Their belief is that if people pray persistently and are not healed, they lack faith.

The New Testament does *not* paint a picture of demonic activity causing *all* illness. Clear distinctions are made between illnesses of demonic origin and illness from other causes. For example:

Jesus went throughout Galilee, teaching in their synagogues, preaching the good news
of the kingdom, and healing every disease and sickness among the people. News about

him spread all over Syria, and people brought to him all who were ill with various diseases, those suffering severe pain, the demon-possessed, those having seizures, and the paralyzed, and he healed them.

Matthew 4:23–24

[Jesus] called his twelve disciples to him and gave them authority to drive out evil spirits and to heal every disease and sickness.

Matthew 10:1

Crowds gathered also from the towns around Jerusalem, bringing their sick and those tormented by evil spirits, and all of them were healed.

Acts 5:16

We believe that, after careful and prayerful discernment, if an illness is believed to be caused by demons, Christians can be confident that the power of God will bring healing. God's power is greater than any demonic power. Referring to evil spirits, John encourages the early believers: "You, dear children, are from God and have overcome them, because the one who is in you is greater than the one who is in the world" (1 John 4:4).

This raises the issue of whether demons can influence Christian believers. Some Christians teach that true believers can be possessed by demons and will only be healed when the demons are cast out from them. A study of New Testament passages by John Christopher Thomas, a scholar from within the Pentecostal tradition, concludes that nowhere in the New Testament is a believer described as being possessed by a demon or in need of exorcism.[2]

However, believers can be oppressed by demons, a situation in which significant suffering can be caused. For example, the healing of Simon's mother-in-law is similar in some ways to the rebuking of evil spirits (Luke 4:38–41). Yet it was very clearly not an exorcism. People therefore can suffer at the hands of demons without being possessed by them. We are informed more clearly that Satan was involved in Paul's affliction with the thorn in the flesh, yet Paul was clearly not demon possessed (2 Corinthians 12:7–10).

We can turn to another gospel passage for an important caution regarding the exorcism of demons. Jesus warns that after a demon is cast out of a person, it may try to return and repossess him or her.

When an evil spirit comes out of a man, it goes through arid places seeking rest and does not find it. Then it says, "I will return to the house I left." When it arrives, it finds the house unoccupied, swept clean and put in order. Then it goes and takes with it seven other spirits more wicked than itself, and they go in and live there. And the final condition of that man is worse than the first. That is how it will be with this wicked generation.

Matthew 12:43–45; see also Luke 11:24–26

To prevent this, the void created by the exorcism should be filled by the true Spirit—the Holy Spirit who indwells all of those who become true Christians.

You, however, are controlled not by the sinful nature but by the Spirit, if the Spirit of God lives in you. And if anyone does not have the Spirit of Christ, he does not belong to Christ. But if Christ is in you, your body is dead because of sin, yet your spirit is alive because of righteousness. And if the Spirit of him who raised Jesus from the dead is living in you, he who raised Christ from the dead will also give life to your mortal bodies through his Spirit, who lives in you.

Romans 8:9–11

These passages have important implications for what are called "deliverance ministries," healing through casting out demons. While deliverance ministries have a definite role in the church, those churches that focus primarily on delivering Christians from demon possession must be seriously questioned.

The Pentecostal scholar Thomas notes that, since only about 10 percent of the infirmities described in the New Testament are attributed to demons, "it would seem wise to avoid the temptation of assuming that in most cases an infirmity is caused by Satan and/or demons. . . . The current specialization in exorcisms by some in the church is misdirected at best."[3]

On the other hand, one of Satan's most effective tactics in the Western world has been to convince people that he does not exist. People who do not believe in his existence will have few qualms about trying spiritual practices. Having lowered their defenses, they will be open to therapies that can be spiritually harmful.

Many contemporary Christians with whom we talk seem stunned to learn that instantaneous healing that is not from God can occur.

Some Illnesses Do Have a Purely Physical Cause

While acknowledging that both demons and God can and do cause illnesses, we must not minimize the physical sources of disease, such as viruses, bacteria, cancers, genetic factors, as well as our overeating and lack of exercise and the environmental factors that are poisoning our bodies.

Contrary to those who claim all illness is punishment from God or the result of demon possession, many biblical accounts of healing simply state that the person was ill. Sometimes illness and death were caused simply by crime and accidents. Sometimes people suffer because they just happen to be in the wrong place at the wrong time.

Now there were some present at that time who told Jesus about the Galileans whose blood Pilate had mixed with their sacrifices. Jesus answered, "Do you think that these Galileans were worse sinners than all the other Galileans because they suffered this way? I tell you, no! But unless you repent, you too will all perish. Or those eighteen who died when the tower in Siloam fell on them—do you think they were more guilty than all the others living in Jerusalem? I tell you, no! But unless you repent, you too will all perish."

Luke 13:1–5

The people who suffered were not worse sinners than those who escaped. Conversely, Jesus often simply healed people, making no mention of sin or demons.

Illness of Unknown Origin

In some cases we may never know with certainty the actual origin (or origins) of a particular illness or tragedy. Constantly asking "Why?" or "Why me?" can make it more difficult to accept the comfort God wants to give us in the midst of suffering. Immediately before his passage on healing, James, in 5:11, reminds us of the example of Job: "As you know, we consider blessed those who have persevered. You have heard of Job's perseverance and have seen what the Lord finally brought about. The Lord is full of compassion and mercy." Yet throughout the terrible suffering endured by Job, he never learned why these tragedies had befallen him. We rarely do either.

Some Illness Is Caused By Our Living in a Fallen World

Sin originally led to the downfall of humanity. When sin entered the world, humans changed—not only spiritually, but mentally, emotionally, and physically. With the entrance of sin, humans lost intimacy with God and became alienated from God (spiritually). This resulted in the progression from health to disease (physically), wholeness to emptiness (emotionally and psychologically), and harmony to anarchy (socially).

Spiritual separation from God, physical disease, psychological dysfunction, and social disorder all find their origin in sin. This is often referred to as "general judgment"—God's judgment of sin against all people.

When the New Testament writers mention people being sick, they rarely associate the illness with sin or demons. The clear implication, therefore, is that much illness is of natural origin and exists simply because people live in a fallen world. We can even gain some hope from the knowledge that the world is not the way God wants it to be, and that he promises us a better future.

We know that the whole creation has been groaning as in the pains of childbirth right up to the present time. Not only so, but we ourselves, who have the firstfruits of the Spirit, groan inwardly as we wait eagerly for our adoption as sons, the redemption of our bodies. For in this hope we were saved. But hope that is seen is no hope at all. Who hopes for what he already has? But if we hope for what we do not yet have, we wait for it patiently.

Romans 8:22–25

Some Illness Sets the Stage for a Display of God's Power

God can and does use illness for some special purpose. In the gospel of John, the disciples encountered a blind man, which gave Jesus the opportunity to address this belief of sin and sickness.

As he [Jesus] went along, he saw a man blind from birth. His disciples asked him, "Rabbi, who sinned, this man or his parents, that he was born blind?"

"Neither this man nor his parents sinned," said Jesus, "but this happened so that the work of God might be displayed in his life."

John 9:1–3

While we readily accept our talents and abilities as gifts from God by which we can glorify him, our disabilities and weaknesses are similarly opportunities by which God can be glorified. God declared to Moses, "Who gave man his mouth? Who makes him deaf or mute? Who gives him sight or makes him blind? Is it not I, the LORD?" (Exodus 4:11). God has the right to make us as he wishes, just like a potter does with his creations (Romans 9:20–21).

God struck Paul blind after he met Jesus on the road to Damascus (Acts 9:8–9). Why? While this may in part have been a punishment for Paul's past sins, it forced him to take some time to think over what he had learned on the road. His subsequent healing at the hands of someone he had sworn to persecute must also have served as important evidence that God was behind Christianity (Acts 9:17–19).

Usually we cannot determine "why" God is allowing or causing illness, but almost always a Christian can determine "what" God is doing in and through an illness. The healthy and biblical question for a Christian to ask is not "Why is God doing this to me?" but "What is God doing in this situation?" The first question often arises from an attitude that "if God loved me he would not allow this to happen!" The second indicates a belief and trust that what a loving God allows to happen can be used for good. It is more in keeping with what Paul said in Romans 8:28: "And we know that in all things God works for the good of those who love him, who have been called according to his purpose."

Jim's case is a good example. Jim had grown up in a small local traditional church, as had his dad and his dad's dad. Going to church every Sunday was just something that people in his hometown did.

The minister was nice, but his ministry and sermons never led Jim to consider something beyond Sunday morning religion—like his need for a personal relationship with God.

Perhaps Jim wasn't led because the minister never had such a relationship himself. The minister had gone to seminary for many of the reasons Christians enter other helping professions. As a pastor he could help other people, have a respectable job, and make a good living. His desire was to *serve* others, not *inspire* them. The pastor and Jim coexisted.

Religion and faith were not on Jim's mind the day he, at his wife's insistence, went for his first routine physical in more than twenty years. During the exam, Jim's family doctor found a lump in his prostate. Further testing confirmed that it was a potentially lethal form of cancer. According to the cancer specialists, radical surgery offered the best hope of curing Jim's cancer. The alternatives, watchful waiting, herbs and vitamins, or radiation therapy could, according to the consultants, mean the spread of the cancer to other parts of his body. Jim was terrified.

Jim remembered a Sunday school lesson on the book of James that taught sick people to see their church elders for prayer and anointing with oil. He didn't think those things could hurt. So Jim talked with his pastor. To his surprise, the pastor laughed.

"Jim," the pastor said, "we haven't done those sorts of healing services in over a century. We know that most of those miracles in the Bible were just made up by Christ's followers after he died. Why should we perpetuate a myth?"

Jim was deeply hurt and disappointed. He hadn't asked for a miracle. All he had wanted was the love and prayers of fellow Christians. His pastor wasn't even offering hope.

The night before surgery, Jim slept fitfully. He said later that his only comfort was knowing that his family physician, a man he trusted, would be assisting during the surgery.

The next morning in the preoperative area, as Jim waited to be taken into the operating room, he became increasingly nervous about the surgery, almost terrified about the possible outcome. He wanted to call out to God . . . he wanted to pray . . . but he didn't know how.

In the midst of this emotional crisis, Jim's family doctor arrived, dressed in green operating room scrubs. "Jim," he said, "I know surgery can be scary. For most of us, it brings up questions about God. Every time I've ever taken patients to the O.R., they've wanted to somehow talk to God and ask for his protection and healing. Sometimes they have important things they want to get reconciled with him. So, would you mind if I had a little prayer with you?"

Jim was dumbfounded. Never had he seen religion like this . . . played out in the workplace. He shook his head. Object? No way!

As the doctor began to pray, Jim reached up and grasped the doctor's hand. As the doctor continued the prayer, Jim felt an unexpected sense of peace and something he could not remember feeling for a long time—tears running down his cheeks. Jim found himself squeezing the doctor's hand as he prayed.

After the prayer, Jim dried his tears, feeling somewhat embarrassed. The doctor asked if he had any other questions. "Just one," replied Jim. "You won't tell anyone, will you?"

"Tell them what, Jim?" inquired the doctor. "That we prayed?"

"No," Jim replied. "That we held hands!"

In the days following surgery, Jim's pastor stopped by his room to check on him. They would talk briefly. It was a nice gesture, but that was all. The pastor's visits weren't helpful—spiritually. And Jim now realized for the first time in his adult life that he needed spiritual guidance. He got it from his family doctor, who suggested that Jim begin looking at what the Bible had to say about health, prayer, and recovery. The doctor's words had meaning and hope—and for a cancer patient, no medicine is sweeter.

Because of his upbringing, Jim always thought of himself as a Christian. But during his physical recovery, he realized he did not have a personal relationship with God. Jim's doctor suggested he read the gospel of John. Verses 12 and 13 of chapter one hit him hard:

Yet to all who received [Jesus], to those who believed in his name, he gave the right to become children of God—children born not of natural descent, nor of human decision or a husband's will, but born of God.

Jim realized he had never had the spiritual birth described here. After he finished reading the whole Gospel, Jim knew he wanted a personal relationship with God. He prayed for forgiveness, he thanked God for Jesus' sacrifice on the cross that paid the penalty for his sins. He pictured Jesus standing at the door, and he invited him in (Revelation 3:20).

Jim's relationship with God blossomed as he grew spiritually. He learned how to pray, and he learned how to begin to heal—not only physically, but spiritually. Jim knew, in the depth of his heart, that without the cancer, his spiritual journey would not have begun. He realized that the cancer, as life-threatening as it was, had become an opportunity for him to receive a very special and soul-saving gift from a very special and soul-saving God. He vowed to help other men in their struggles, both with cancer and with finding a personal relationship with God.

God could have healed Jim's cancer miraculously—but he chose not to. Instead, God allowed Jim to grapple with his cancer so that God could bring about the ultimate healing: spiritual restoration of Jim's relationship with God.

We don't believe God would have been pleased if Jim had pursued any and every form of healing, regardless of its spiritual price.

God can use disease to draw people who don't know him to himself, and as a means of discipline for some who know and worship him. How we respond to disease or disorders that he causes or allows is very important to him. According to the Bible, he uses these experiences (illness and injury) to refine or purify his people.

We also rejoice in our sufferings, because we know that suffering produces perseverance; perseverance, character; and character, hope. And hope does not disappoint us, because God has poured out his love into our hearts by the Holy Spirit, whom he has given us.

Romans 5:3–5

Notes

1. John Christopher Thomas, *The Devil, Disease and Deliverance: Origins of Illness in New Testament Thought* (Sheffield: Sheffield Academic Press, 1998), 63–64.

2. Ibid., 301.

3. Ibid., 317.

5

How to Pursue Good Health – the Basic Principles

Tom, a master chef in New York, worked at least sixty hours a week for the owner of an upscale Manhattan restaurant. He loved the work and was delighted that his skills were appreciated by his employer and the sophisticated diners who came to the restaurant.

But the work was strenuous. Tom's body ached from the constant handling of the large pots, pans, and other implements in the commercial kitchen. He ate properly when he ate, but he was often too busy and skipped meals. He always skipped breakfast just to get a few more minutes in bed.

Tom knew he needed a change, to treat himself better, so when he was recruited to be the private chef for a wealthy family, he left the restaurant. Soon Tom was eating right, getting enough rest, and taking long walks every afternoon. He began to feel better than he had in months. His achiness and fatigue diminished drastically, but did not disappear.

Friends suggested an array of vitamins and herbal supplements. They were all natural, "safe," his friends told him, available in any health food store. Tom thought they might help. But he decided to first see his doctor, get an expert's opinion. The physician praised Tom's lifestyle changes, but he recognized that Tom's symptoms were a concern. He was right. Extensive testing revealed that Tom was in the early stages of multiple sclerosis.

That early diagnosis probably prolonged Tom's life. Multiple sclerosis is much easier to treat in its early stages. Tom's increase in exercise, improved diet, and regular rest strengthened him for the long fight to come. There's a good chance he will lead a rich, full life, with the disease progressing slowly enough to be little more than a tolerable burden to which he can adapt. To Tom's surprise, his physician suggested he take some of the nutritional supplements recommended by his friends.

Had Tom tried to be his own physician, treating himself first with the nutritional supplements, his multiple sclerosis might have progressed untreated to where it could no longer be dismissed as mild fatigue, and the potential for his future would likely have been far bleaker.

What Does It Take to Keep You in Good Health?

Good health, to most people, is one of the most desirable aspects of life. Anyone who has experienced chronic illness or long-term disability is likely to say that if they had a choice between being rich and being healthy, they would pick being healthy.

Certainly this is verified every day by the millions of people spending billions of dollars for everything from herbal remedies and vitamins to health spas, the latest high-tech scanners, lasers, and surgeries. People choose to stay in jobs they dislike because of the medical benefits.

Both conventional health care providers and alternative medicine practitioners consider themselves to be in the business of keeping you healthy. The motives of both groups are generally to provide the best care for the patients who choose to come to them.

But God also plays a role in healing, though it often has been neglected. Over the years, with the great successes and advances of medical science, the church has been left to care for people's spiritual needs while medicine takes care of physical healing. In general, only when medicine can do no more do people turn to God for a miracle. And when there is no miracle, they question God and even turn away from him—again.

God rarely gets credit for illnesses medicine can cure, but gets blamed for illnesses that medicine can't cure. How often have we heard people wonder why God would strike someone down with cancer or AIDS?

God's successes in healing also prompt questions. Stories of people who apparently have been miraculously healed cause others, some with the same illness, to wonder, "If God would heal them, why not me?"

Many people expect medicine to have a cure for everything. When one doctor cannot cure an ailment, they turn to another. And another. They search among alternative therapies, believing the books and advertisements that offer hope, a cure. Some demand that nature or medicine or God remove all discomforts and limitations, even those that most people accept as a normal part of aging. They seek the latest miracle cure or health fad in order to extend their life expectancy—to "cheat death" and "live longer," "look younger."

Our Mysterious Modern Ailments

At the beginning of the twentieth century, physicians faced the challenge of trying to treat numerous diseases that had no known cures. Influenza took the lives of millions of Americans. Pneumonia, diarrhea, chicken pox, measles, and scarlet fever were deadly threats to children whose chance for survival into adulthood in some communities was as low as 50 percent. Cancer in any form was usually a death sentence. Heart disease guaranteed that many men would not see their fiftieth birthday. And hospitals were places most people went to die.

At the beginning of the twenty-first century, it might be argued that the biggest challenge society faces is the problem of symptoms in search of a disease. Pharmaceutical companies and companies making herbal remedies are getting rich from the sale of products to fight sleep disorders, elevate mood, and relax tense nerves for reasons that may not be related to physical illness. Fatigue, lethargy, and a sense of spiritual emptiness are more likely to reduce on-the-job performance and interfere with personal relationships than any biological malady.

Busyness and Stress Contribute to Signs of Illness

What is behind these vague symptoms? One contributing factor is that people spend more hours on the job. Salaried employees are being asked to tackle extra work as corporations trim the number of employees to lower overhead and earn higher profits. Jobs that once were hourly are now salaried since a salaried employee does not receive overtime pay. Additional work does not require additional compensation. Service jobs, where pay remains hourly, often pay workers little more than minimum wage. Most of these workers are forced to work a second job in order to meet their expenses.

Working longer hours leads to a series of complications. Few working couples get adequate rest during the week. To do *something* different from the regular workday, we rob a half hour, an hour, or even more from the sleep we need to watch television, play on the computer, or spend more time with our children (keeping them awake too long as well).

Most people are sleep-deprived, a fact reflected in highway accident statistics. Law enforcement agencies increasingly warn that overtired drivers falling asleep at the wheel may be as great a problem as drunk driving.

Family interaction, once an essential and enjoyable aspect of every day, is increasingly seen as an intrusion into other activities now viewed as more important. The shared breakfast or evening meal is now a weekly event at best. Job requirements for parents and teenagers, extracurricular school activities, sports, exercise, music, etc., etc., all mean that most families rarely spend more than a few minutes a day together, and those few minutes are often filled with tension. The push is to get ready for the next event, not be together as a family.

Christians active in their churches add a list of other activities to their schedule. An appropriate focus on our spiritual health and that of our loved ones commits us to activities that can further isolate family members from one another. Church services, Bible studies, youth programs, weekend retreats, and serving the needy can result in even less time with loved ones who also need our spiritual support and encouragement. All these are important, but we need balance.

Some adults add to their stress by combining too many unrelated activities. There was a time when parents would attend their children's athletic events, school plays, and Christmas pageants with nothing more on their minds than enjoying the diversion and encouraging their children. Today it is difficult to go to such an activity without seeing adults using cell phones, Palm Pilots, and other electronic devices. Soccer, baseball, and football practice fields often have parents using laptop computers in their cars or on the bleachers. They glance up from time to time, waving vaguely in the direction of their sons or daughters, trying to give the impression they are watching, yet fooling no one, especially not their children.

Our point is not that any of these activities are wrong, in and of themselves. Nor are we saying that being busy is wrong. The Gospels record that Jesus had a very busy schedule during his public ministry. Paul covered many hundreds of miles in his missionary journeys, preached often, discipled many, and allowed the burdens of many people to weigh heavily on his heart (2 Corinthians 11:28–29). Christian servants throughout history have led active lives and done much to further the kingdom of God.

But there is something wrong when the first thing everyone comments on these days is how busy and stressed out they are. The problem is not that we are busy, but how we balance our activities with times of empowerment. The problem has less to do with what we're doing, and more to do with the mindset with which we approach our activities. If we don't get this right, the consequences can be serious.

Overactivity can lead directly to health problems. Excessive busyness also negatively impacts our significant relationships: with God, with our spouses, with our children, and with those few really close friends we all need. This lack of critical interaction with others can affect our health. Doctors know that a loving touch combined with leisure time spent with a loved one usually reduces stress, lowers blood pressure, and can have a positive effect on the immune system. If you are a parent who has held a sick child when he or she awakens frightened, feverish, and confused, you have experienced the slower heart rate and more relaxed breathing that come from the simple act of being enveloped in love. The child is still sick, but the symptoms seem to ease as he or she falls asleep in your arms.

The Negative Effect of a Sense of Isolation

Isolation also has a negative impact. Many of us are isolated from family members, living in different cities, different states, even different countries. We've lost the old-fashioned connection with neighbors. The isolation from neighbors started innocently enough with the proliferation of televisions that took people off their porches and stoops. It reached a new level with the invention of the Walkman-type tape player. For the first time, you could walk down the street wearing earphones, enjoying music or a book on tape. The social nicety of acknowledging a passerby was no longer necessary because the sight of the earphones alerted everyone that you were lost in a diversion only you could hear. What used to be rude became acceptable.

We gradually abandoned other forms of casual conversation. When was the last time you shared a sales clerk's joy at her daughter being accepted into college or her son making her a grandmother? When did you last extend your sympathies to another supermarket regular who had just lost a spouse? When did you last see anyone offering commiseration and an old family home remedy to a cold sufferer wandering the aisles of the neighborhood pharmacy?

These were the familiar strangers of daily life, the momentary interactions providing a respite from troubles, a sense of community, an awareness that, if ever so briefly, we all matter in someone else's life. For some elderly living alone, this tenuous community can be the incentive to get out of bed and go for a daily walk. This sense of community is the reason some people mourned the demise of the old five-and-dime with its lunch counter as they would mourn the passing of a loved one. The longtime waitresses, the men and women who stopped in for coffee and doughnuts all became a family of sorts. They shared casual conversation. And everyone felt as though they mattered.

The shopping mall food court became a substitute. But it requires a car or bus to get to the mall. It's not part of a casual stroll in the neighborhood. Coffee shops also are filling this void to a degree. Unfortunately, they're creating an environment that partially perpetuates the trend they could have countered. Many have added rental computer terminals with Internet access so patrons have the illusion of community while focusing solely on the screen, oblivious of anyone nearby.

How the Invasion of the Computer Affects Health

And that leads to another challenge to our physical and emotional health—the lengthy use of the computer. In just a few years, the Internet went from being a link among colleges, universities, and government agencies, all engaged in research, to a significant tool of business, interpersonal communication, entertainment, and relaxation. Individuals who have escaped the computer on the job (a rapidly diminishing number) have one at home for Internet access and email.

For some workers, a free personal computer for home use is a perk of their job. Ostensibly the employer-provided computers upgrade the technical skills of the employees and their families. Practically, these computers seductively enter the home, and work hours are extended into leisure time.

Computers not only further our isolation from one another, they have also created health problems. Some are placed on desks never meant to hold them. Keyboards and mouse pads are often in the wrong position for proper use, resulting in the pain and disability of carpal tunnel syndrome—now the most common workplace disability in America. We are also likely to resort to poor posture in an effort to compensate for the bad angle of the keyboard and, in many instances, the monitor, increasing the risk of low back pain, shoulder and neck pain, headaches, and other similar discomforts.

Adding to our problems is room lighting that is either standard tungsten or fluorescent bulbs. We are deprived of full-spectrum light, the type found outdoors at noon. Such light stimulates our body's production of a natural tranquilizer and mood-elevating brain hormones. When you spend your day indoors, staring at a computer screen, without any sunlight, you may feel depressed for seemingly no reason. You are likely to feel emotionally uplifted if you take at least a brisk fifteen- to twenty-minute walk outdoors.

Computer use has also altered our eating habits in much the same way that early television use changed mealtime. The newness of television led many families to make TV-watching the focus of their lives. The dinner hour was shared with television news programs. Since many sets were placed in the living room or family room, dinners were moved to be near the sets. Family members, eating dinner from plates set on TV trays, abandoned conversation in favor of watching TV.

Soon normal preparation of food was considered a time-consuming nuisance and the TV dinner—a frozen meal of meat, a vegetable, potato, and dessert—entered the home. The nutritional quality was questionable, but the convenience was undeniable.

Fast-food restaurants and takeouts are offering another time-saver that has had a negative impact on the diet. Between 1978 and 1995, people in the United States more than tripled the percent of calories they got from fast-foods, and almost doubled the percent they got at restaurants in general.[1] Restaurants can serve healthy food, but what people order has more fat, sodium, refined sugars, and calories than what people cook at home. Diets with nutritious meals are sabotaged by overindulging in caffeinated beverages and snack foods—pastries, chips, and ice cream. Sugar and caffeine are stimulants that enable people to work longer hours than are healthy, increasing the risk of heart disease, hypoglycemia, diabetes, and obesity.

Today's Internet has created the illusion of friendship and community. We can instantly write messages and keep up a form of personal contact through chat rooms and email, all without any face-to-face contact. You cannot see a smile or a tear. You cannot get a hug or hold a hand, share a kiss or walk together in silence. Real interaction is missing. The sense of community and caring that can reduce blood pressure, slow the pulse rate, and trigger what has been called the "relaxation response" is gone.

Participation in a real community can lead to a longer life, regardless of other factors such as diet and exercise. In 1983, a study of the residents of Alameda County, California,[2] showed that people who eat right and exercise regularly, yet are basically loners, frequently have shorter life spans than those who may not take such good care of their bodies, yet feel they are needed, wanted, and loved as part of a community. We may instinctively sense this but let the popular culture lull us into an increasingly isolated way of living and working.

We could go on and on about how modern lifestyles contribute to unhealthy habits. Because of the quality of air circulated on airplanes, frequent flyers know they might experience headaches and more than their share of airborne viruses. "Weekend warriors"—sedentary workers active in sports on weekends—know their muscles will ache on Monday. The late-night movie watcher expects to be tired the next morning.

Physicians are seeing the common complaints linked to these lifestyle changes. Patients say they are tired. Many have headaches or chronic back pain. Depression is frequently mentioned, and many admit their relationships are strained. Many visit doctors asking for a sleeping pill or an antidepressant. Others seek a stimulant. Still others want a tranquilizer. Some worry that they might have Chronic Fatigue and Immune Dysfunction Syndrome (CFIDS), Fibromyalgia Syndrome (FMS), or the early stages of heart disease or cancer. If a doctor asks about their spiritual life, they smile, a bit sheepishly, and say that Sunday is often their only day of rest—unless their children have a baseball game, a soccer game, a...

How Can You Change Your Lifestyle?

Perhaps you see yourself in this situation. You probably have seen it in friends and coworkers. You wonder what you can do. You may have heard that some have found relief from a particular pharmaceutical, an herbal supplement, acupuncture, or some other form of health care. What you may not have heard is that all of these therapies, conventional and alternative, may be helping people avoid their true need while, in some cases, putting them at further risk. These remedies may bring relief for the moment, but something more fundamental may need to change. The person may have a real medical problem that is being ignored. The lifestyle may even be compounding existing medical problems.

Before we look at how to analyze your lifestyle to determine if anything is adversely affecting your health, consider the following principles.

First Do No Harm

Perhaps the classic story of the man who ignored medical advice is that of runner and author James Fixx. The author came from a family of men with a history of heart disease that killed them when they were in their early forties. All had been overweight and underexercised, so Fixx decided to be the exception.

Fixx changed his diet and began running. At first he could pass only a couple houses before becoming so winded he'd have to slow to a walk. After a while he could run from one end of his suburban street to the other before having to catch his breath. Then he went around the block. Over time his distances increased and his weight decreased. He became fit, trim. He began writing best-selling books showing others how they could do what he did.

He also stopped seeking medical advice even though, because of his genetic heritage, Fixx remained at high risk for heart problems. When he began experiencing mild chest discomfort while running, his doctor recommended tests to determine whether he needed medicine, surgery, or both to treat his heart problem. His prognosis, with treatment, was excellent.

Instead of keeping the appointment, Fixx decided to run out the pain. Most athletes experience a certain amount of discomfort in the early stages of exertion. Then their bodies begin producing beta-endorphins, natural painkillers that allow them to continue their activity without further problems. Long-distance runners know that once they get "through the pain" and "into the zone" they'll feel better and be able to continue for a few more miles. This phenomenon is called "the runner's high."

Beta-endorphins are a natural reaction to discomfort. They are not some naturally produced medication that can heal what is wrong with the body. If anything, they mask the seriousness of a symptom.

Fixx apparently believed his natural beta-endorphins could deal with his chest pain and continued running. His body was found by the side of the road. He died, like other men in his family, in his forties from a heart attack. The sad part of the story is that if Fixx had combined his admirable new lifestyle with a medically appropriate program designed specifically for his damaged heart, his life might have been dramatically prolonged.

Before Making Any Changes, Rule Out Any Medical Problems

What does all this mean for you? Before you embark on any lifestyle changes, especially any alternative therapies or remedies, see a doctor to rule out any medical problems, whether you have any symptoms or not. Early diagnosis and proper treatment can mean the difference between life and death. That initial medical review should include the following:

- Have a physical exam to learn if you have any health problems that must be addressed in conventional ways.
- Examine your lifestyle to determine how it might be creating or contributing to any "symptoms" or ailments.
- Inform your physician (one you can trust) of your entire lifestyle—exercise, diet, and unusual stress factors (divorce, loss of a loved one, loss of a job, a new marriage or child).
- Ask your physician to review all prescription medications as well as the vitamins, supplements, herbal products, and over-the-counter medications you take.
- Talk with your pharmacist about possible interactions between medications and nutritional supplements you take, even any infrequently taken over-the-counter products.

Take the Lifestyle Exam

Examining your lifestyle may be just as important for your health and sense of well-being as having a periodic exam by a physician. Lack of rest, lack of adequate daylight exercise, a faulty diet, concerns about your job, pressures from family and friends and even church may all have a negative effect on your health.

As you plan for making lifestyle changes, ask yourself the following questions. There are no right or wrong answers. These questions are meant to focus your awareness on issues that may be impacting your stress level and affecting your health. Some may not apply to you. Others could be the key.

1. What is the average time you spend walking outdoors during daylight hours each day? Include going to and from a parking lot or public transportation pickup point if the distance is at least a half mile. Include lunchtime activity, though not if you regularly pause at store windows or go in and out of shops to briefly check merchandise. The ideal is at least a twenty-minute, uninterrupted walk each day during daylight hours.
2. Do you regularly take the stairs at work? If you are on an upper floor of your building, do you walk up at least one flight of stairs? You might walk a flight and then catch the elevator or take the elevator to a floor just below your own. You might also walk up one flight from your office, then catch the elevator to go down to the lobby. However you do it, walking up at least one flight of steps enhances your cardiovascular system.
3. What type of lighting do you have at work and at home? Is it bright or subdued? Do you have full-spectrum bulbs or traditional fluorescent or incandescent lights? If the latter, arrange to replace the bulbs with full-spectrum lights or add a light to your desk that will use such bulbs.

4. Can you open windows where you work or do you work in a building that is sealed and recycles air? Sealed buildings, even with cleaned, recycled air, can pose health problems that don't occur in buildings with fresh air.

5. How many hours a week do you spend watching television? How long do you use a computer in any manner—from work to the Internet to using a DVD drive to enjoy a movie?

6. Do you live alone or in an emotionally unsatisfying relationship?

7. Do you feel loved and needed by a spouse, other family members, friends, or coworkers?

8. Do you enjoy activities with others? These might include attending religious services and programs, such as Bible study, social clubs, athletic leagues. Do you participate on a regular basis or just on occasion?

9. How many times a week do you eat convenience foods? Include meals in fast-food restaurants, snack foods, and prepackaged meals.

10. How many times a week do you eat fresh fruits and vegetables?

11. When you go out to lunch in a restaurant or coffee shop, do you focus on sandwiches and fries or do you order salads and lunch specials that include a vegetable and lean meat, poultry, or fish?

12. Are you in a caretaker position for a loved one with a chronic illness such as Alzheimer's?

13. Do you have financial concerns you worry you cannot handle?

14. Do you work in a job requiring extensive overtime?

15. Do you work more than one job, either full- or part-time?

16. Do you regularly attend a religious service where you feel a part of the congregation?

17. Do you participate in spiritual activities with others, such as Bible study, prayer groups, food programs?

18. Have you recently relocated, changed your job (or retired), had an illness, or lost a loved one?

19. How much restful sleep do you get on an average night?

20. How many mornings a week do you awaken feeling tired?

21. Do you drink several glasses of water a day (excluding soda, coffee, and other beverages), or do you regularly feel thirsty, as though you have cotton balls in your mouth?

22. Do you keep putting off activities that give you pleasure because you feel you should use that time in some other "useful" way?

23. Do you have any personal space at home or at work? This is an area that might have flowers or pictures, personal mementos or special collectibles, handicrafts from children—items that can make you smile, remind you of loved ones, help you relax.

24. How often do you have a quiet time with the Lord, and how often do you take time to read the Bible and pray—alone?

25. Do you feel overly obligated to others? Do you feel you should say "no" more often but cannot bring yourself to do it?

26. Do you serve others in a regular way? This is important among friends and family and those we don't know. When you do serve others, are you grateful for the opportunity or resentful?

27. Are you your own harshest critic, or do you have a healthy appreciation for the unique and special person you are in God's eyes?

28. Do you see the role God has for you in life, and the gifts and talents he has given you that bring purpose to your life?

29. When you spend time with your spouse or children, are you happy to be with them or worried about your busy schedule? What would they say?

30. Do you have any friend who knows your loftiest dreams and your deepest fears? Do you know what they are? Does anyone know what character issue God is working on in your life at the moment? Do you know?

Did you recognize other areas that are negatively impacting your physical, spiritual, and emotional well-being? Consider how you can modify your lifestyle to improve your quality of life. If you're tired, can you get more sleep? If you're overweight, can you modify your diet and get more exercise? For most people, a change in lifestyle alone will result in at least some improvement in their health.

But if you also need some form of aggressive medical treatment, don't make the mistake Jim Fixx—and too many others like him—have made. For anyone with a medical problem, lifestyle changes must be a part of proper treatment, as prescribed by a doctor.

Taking a Look At What the Alternatives Can Offer

You've seen your doctor, who finds no medical problems. You've changed your diet, cutting down on fats and adding more vegetables and fruits, more whole grains. You now walk four times a week. And you've become an active member at church, gaining a few friends you see regularly.

But you wonder if there's more you can do, should do. Alternative medicine seems to have so much to offer. You hear about the megadoses of vitamins and herbal remedies that people are taking to prevent a laundry list of ailments, the "therapist" who helped a man with back pain.

In the next chapters, you'll find some important cautions and guidelines. Our specific reviews of the various therapies and remedies are in part 4.

Notes

1. Bonnie Liebman and David Schardt, "Diet & Health: Ten Megatrends," *Nutrition Action Health Letter* 28, no. 1 (January/February 2001), 4–12.

2. Lisa F. Berkman and Lester Breslow, *Health and Ways of Living: The Alameda County Study* (New York: Oxford University Press, 1983).

PART THREE

EVALUATING ALTERNATIVE MEDICINE

6

What You Need to Know About the Alternatives

Mary, a secretary for the president of a large department store, began having backaches that seemed to start for no particular reason, though she realized she had poor posture when working at her computer. The backaches got worse after the man Mary thought might propose marriage broke off the relationship. She also began working a lot of overtime. Sleeping became difficult.

Mary went to a new wellness center, recommended by a woman at church who said the center had helped a relative with arthritis. Mary was advised to make some simple changes to her work area and begin taking walks outside, in sunlight, to alter her mood. Encouraged by her improvement, Mary tried a healing technique called Reiki that the center said was similar to the laying on of hands, only older. The practitioner told Mary her body had "energy blockages" that he would "unblock" by using his hands to direct energy to her. "I did feel better after the treatments, though I later realized I felt no better than after I changed my lifestyle," Mary said.

"I also had the feeling that this Reiki was some New Age practice that had nothing to do with God. When I asked the practitioner, he said if I wanted to believe that Universal Life Energy was God, I could. It would not hinder my healing."

Mary stopped the treatments. She was afraid some practices went against Christian teachings. The woman who had recommended the center held a different view, saying if Mary felt better, the treatment must be good. "After all," she said, "we know that all healing comes from God."

All Healing Is Not from God

How we pursue health and healing is very important. Our concern, as Christians, is that there are wrong ways (or even evil ways) by which people can pursue and even receive healing. We wish to make the case that healing achieved by inappropriate means is healing that is not good and, in our view, is healing that is not from God.

This is most important when it comes to the spiritual aspects of some alternative therapies. We believe that certain therapies may have spiritual roots that make their pursuit inappropriate for Christians. Any type of healing that might occur via these therapies is not worth the spiritual cost. Therefore, from a biblical perspective, some forms of therapies are *always* wrong. Further, any seeking of healing, even "good healing," for the wrong reasons or for the wrong motives, may be wrong.

Before we discuss any specific therapies that we believe the Bible disapproves of, we must note that not all Christian theologians and health care providers agree with our interpretation of Scripture. The people of God come from different traditions. They read different translations of the Bible. They come to different conclusions about the meaning of certain words in the translation they are reading. They even differ on the meaning of certain words used in the original language.

We therefore believe it is essential that we explain our thinking and give the biblical basis for our reasoning. We also provide, in part 4, information on the origins of many alternative therapies. We believe this knowledge will help you to understand why some Christian physicians, theologians, and pastors are so concerned about certain aspects of alternative medicine.

Questions to Ask Yourself Before Pursuing Alternative Therapies

For Christians, no amount of physical benefit should make it worth pursuing a therapy that violates biblical ethics or brings spiritual harm. Here are a few questions to ask yourself before deciding to pursue any form of therapy.

- What spiritual beliefs and values underlie the therapy or are held by the therapist?
- What financial and other resources are required for me to obtain this therapy?
- Should I be spending resources on unproven therapies?

People who believe that their physical and emotional health, as defined by themselves, is the most important thing in life are willing to try any therapy. They often ignore valid and rational medical concerns about specific therapies. They pursue useless therapies and potions, expending large sums of money and time in the hope that they can regain their health.

Know the Power Behind the Healing

It's important to know the background of a therapy before you agree to submit to any treatments. Alternative medicine as a whole is not rooted in any religious tradition, but some therapies are. A number of healing rituals and traditions are part of the Wiccan religion (also called "white witchcraft"). Eastern religions often view healing as dependent on the movement of "life energy" through nonphysical channels that coincide with the physical body. Native-American religion uses herbs as part of its religious healing rituals. In a number of nature religions, shamans contact spirit beings or guides to get advice on how to treat and heal those under their care.

Part of the attractiveness of alternative medicine is its emphasis on the holistic nature of health and healing, which for many includes the acceptance of *all* things spiritual. With this interest in holistic healing has come concern for spirituality in health. Spirituality in today's culture tends to mean many different things. According to many, the meaning of spirituality "can be whatever the individual wants it to mean." What *is* important, this new approach to health care says, is that a person be on *some* spiritual path. When it comes to healing, any therapy can be pursued for its potential benefits. All that matters is whether it works. And if others claim it works, it's worth a try.

Many in the alternative medicine camp teach that "there is no such thing as objective reality." For them a cardinal sin is to claim objectivity. This leads to a strong emphasis on "personal experience" being the deciding factor for what is preferable. As the developer of Therapeutic Touch stated: "Therapeutic Touch works. . . . You can do it; everyone who is willing to undertake the discipline to learn Therapeutic Touch can do it. You need only try in order to determine the truth of this statement for yourself. So, I invite you: TRY."[1]

The problem that Christians *should* have with this approach is that the Bible tells us not to engage in certain practices. Certain forms of healing are always wrong because they are accomplished via prohibited methods. Not only have certain rituals and practices been closely guarded secrets, they have also been consistently condemned by God in the Bible. Prohibited are divination, necromancy, mediumship, spiritualism, witchcraft, magic, and sorcery. The most complete list of prohibitions is found in Deuteronomy 18:9–14, although each practice is prohibited in many other passages. (See also 1 Corinthians 10:18–21.)

Many of these practices have been incorporated into certain alternative therapies. Divination covers a variety of practices used to discover information by supernatural means (Leviticus 19:26; 2 Kings 21:6; Jeremiah 14:14). Also included as divination would be tarot cards, reading or interpreting omens, crystal gazing, and any technique which attempts to discern information transmitted from the spiritual realm through natural objects. Divination also includes direct attempts to contact the spirit world for information, as in the use of spirit guides and shamanism.

Astrology is based on the same principles as divination and is denounced as a waste of time by Isaiah.

> *All the counsel you have received has only worn you out!*
> *Let your astrologers come forward,*
> *those stargazers who make predictions month by month,*
> *let them save you from what is coming upon you.*
> *Surely they are like stubble;*
> *the fire will burn them up.*
> *They cannot even save themselves*
> *from the power of the flame.*

Isaiah 47:13–14; see also Jeremiah 10:2

Necromancy is the act of calling up the spirits of the dead, often called "channeling" within the New Age movement. Again, Isaiah is specific in his denunciation of this practice, but not because it doesn't "work." Rather, necromancy, as with all these practices, displays an attitude of rebellion against God by refusing to do things his way: "When men tell you to consult mediums and spiritists, who whisper and mutter, should not a people inquire of their God? Why consult the dead on behalf of the living?" (Isaiah 8:19). Mediums and spiritists are those who possess the ability to contact the spirits of the dead (Leviticus 19:31; 20:6, 27; 1 Samuel 28; 2 Kings 21:6; 1 Chronicles 10:13–14).

Witchcraft is the use of magical spells and charms to obtain desires through supernatural or psychic powers.

> *Now, son of man, set your face against the daughters of your people who prophesy out of their own imagination. Prophesy against them and say, "This is what the Sovereign LORD says: Woe to the women who sew magic charms on all their wrists and make veils of various lengths for their heads in order to ensnare people. Will you ensnare the lives of my people but preserve your own? I am against your magic charms with which you ensnare people like birds and I will tear them from your arms; I will set free the people that you ensnare like birds. I will tear off your veils and save my people from your hands, and they will no longer fall prey to your power. Then you will know that I am the LORD."*
>
> Ezekiel 13:17–21; see also 2 Kings 21:6; Acts 19:18–19

Sorcery is the ability to use magical spells, an ability usually obtained through contacting evil spirits. The prophet Micah brought this message from God to those who in his day dabbled in these occult practices: "I will destroy your witchcraft and you will no longer cast spells" (Micah 5:12; see also Galatians 5:20).

These practices are all condemned because they lead people away from the true God and entrap people in false ways. The use of magic and charms to influence the future reflects a lack of trust in the goodness of God to bring about what is best in a situation. Instead of trying to manipulate the future, we are called to trust in God's trustworthiness.

Occult practices should always be avoided. Clearly, great discernment must be exercised before dabbling in alternative therapies associated with occult and New Age ideas.

Performing spiritual acts with good intentions and getting good results does not excuse being unaware of the source of the power behind those acts. The Bible clearly teaches that good and evil spiritual forces exist. This teaching is contrary to New Age and postmodern claims. Scripture states that evil spiritual forces are powerful and dangerous and should not be dabbled with (Ephesians 6:12; 1 Peter 5:8; 1 John 4:4). It is, in our opinion, naïve and dangerous to think or teach that Satan would not use his powers to heal people, especially since healing is such an important sign of the Messiah. Satan will resort even to "good deeds" to deceive people and draw them away from God. Jesus warned us: "For false Christs and false prophets will appear and perform signs and miracles to deceive the elect—if that were possible" (Matthew 24:24; Mark 13:22).

Biblical Characters Condemned for Pursuing Certain Forms of Healing

The Bible recognizes the great temptation inherent in healing by evil spirits and illicit healers. The Old Testament describes an intense conflict between legitimate and illegitimate approaches to healing and spirituality. An incident involving King Ahaziah, the eighth king of Israel, clearly demonstrates this.

> *Now Ahaziah had fallen through the lattice of his upper room in Samaria and injured himself. So he sent messengers, saying to them, "Go and consult Baal-Zebub, the god of Ekron, to see if I will recover from this injury." But the angel of the LORD said to Elijah the Tishbite, "Go up and meet the messengers of the king of Samaria and ask them, 'Is it because there is no God in Israel that you are going off to consult Baal-Zebub, the god of Ekron?' Therefore this is what the LORD says: 'You will not leave the bed you are lying on. You will certainly die!'" So Elijah went.*
>
> 2 Kings 1:2–4

In contrast, King Hezekiah of Judah became deathly ill and was told by the prophet Isaiah that he would not recover. Hezekiah responded differently, which resulted in God healing him.

> *Hezekiah turned his face to the wall and prayed to the LORD, "Remember, O LORD, how I have walked before you faithfully and with wholehearted devotion and have done what is good in your eyes." And Hezekiah wept bitterly. Then the word of the LORD came to Isaiah: "Go and tell Hezekiah, 'This is what the LORD, the God of your father David, says: I have heard your prayer and seen your tears; I will add fifteen years to your life.'"*
>
> Isaiah 38:2–5; see also 2 Kings 20:2–6

Interpretation of another incident has sparked controversy on the role of physicians. King Asa was a godly king in Judah during the early years of his reign. However, "In the thirty-ninth year of his reign Asa was afflicted with a disease in his feet. Though his disease was severe, even in his illness he did not seek help from the LORD, but only from the physicians. Then in the forty-first year of his reign Asa died and rested with his fathers" (2 Chronicles 16:12–13).

Some conclude from this passage that the Bible condemns using physicians and calls on people to seek only healing from God. Yet Scripture refers to physicians and their role in healing (Jeremiah 8:22; Matthew 9:12), and Luke, the author of a Gospel and of Acts, was a physician (Colossians 4:14). Even the context of the passage about Asa makes it clear that Asa's primary problem was not his use of physicians but his refusal to ask God for help. It is most likely that the physicians Asa relied on were Gentiles who practiced pagan magical healing.[2] Support for this view comes immediately after Asa's death, when his son, who succeeded him as king, is praised because he followed God and "did not consult the Baals" or carry out the idolatrous practices of Israel (2 Chronicles 17:3–4). Biblical examples show the need for discernment regarding where we turn for healing.

'Life Energy' Forces May Be a Link to 'Medical Magic'

Alternative therapies based on "life energy" use principles just like those generally believed in the Bible to constitute magic. Although "magic" is difficult to define concisely, magical practices do have some common features. Magic involves specific techniques or rituals by which people attempt to manipulate supernatural powers to meet their immediate needs.[3] Practitioners of energy medicine claim they can manipulate a supernatural force using certain techniques to bring about healing or relaxation in an individual.

Christians who use, promote, or support energy medicine should reflect on the incompatible, irreconcilable natures of magical healing versus divine healing. Many magical incantations that used Christian terms have survived from the first centuries of the church and are characterized by the same common features found in magic today. As one authority noted, "There is never anything humble about the requests addressed to supernatural agents."[4] In magic, a healing is demanded. "In magic a ritual is performed and if it is correct in every detail, the desired result must follow unless countered by stronger magic."[5] The focus is on the present-day desires of the individual, and not on any long-term goals or the needs of the community.

Magic and the Occult Can Cause Harm

Often, the magic doesn't work, but it can still do harm. It wastes precious time, time that could have been used to seek proven, effective remedies. Instead, a cancer continues to grow. Diabetes and high blood pressure go untreated and continue to do damage.

An even bigger problem arises when magical practices do work! Long associated with occult traditions, many of these practices can lead people into all sorts of entanglements with occult forces of evil. Kurt Koch, a Christian theologian and an authority on the occult, recounts many stories of people being healed by alternative therapies without knowing of the occult connections. One young man went to an iridologist who diagnosed his illness and suggested some treatments.[6] (See Iridology, page 235.) Soon afterward, this young man recovered completely from his illness. But then he noticed some disturbing changes. Every time he tried to enter a church, he experienced physical pain. The same thing happened whenever he tried to read a Bible or sing a Christian hymn. He rapidly became severely depressed, started abusing drugs, and eventually had a complete emotional breakdown. Certainly, not all iridologists (or alternative practitioners in general) are connected with the occult, but this particular one was.

We acknowledge that this story has all the limitations of testimonials that we describe elsewhere in our book. But it fits the pattern of stories where people inadvertently received an occult healing and paid for it with their emotional and spiritual health.

Be suspicious of any practitioner who accurately diagnoses illnesses by "extraordinary" means, or who knows things about others through some "amazing" intuition. Those powers must come from somewhere. The chances are that they are supernatural powers. Great caution and discernment are necessary to ensure they are not occult powers.

The Gray Area of Alternative Medicine for Christians

Alternative therapies are practiced in different ways by different people. When Julie, a Christian who feels called to teach others about some alternative therapies, practices Therapeutic Touch, she prays to God and asks him to bring about healing. She honestly believes she is getting in touch with the power of God and being used by him to minister to those she treats. Yet many others trained in the same technique call upon a universal life energy to bring healing.

Meditation can be practiced as a way to get general spiritual guidance, to become more at peace with one's inner self, to simply relax—or to contact spirit guides. Meditation is taught by both practitioners of the occult and by the Bible! How are we to discern which is which? How can we know whether an alternative therapy violates the biblical commands to avoid inappropriate spiritual influences?

Biblical Principles on Which to Base Decisions

Scripture gives us some clear principles to rely on when making decisions in these areas. First, most of the above passages condemning occult practices come from the Old Testament. Most theologians teach that Christians are not bound by many of the Old Testament laws, such as those related to worshiping in God's temple.

Does that mean that prohibitions of divination and magic no longer apply to Christians? Paul makes it clear that events described in the Old Testament remain important teaching tools for Christians. "Now these things occurred as examples to keep us from setting our hearts on evil things as they did. . . . These things happened to them as examples and were written down as warnings for us, on whom the fulfillment of the ages has come" (1 Corinthians 10:6, 11).

We should learn from the Old Testament accounts. Occult practices are denounced in the most forceful language possible. Nowhere in the New Testament are we told that these practices are now permissible or that God has changed his perspective on them. The occult practices forbidden in the Old Testament remain forbidden. The Old Testament accounts of Israelites conducting these practices stand to their shame and detriment and remain as examples to us of things not to be practiced under any circumstances, even in the pursuit of healing.

The second general principle found in 1 Corinthians 10 is that Christians were to have no involvement whatsoever in sacrifices made to idols or demons. "No, but the sacrifices of pagans are offered to demons, not to God, and I do not want you to be participants with demons. You cannot drink the cup of the Lord and the cup of demons too; you cannot have a part in both the Lord's table and the table of demons" (1 Corinthians 10:20–21).

Any alternative therapy involving contact with any spirit other than God is forbidden. Shamanism, Reiki, channeling, divination, and any other "therapy" which attempts to bring knowledge or healing from other spirits or spirit guides should be avoided.

Are Homeopathic and Herbal Remedies Spiritually Tainted?

Some homeopaths and herbalists invoke various spirits when preparing their remedies. Christians should avoid seeing these sorts of practitioners, or using their particular remedies. But what if a Christian happens to use one of these remedies? Have they spiritually "contaminated" themselves? We believe that Christians need not fear that a remedy prepared by a homeopath or herbalist is somehow contaminated with evil spirits, regardless of what means were used in the preparation.

We come to this conclusion because Scripture provides guidance on a similar issue faced by the early church. In those days, meat would be sacrificed to idols in pagan temples and later sold in the marketplace. There was debate among Christians whether eating this meat was involving oneself in occult activities (Romans 14; 1 Corinthians 8; 10). But Paul said, "Eat anything sold in the meat market without raising questions of conscience, for, 'The earth is the Lord's, and everything in it.' If some unbeliever invites you to a meal and you want to go, eat whatever is put before you without raising questions of conscience" (1 Corinthians 10:25–27).

Some homeopaths believe they spiritually vitalize their preparations as they make them. Dana Ullman, president of the Foundation for Homeopathic Education and Research, wrote: "Homeopaths conceptualize a 'life force,' or 'vital force,' they describe as the inherent, underlying, interconnective, self-healing process of the organism. This bioenergetic force is similar to what the Chinese call 'chi,' the Japanese call 'ki,' yogis call 'prana,' Russian scientists call 'bioplasm,' and Star Wars characters call 'The Force.' Homeopaths theorize that this bioenergetic process is sensitive to the submolecular homeopathic medicines. The resonance of the microdose is thought to affect the resonance of the person's life force."[7]

Some believe herbal remedies are effective because of the nature spirits they say dwell in them. Rosemary Gladstar, an herbalist, says she decides which herbs to use by first examining a patient, "Then I pray and let the spirit of the herbs guide me."[8]

Just because some people use acupuncture needles to manipulate life energy does not automatically mean Christians should have nothing to do with acupuncture. A remedy may be acceptable if the physical components can be separated from the underlying belief system, analogous to how Paul separated the meat from the idolatry.

We must also remember that Paul was talking about food, not remedies and therapies. When applying these verses to alternative medicine, we must ensure that the issues of concern are analogous in all important ways. The freedom to use remedies would, we believe, apply only to those that involve physical matter. A physical basis for some benefit then exists, independent of whether the item was put through some spiritual ceremony. Meat that had been sacrificed in a pagan ceremony would still have nutritional value, and may be considered similar to taking an herbal remedy or using an acupuncture needle. Only remedies with demonstrated benefits (and devoid of any divination, necromancy, mediumship, spiritism, witchcraft, or sorcery) should be used. The physical benefits of all remedies are then best evaluated by scientific criteria.

The principles developed here apply differently when discussing alternative therapies that do not incorporate physical materials. Knowledge of the precise details of the therapy is needed. Alternative therapies like shamanism and Reiki may "work" because they contact spirit guides, and therefore, according to God's Word, should not be used under any circumstances.

Other therapies, especially various meditative and consciousness-altering practices, are not as clear-cut. Included here would be such things as mediation, yoga, visualization, and guided imagery. These are sometimes used for relaxation, but other times they are methods for getting in touch with the "inner self" or some spirit being. This is sometimes viewed as a source of healing in and of itself, and other times it is seen as a means to gain insight and guidance into health-related issues. Before trying any of these types of practices, investigate them thoroughly. Find out what sort of teaching you will be exposed to. Ask others who attended exactly what the sessions involved. (See discussion under each therapy in chapter 12.)

Look to the Bible, Not Inner Voices, for Guidance

When investigating an alternative therapy, many will claim you should follow your instincts and listen to your guiding voice. Guidance by intuition and inner voices has become more in vogue today than guidance through reason and objective evidence. Postmodernism has contributed to this acceptance with its notion that we all create our own reality, that whatever we believe is OK. Christians may even be attracted to these ideas because of our belief that God reveals his will to us through Scripture and the Holy Spirit. If Christians believe they are being led by the Holy Spirit to practice a certain therapy, should we question them? If during meditation or visualization someone gets a strong feeling that God is telling them that a certain practitioner can help heal them, should we say anything more?

Again, Christians must look to the Bible for guidance. The Old Testament was clear that anyone claiming to have a message from God, that is, to be a prophet, was to be put to the test. "You may say to yourselves, 'How can we know when a message has not been spoken by the LORD?' If what a prophet proclaims in the name of the LORD does not take place or come true, that is a message the LORD has not spoken. That prophet has spoken presumptuously. Do not be afraid of him" (Deuteronomy 18:21–22).

It is clearly appropriate, even necessary, to evaluate claims. This is especially important when it comes to information received in an altered state of consciousness. Occult activities and healing rituals have always used a variety of ways to induce meditative states and altered states of consciousness. Through meditation, occultists claim that details concerning what to do during a healing treatment "will soon come 'intuitively' to the healer. Do not be afraid to follow your intuitive sense in this direction."[9]

One occultist claims that students of white witchcraft are unsuccessful as healers when "they fail to act in detail as their inner voice tells them; they leave undone certain things which they are prompted to do in their moments of meditation."[10]

Stemming from these ideas comes encouragement from one of alternative medicine's popularizers, Deepak Chopra, M.D., to "experience the effortless way that intentions can get fulfilled, bypassing the ego and the rational mind."[11] Larry Dossey, M.D., another popular author, encourages us to trust what we feel led to do even though our unconscious mind may lead us to "violate the values we hold dearest in our aware, conscious life, such as our moral and ethical codes, in order to help us."[12]

Underlying these ideas are three core beliefs that contradict clear biblical teaching:

- Personal autonomy is of supreme value.
- Humans are innately good.
- Humans are potentially or actually divine.

Within the world views that hold to these beliefs, meditative practices bring healing by enlightening us to our true nature. Transcendental Meditation (TM), which underlies numerous alternative therapies, claims that, "On the level of the Transcendental Consciousness we are Divine already."[13] All our problems arise, according to TM, because we don't realize this. "Although we are all 100% Divine, consciously we do not know that we are Divine."[14] TM misuses Psalm 46:10 by claiming that God's statement about himself applies to all people. To quote TM's founder, the Maharishi Mahesh Yogi: "Christ said, 'Be still and know that I am God.' Be still and know that you are God and when you know that you are God you will begin to live Godhood, and living Godhood there is no reason to suffer, absolutely no reason to suffer, Man is not born to suffer."[15]

Apparently, this "prophet" is not aware of the teachings in the Bible. Paul taught, "But join with me in suffering for the gospel, by the power of God" (2 Timothy 1:8). Peter instructed us, "Dear friends, do not be surprised at the painful trial you are suffering, as though something strange were happening to you" (1 Peter 4:12).

Chopra claims that the healthy person is the one who believes and affirms that "I know myself as the immeasurable potential of all that was, is and will be. . . . There is no other I than the entire universe. I am being and I am nowhere and everywhere at the same time. I am omnipresent, omniscient; I am the eternal spirit that animates everything in existence."[16]

Nothing could be further from the truth, according to the Bible. There is one God, one Creator, who is completely distinct from his creation. "For there is one God and one mediator between God and men, the man Christ Jesus" (1 Timothy 2:5). Using meditation to bring us in touch with our inner voice is fundamentally flawed because of the biblical teaching about human nature. Humans are not divine or perfect: "The heart is deceitful above all things and beyond cure. Who can understand it?" (Jeremiah 17:9).

Humanity throughout the ages has sought insight through various meditative practices and altered states of consciousness. It was commonly done during Old Testament times, and was consistently condemned by Scripture. At least three reasons are given for rejection of these practices.

1. They can bring people into contact with the demonic realm, which is spiritually and physically dangerous for people.

2. The knowledge that would be obtained in these states was unreliable. The false prophets of Israel claimed to get reliable information through visions, trances, dreams, and altered states of consciousness. Scripture labels the information obtained by these "prophets who wag their own tongues" as "false hopes," "delusions of their own minds," "false dreams," and "reckless lies" (Jeremiah 23:16–32). These ways of gaining knowledge lead to deception, not true insight. "Woe to the foolish prophets who follow their own spirit and have seen nothing! Your prophets, O Israel, are like jackals among ruins. . . . Their visions are false and their divinations a lie" (Ezekiel 13:3–6).

3. The third reason for rejecting insight gained from our intuition and inner selves is moral. At its root, New Age beliefs hold that human nature is good and perfect— divine, in fact. According to these views, a student of white magic "has to learn to do the right thing as he sees and knows it. . . . He must depend on himself. . . ."[17] The Bible holds that dependence on self is the root of humanity's problems.

Be Careful of the Impact Your Decisions May Have on Others

Christians must be concerned about more than their own freedom to choose; they must consider the impact their choices have on others, how others will interpret their actions. If a Christian uses a therapy or remedy with links to the occult, their example may cause others to follow that lead. In 1 Corinthians 8:12, Paul uses very strong language to condemn such actions by calling them a "sin against Christ."

The impact of how others view our involvement in these practices should always be taken into consideration. Our witness to the power of Christ may be damaged in the eyes of the world if we are feverishly chasing after ineffective or spiritually dangerous remedies.

Notes

1. Dolores Krieger, *Accepting Your Power to Heal: The Personal Practice of Therapeutic Touch* (Santa Fe, N.M.: Bear & Company, 1993), 8.

2. Darrel W. Amundsen and Gary B. Ferngren, "Medicine and Religion: Pre-Christian Antiquity," in *Health/Medicine and the Faith Traditions: An Inquiry into Religion and Medicine*, ed. Martin E. Marty and Kenneth L. Vaux (Philadelphia: Fortress, 1982), 53–92.

3. Howard Clark Kee, "Magic and Messiah," in *Religion, Science, and Magic: In Concert and In Conflict*, ed. Jacob Neusner, Ernest S. Frerichs, and Paul Virgil McCracken Flesher (New York: Oxford University Press, 1989), 121–41.

4. Kee, "Magic and Messiah," 126.

5. John Ferguson quoted in Kee, "Magic and Messiah," 123.

6. Kurt E. Koch, *Occult ABC* (Grand Rapids: Kregel, 1986), 104.

7. Dana Ullman, *Discovering Homeopathy: Medicine for the 21st Century*, rev. ed. (Berkeley, Calif.: North Atlantic, 1991), 15.

8. Rosemary Gladstar, *Herbal Remedies for Children's Health* (Pownal, Vt.: Storey, 1999), 24.

9. Yogi Ramacharaka, *The Science of Psychic Healing* (Chicago: Yogi, 1909); A. E. Powell, *The Etheric Double: The Health Aura of Man* (1925; reprint: Wheaton, Ill.: Theosophical Publishing House, 1969), 70.

10. Alice A. Bailey, *A Treatise On White Magic*, 6th ed. (New York: Lucis, 1963), 586.

11. Deepak Chopra, *Ageless Body, Timeless Mind: The Quantum Alternative to Growing Old* (New York: Harmony, 1993), 99.

12. Larry Dossey, *Healing Words: The Power of Prayer and the Practice of Medicine* (New York: HarperSanFrancisco, 1993), 61.

13. Maharishi Mahesh Yogi, *Meditations of Maharishi Mahesh Yogi* (New York: Bantam, 1968), 177.

14. Ibid., 177.

15. Ibid., 178.

16. Deepak Chopra, *Escaping the Prison of the Mind: A Journey from Here to Here* (San Rafael, Calif.: New World Library, 1992), audiocassette.

17. Bailey, *Treatise On White Magic*, 586.

7

Alternative Medicine and Children

The growing interest in alternative medicine among adults has carried over to children and into the offices of pediatricians and family practitioners. If a parent is taking echinacea, a popular remedy for preventing colds that we consider to be scientifically unproven though apparently safe for many people, should a child with a runny nose be given it? Is garlic oil a better eardrop than commercial products made specifically for children? What about acupuncture for children with cerebral palsy, or megavitamin therapy for children with Attention Deficit Disorder (ADD) or Attention Deficit Hyperactivity Disorder (ADHD)?

A survey by the American Academy of Pediatrics found that 93 percent of pediatrician members reported being asked about alternative therapies by the parents of their patients.[1] A study at a pediatric outpatient clinic in a Canadian university hospital found that 11 percent of the children had previously been to an alternative medicine practitioner (most commonly a chiropractor or homeopath).[2] This survey didn't evaluate overall interest, since many alternative therapies do not involve visiting a practitioner. Other studies have asked parents who have children with chronic or recurring illnesses whether they use alternative therapies. As many as 70 percent of these parents said they use these therapies in addition to conventional therapies.[3]

Herbal Remedies Increase Some Risks for Children

Kathi J. Kemper, M.D., an associate professor of pediatrics at the Center for Holistic Pediatric Education and Research at Harvard Medical School, has published numerous articles on the use of alternative medicine in children. In particular, she has been concerned about children who have surgery after taking herbal remedies. She has noted that some herbal remedies increase bleeding during surgery.[4]

Other concerns involve interactions between popular herbal remedies and drugs critical for sustaining life. For example, St. John's wort, the enormously popular antidepressant that has proven to be effective for people with relatively mild depression, may be potentially life-threatening when used with certain medications for the treatment of AIDS and other conditions.[5]

Parents use alternative therapies and herbal remedies for their children for the same reasons they use them on themselves. Parents believe they are cheaper, safer, and have little risk of side effects. What is sometimes forgotten is that the reason herbal remedies work, when they do, is because they alter the body's chemistry. A product that can safely affect an adult's health might be overwhelming for a child. The child's immune system might be compromised. The child may have an adverse reaction. We have little information on dosage and effectiveness of herbal remedies in adults; we have even less on children.

Some Procedures Are Generally Safe for Children

Some procedures may be harmless to try. Acupressure and acupuncture are felt by many practitioners to be generally safe in children, though whether they will be effective for the problem a child is having is questionable. One estimate claims that the number of children being treated by chiropractors increased 50 percent between 1997 and 2000.[6] While many adults seek chiropractic care for musculoskeletal problems, children are commonly treated by chiropractors for ear infections, allergies, asthma, colic, and bed-wetting. Very few randomized controlled trials of chiropractic exist for any pediatric condition, with one of the first finding it was no more beneficial than a placebo for children with asthma.[7] The lack of value placed by some chiropractors on the importance of research evidence has also been of concern. Thus, for example, only 30 percent of chiropractors in the Boston area promote immunization, the effectiveness of which is supported by high-quality studies, while 70 percent recommend herbs and dietary supplements with little or no research support.[8]

In contrast, the use of martial arts to help children learn self-control may be a valid approach to helping some hyperactive children. Anecdotal evidence is so strong that many school systems suggest this form of physical activity to parents of children being treated for ADD or ADHD. [Note: While most schools are concerned with martial arts as a sport or for self-defense, some have instructors steeped in traditional Chinese medicine (see Traditional Chinese Medicine, page 279). This may expose children to a philosophy of life quite opposed to Christian teachings. Before enrolling a child in any form of karate or judo, parents would be wise to sit in on several classes, both exclusively for children and for adults, to hear and see what is being taught.]

The University of Arizona Medical Center has been experimenting with aspects of alternative medicine for children.[9] While nothing is conclusive at this writing, some therapies are starting to show some positive results. For example, hypnosis is proving to be helpful in relaxing the muscles of children with cerebral palsy. This appears to reduce or delay the deterioration that inevitably comes with the disease. See the entry on hypnosis in chapter 12 for the concerns we have about hypnosis in general.

At this writing, the field of pediatric alternative medicine is just beginning to be exposed to the scientific method. Yet we are already seeing active promotion of alternative therapies for children. Rosemary Gladstar is an herbalist who has written numerous popular books, one of which promotes herbal remedies for children.[10] She claims herbal remedies are safe for children, stating, "Contrary to what you may have heard or read, my experience has been that almost any herb that is safe for an adult is safe for a child so long as the size and weight of the child are accounted for and the dosage is adjusted accordingly."[11] But she acknowledges that herbs affect people differently and could cause serious adverse reactions.

Gladstar bases her claims on her years of experience using herbal remedies. She does not refer to any controlled scientific studies as support for her decisions. On the contrary, she points out that "most herbalists rely on years of experience and intuition." Her view of scientific research is summed up in the following statement: "If a plant has been found safe and effective for a thousand years of human use, it may be wise to question the validity and applicability of the scientific tests now being used. There is generally some unidentified magic in the plant in the form of another chemical or an innate natural wisdom that allows the medicine, when taken as a whole, to function in a safe and beneficial manner."[12]

After examining a child, Gladstar says she will "pray and let the spirit of the herbs guide me. This, of course, is balanced with a thorough understanding of the herbs I am using, plus many years of experience."[13] We have scientific concerns about Gladstar's approach, especially when people without her experience use herbs for children.

Her approach also demonstrates why Christians need both spiritual and scientific discernment when investigating alternative therapies. Herbalism teaches that the healing power of herbs comes as much from spirits that reside throughout nature as it does from chemicals in the plants. In contrast, herbal medicine refers to the "secular" approach to herbs: the idea that they work naturally through the chemicals they contain. Taking children to an herbalist could expose them to teachings that contradict the Bible and may expose them to spiritual activities that could be harmful.

Some Remedies Should Never Be Used for Children

We also believe that reliance on experience and intuition may lead to physical harm. For example, Gladstar claims children can use "gentle herbs" like borage and licorice "with no residual buildup or side effects," and also use "stronger" herbs like comfrey and chaparral.[14] In chapter 13, we discuss clinical evidence that these particular herbs have all caused serious side effects in adults. We believe this is strong evidence that they should never be used in children.

Homeopathic remedies (another form of alternative medicine) are commonly given to children. One study found that children comprised a third of all the patients seen by homeopaths.[15] Before they are three years old, most children will get at least one ear infection. Some parents try homeopathic remedies. While at least three-quarters of all ear infections in children go away on their own, some infections can progress to more serious conditions, most of which can be treated effectively with antibiotics.

Given the high rate of spontaneous remission of these ear infections, use of homeopathic remedies frequently appears to be successful, so some will claim that homeopathy can cure ear infections, but a review of reports found "there is no published evidence to support this claim."[16] This review of all relevant research found only two studies involving homeopathy and ear infections. Even though both studies showed positive results for the homeopathic remedies, the design of the research made it impossible to place any confidence in these results. These studies were not blinded, nor were they properly randomized. One compared homeopathy with conventional medicine, but the children using conventional medicine had infections that had already proven to be more difficult to treat. Results of more recent, better designed research on homeopathy for a variety of other conditions have tended to find that homeopathy is no more effective than placebo.[17] Reviewers of these studies have also noted "that more rigorous trials have less-promising results."[18]

Not Enough Is Known About What Works in Children

It will be many years before a broad range of therapies and herbal remedies can be adequately tested to assure the safety and effectiveness of their use with children. Until then, parents might limit their exploration of alternative treatments to those that do not alter the body's chemistry—such as acupuncture and acupressure. Children should never be given herbal remedies or megadoses of vitamins in the belief that they are safer than pharmaceuticals. We still know too little about what works, what doesn't, the appropriate preparation, and the proper dosage for age and body weight to be able to trust such potentially dangerous products as herbal remedies for children. We also do not know whether a child's growing body will react quite differently from that of an adult.

Gladstar's approach is simply to treat children as small adults. She describes two "rules" for calculating doses for children based on their ages and the adult dose.[19] One she calls Young's Rule, which calculates that a four-year-old should be given one-quarter the adult dose. The second she calls Cowling's Rule, which calls for a four-year-old to be given one-sixth the adult dose. Yet Gladstar's own dosing recommendations call for a four-year-old to be given less than one-twentieth of the adult dose. Such inconsistency reveals how little is known about dosage of herbal remedies for children.

Conventional medicine has learned through tragic experience that the approach of just reducing the adult dosage can be dangerous for children. Reye's syndrome, a condition that can cause permanent disability or death, is just one example. Until the 1980s, hundreds of children in the United States got this disease every year.[20] The culprit: aspirin. A link was discovered between aspirin and Reye's syndrome, leading to much publicity discouraging aspirin use for children seventeen years of age or younger. By the late 1990s, only two cases of Reye's syndrome were being reported per year. We now know that the developing body chemistry of children is very different from the body chemistry of adults. This success story should serve as a precaution against giving children any medicine without knowing how safe it is—for children.

Parents considering treating their children with alternative therapies should keep in mind that many alternative medicine practitioners have little conventional medical training. In Massachusetts half of the homeopaths involved in one study had no medical training, and their training in homeopathy ranged from twenty years to only *three weeks*.[21] All practitioners should know their limitations and when to seek input from others. The Massachusetts homeopaths stated they would, on average, treat a child for three to four months before deciding their therapies were not working. Only half of the nonphysician homeopaths would refer a two-week-old child with a fever of 101.5° F to a physician even though any newborn with such a high fever needs to be seen immediately by a physician.

In this same study, less than a third of the homeopaths recommended immunization, and almost 10 percent actively opposed immunization. In England, the most common reason given for not having children immunized is the recommendation the parents received from a homeopath.[22] While all vaccines carry a small risk of adverse effects, lack of immunization carries significant risks. Children in the United States who were not immunized against measles were between 22 and 35 times more likely to contract the illness than those who received the measles vaccine.[23] As more people refuse to be immunized, the health of the community can be affected negatively. During the 1970s and 1980s concerns about alleged side effects from the *pertussis* vaccine led to reduced usage, resulting in a major resurgence in whooping cough (also called *pertussis*). This infection can be very serious in young children, which is why those alternative therapists who preach against established immunization programs do not have scientific support.

Talk with your child's physician about any alternative, complementary, or herbal remedies that you are considering for your child. Most physicians who care for children are happy to discuss this topic. In fact, more than half of the pediatricians in one study reported that they already have such discussions with the parents of their patients.[24] However, keep in mind that as limited as the testing of alternative products sold for adult use has been, there are far fewer tests, if any, concerning children. And since children are not just miniature versions of adults, information on the appropriate dosage and preparation may not be available.

Risks Generally Are Too Great for Children

In general, we believe that alternative medicine is inappropriate for the vast majority of children. The potential risks are too high. Until studies are performed showing that a particular alternative therapy is safe and effective for children, that therapy should, in our opinion, be avoided.

Equally important, keep in mind that many minor illnesses play an important role in early childhood development. They challenge the body and help build the immune system we need as healthy adults. Compromise the immune system in a child, and you may have an adult with a chronic condition that could readily have been avoided by letting a minor illness run its natural course during childhood.

Notes

1. Report by Kathi J. Kemper, M.D., M.P.H., associate professor of pediatrics at Harvard Medical School, in *AMNews* (American Medical News), March 27, 2000.

2. Linda Spigelblatt, Gisèle Laîné-Ammara, Barry Pless, and Adrian Guyver, "The Use of Alternative Medicine by Children," *Pediatrics* 94, no. 6 (December 1994): 811–14.

3. Anju Sikand and Marilyn Laken, "Pediatricians' Experience With and Attitudes Toward Complementary/Alternative Medicine," *Archives of Pediatric and Adolescent Medicine* 152, no. 11 (November 1998): 1059–64.

4. Paula Gardiner and Kathi J. Kemper, "Herbs in Pediatric and Adolescent Medicine," *Pediatrics in Review* 21, no. 2 (February 2000): 44–57.

5. Stephen C. Piscitelli, Asron H. Burstein, Doreen Chaitt, Raul M. Alfaro, and Judith Falloon, "Indinavir Concentrations and St John's Wort," *Lancet* 355 (February 2000): 547–48; Frank Ruschitzka, Peter J. Meier, Marko Turina, Thomas F. Lüscher, and Georg Noll, "Acute Heart Transplant Rejection Due to Saint John's Wort," *Lancet* 355 (February 2000): 548–49.

6. Anne C. C. Lee, Dawn H. Li, and Kathi J. Kemper, "Chiropractic Care for Children," *Archives of Pediatric and Adolescent Medicine* 154, no. 4 (April 2000): 401–7.

7. Jeffrey Balon, Peter D. Aker, Edward R. Crowther, Clark Danielson, P. Gerard Cox, Denise O'Shaughnessy, Corinne Walker, Charles H. Goldsmith, Reic Duku, and Malcolm R. Sears, "A Comparison of Active and Simulated Chiropractic Manipulation as Adjunctive Treatment for Childhood Asthma," *New England Journal of Medicine* 339, no. 15 (October 1998): 1013–20.

8. Lee, Li, and Kemper, "Chiropractic Care for Children," 401–7.

9. *AMNews* (American Medical News), March 27, 2000.

10. Rosemary Gladstar, *Herbal Remedies for Children's Health* (Pownal, Vt.: Storey, 1999).

11. Gladstar, *Herbal Remedies*, 10.

12. Rosemary Gladstar, *Herbal Healing for Women* (New York: Fireside, 1993), 25.

13. Gladstar, *Herbal Remedies*, 24.

14. Ibid., 11.

15. Anne C. C. Lee and Kathi J. Kemper, "Homeopathy and Naturopathy: Practice Characteristics and Pediatric Care," *Archives of Pediatric and Adolescent Medicine* 154, no. 1 (January 2000): 75–80.

16. E. P. Barrette, "Homeopathy for Acute and Chronic Otitis Media," *Alternative Medicine Alert* 3, no. 4 (April 2000): 39.

17. Klaus Linde, Michael Scholz, Gilbert Ramirez, Nicola Clausius, Dieter Melchart, and Wayne B. Jonas, "Impact of Study Quality on Outcome in Placebo-Controlled Trials of Homeopathy," *Journal of Clinical Epidemiology* 52, no. 7 (July 1999): 631–36.

18. Linde et al., "Impact of Study Quality," 631–36.

19. Gladstar, *Herbal Remedies*, 25–26.

20. Ermias D. Belay, Joseph S. Bresee, Robert C. Holman, Ali S. Khan, Abtin Shahriari, and Lawrence B. Schonberger, "Reye's Syndrome in the United States from 1981 through 1997," *New England Journal of Medicine* 340, no. 18 (May 1999): 1377–82.

21. Lee and Kemper, "Homeopathy and Naturopathy," 75–80.

22. Neil Simpson, Simon Lenton, and Robina Randall, "Parental Refusal to Have Children Immunised: Extent and Reasons," *BMJ* 310 (January 1995): 227.

23. Daniel R. Feikin, Dennis C. Lezotte, Richard F. Hamman, Daniel A. Salmon, Robert T. Chen, and Richard E. Hoffman, "Individual and Community Risks of Measles and Pertussis Associated with

Personal Exemptions to Immunization," *Journal of the American Medical Association* 284, no. 24 (December 2000): 3145–50; Daniel A. Salmon, Michael Haber, Eugene J. Gangarosa, Lynelle Phillips, Natalie J. Smith, and Robert T. Chen, "Health Consequences of Religious and Philosophical Exemptions from Immunization Laws: Individual and Societal Risk of Measles," *Journal of the American Medical Association* 282, no. 1 (July 1999): 47–53.

24. Sikand and Laken, "Pediatricians' Experience," 1059–64.

8

The Gurus: Fraud, Quackery, or Wisdom?

Evaluating the philosophy of a popular writer in the field of alternative medicine is never an easy task. The vast majority of these writers are fervent evangelists for what they believe to be the truth about healing and wellness. Most are well educated. We believe that most of these writers are sincere.

We also believe that some are sincerely wrong. Their ideas are spiritually questionable or medically unsound—or both. They're not necessarily or knowingly trying to mislead anyone. They care about their patients and the public at large. They believe conventional medicine (and sometimes an alternative medicine approach they have witnessed) is naïve or even dangerously wrong. After experimenting with different forms of health care, they have developed an approach that—when you listen to the stories of success they tell—seems excellent.

What separates these writers—this type of health care practitioner or adviser—from others who may share some or all of their beliefs is their popularity. They've written a popular book or established a strong Internet presence. Their notoriety gives them credibility in the eyes of many. Their written words lay out a case so compelling that many readers blindly and trustingly try the recommendations. Many are not concerned about what their physician might think or whether the suggestions have been scientifically evaluated.

Perhaps the practitioner is charismatic and has built up a following through appearances on radio and television. It's easy to believe someone who seems so honest and compassionate, who looks attractive and even has a pleasant voice. Especially drawn to this type of expert are those who have experienced a conventional medical practitioner who, despite great skill and knowledge, has a terrible bedside manner and little or no apparent gentleness or tenderness.

Also vulnerable are those with little hope of a cure, who have been told there is no treatment. Perhaps a spinal cord injury is restricting a once-active person to life in a wheelchair.

A cancer has so riddled a man's body with disease that he now has only months to live. A young woman, crippled from birth, knows that no amount of conventional surgery can fix her body. Then there are those who suffer from chronic fatigue syndrome or fibromyalgia or some other chronic pain syndrome for which there is no cure and little relief.

Desperation can drive such individuals to try anything that offers hope—a tiny miracle—even a small reduction in their suffering. "What have I got to lose?" they ask. They're drawn to anyone who offers the promise of a better tomorrow—no matter how unlikely, how expensive, how outlandish the claims—because they can no longer stand the pain or aren't ready to accept the severe limitations of their physical world.

When people are desperate, they don't care about objective evaluation of remedies. They want help. And that's when they are prone to fall prey to frauds, quacks, or those who are true believers in what is truly wrong. These terms are not easy to clearly distinguish from one another. People don't agree on precisely how to define each one. But any discussion of alternative medicine is sure to eventually raise at least one of these terms. Therefore, we need to discuss what they generally mean, and how we will be using them.

Medical Fraud Knowingly Uses Worthless Treatments

Fraud is set apart from the other terms when the practitioner uses a medical treatment that he or she knows is worthless. Good examples of medical fraud are a variety of electronic devices used over the years to "treat" cancer, heart disease, arthritis, and numerous other conditions. The precise type of device and the claims vary, but what they often have in common is a "box" that looks scientific. The gauges, dials, lights, and switches all appear to function, but in reality do nothing. The more complex the box appears and the more knowledgeable the health care provider seems to be about the device, the more confident a patient is that the treatment works.

In fact, many patients exposed to such devices will likely leave a session feeling better. The reason: they've received the concentrated attention of a seemingly caring individual who has carefully listened to their complaints, commiserated with their suffering, and strongly suggested that healing will take place.

Patients also hear of others who have received the therapy and say it works. Perhaps their pastor or other respected church leader claims the therapy is effective—it may even have helped the pastor or a close relative. Commercials on local Christian radio stations suggest that hundreds or even thousands have been helped by the therapy. Reference is made to reputable "scientific studies" that "prove" the therapy works. Books, magazine articles, and a Website may all praise the therapy, giving the sufferer hope and a feeling of enthusiasm.

But when all the claims are bogus, it's fraud. Any good results are due in part to the placebo effect, part to wishful thinking. Although the improvement or relief may be real, it's only temporary. The people offering the therapy know the treatment itself does *not* work. They exaggerate the benefits. They make up some of the stories about the people who have benefited. They leave out the stories of those who have been unhappy with the product.

What Quacks Don't Know Could Harm You

We see quackery as different—at the level of the practitioner's motivation—from fraud. Fraud is intentionally selling therapies the practitioner knows can't do what is claimed. Quacks don't know the therapies they're promoting can't work. We use the term quackery to describe what might be considered medical nonsense, but sometimes it also refers to medical incompetence. The word is shortened from *quacksalver*, which originally referred to untrained persons who practiced medicine.

The problem with quackery is that the gurus—the seemingly wise experts who present their ideas to the public—believe what they are saying. Generally they're not trying to mislead anyone. They genuinely feel that what they are doing and recommending helps patients, and they have anecdotal evidence for support. None of this lessens their responsibility to check the accuracy of their claims. A person providing a worthless treatment may have been duped by someone who knew the therapy was fraudulent. Quacks are convinced their therapies work. Even when there's plenty of evidence that a therapy is useless, they continue to hold on to their false beliefs and offer their therapies. They don't want to know about the evidence that proves their therapy is worthless.

Quacks are often inspired by misunderstood geniuses of the past who fought against the establishment every step of the way until they finally achieved some radical breakthrough. Some were even vilified when reporting their findings. Yet in the end, these geniuses were shown to have been right. What was viewed as outlandish and impossible in their day eventually became "obvious" and routine. Many quacks see themselves as the heirs to the misunderstanding and ultimate triumph of those historical figures.

They love to quote Arthur Schopenhauer, the nineteenth-century German philosopher, who stated:

> All truth passes through three stages.
> First, it is ridiculed.
> Second, it is violently opposed.
> Third, it is accepted as being self-evident.

Indeed, some of today's quackery may contain some grains of truth that will prove useful in tomorrow's medicine. But we think a close examination will reveal the difference between a medical breakthrough and most quackery. For example, in the 1970s a medical professional promoted the idea that a healthy diet was determined by eating only vegetables arranged by color. He had an elaborate theory that he personally followed. His health was excellent, his vitality the envy of much younger men and women. For a while he lectured to select employees of major corporations—divisions of IBM, General Motors, and others. At home, he had his wife arrange a vegetable platter with careful attention to green, red, and other colors.

He was serious. He was certain that if he could disseminate his information widely enough, he would improve the health of people everywhere, that his theory would become part of mainstream medicine. Yet no evidence from controlled studies has demonstrated that his approach to nutrition works. We are fairly certain that his claims meet our definition of quackery.

Sniffing Out Frauds and Quacks

How can you tell if something is a fraud? Or quackery?

First, look at the claims. If something seems too good to be true, it probably is. Or if someone is offering a cure-all, a panacea, giving a laundry list of ailments that are all guaranteed to be cured by the same remedy, it's almost certainly deliberate fraud.

A good example of a too-good-to-be-true advertisement is a booklet distributed recently through the mail that was offering information on old remedies.[1] On the front cover were the words "Read This or Die." The back cover stated, in part: "After you read this bulleti . . . you probably won't die of cancer, won't die from a heart attack, won't die of a stroke, won't die of diabetes—or any common condition." The fine print promised even more: "And I'm fairly certain you'll never suffer from arthritis, osteoporosis, high blood pressure, insomnia, cataracts, glaucoma, memory loss, Alzheimer's, impotence, depression, candida, or any long-term viral disease." The brochure claimed, "Doctors have usually ignored or suppressed the truly great discoveries—for about 50 years, on average." Information on these "truly great discoveries" was offered via a subscription to a newsletter that promised to lead readers to the best sources for "effective treatments and cures for every major disease troubling mankind." Some of the products listed are available from only one supplier, according to the booklet.

Sound too good to be true? Then it probably is. Writers of such brochures often play up the popular, though erroneous, idea that there is a conspiracy to keep the public from learning about some simple way to become and stay healthy. The booklet states that although people throughout the world have found ways to stop "every killer disease and chronic illness . . . you just haven't been told about their solutions yet."

The implication of these sorts of claims is often that physicians and pharmaceutical companies have a financial stake in keeping you sick. The realities of the health care industry would even seem to confirm what they claim. Dozens of companies manufacture pharmaceuticals. Most make money selling medicines only if you are sick. Physicians are healers. They, too, are called most often when there is sickness or injury. If there is nothing to heal, the conspiracy theorists reason, the physicians have no job. No money.

Many people buy this argument. The pitch is selling a dream, a hope: to be disease-free until death from old age. So they order and start using a "simple" and "natural" preparation. Many times it costs "only a few dollars" a month—although some frauds can be very expensive. It's money, they reason, that would have gone to "doctoring" or "the medical establishment" anyway. Besides, they expect to save money. They'll no longer need to belong to an HMO or buy health insurance. If everyone would use this "miraculous product," the billion-dollar health care industry would simply collapse.

Promises like this are nonsense, fraud. No one product can cure or prevent all ills. Period! Promoters of such claims find it a lucrative way to make a lot of money.

For Opportunists, Timing Is Everything

Opportunists and frauds are usually out to make big bucks off of your ignorance and blind faith. They take what is still unproven and hype it as the latest breakthrough. They pick up on major newspaper reports of a promising new therapy in the early stages of scientific testing and promote it as the answer to whatever ailment is current in the media.

For example, an ideal situation for the opportunist would be reports that an herbal remedy seems to slow tumor growth in mice. We're talking about herbs (which are unregulated), and cancer (a universal fear), and research suggesting the herbal remedy offers some hope to cancer victims. Timing is crucial. The opportunist's sales pitch gives all the positives from the initial finding and none of the negatives.

Opportunists don't mention that the initial test has not been repeated. Those "promising results" reported with such certainty may either turn out to be an error or may never be proven in humans.

They don't say that the idea of the herb, or some component in it, providing a safe preventive for cancer is just a theory—a hope—based on a preliminary finding. What's still needed are careful studies, first with animals, then with humans. The product is years away from being reported in reliable medical journals, another fact ignored by the opportunist. They also fail to mention that no one knows the side effects of taking the herbal remedy, or what drugs or foods might interact with it, or even who might benefit from taking the product, and how.

The opportunist gives no warnings. There is no "buyer beware."

The opportunist, once the product is on the market, enlists others to sell the product. Thus the people we meet selling these products sincerely believe that the product does what they claim it will do. They believe it. They want you to believe it too. But this sales force often has the tell-tale signs of the quack: little or no training in medicine or any health care field related to what they are selling. If you place your faith in them and their remedies—and they're wrong—you may have made a costly mistake—risking your health and throwing away your money.

Warning Signs of Quackery and Fraud

Suspect quackery? Fraud? What are the warning signs? When evaluating a medical claim, here's what to look for. We don't claim this is an original list as we have heard these warnings from many people over the years. We've modified and combined these ideas and added some of our own. We hope that as you evaluate a new remedy, you'll stay clear of the ones that are advertised along the lines of what we view as "quack ads."

1. Watch out for products and practices promoted as a "Major Breakthrough," "Revolutionary," "Magic," or "Miraculous." The real value of a medical therapy is rarely known until after it has been in use for many years. Only after a large segment of the population has received the therapy can a profile of the ideal patient be known. It often takes years to uncover the common side effects. Only after many people have used a therapy can we know with some certainty that it is truly effective.

Aspirin could fit into this category as a "miracle" drug. Just ask any arthritis sufferer who has tried it. However, over the years since its introduction in 1899, physicians have learned that up to 25 percent of the population may not be able to safely use aspirin. It can cause serious internal bleeding. Some may have an allergic reaction to it. And in a small number of children (up to age seventeen), aspirin use is associated with the potentially fatal Reye's syndrome. The passage of time has enabled physicians to standardize the dose of aspirin, understand who should and should not use it, and take advantage of its anti-inflammatory, antifever, antipain (analgesic), and anticlotting properties. We're still learning about the benefits (and dangers) of aspirin. Only recently have doctors started recommending aspirin as an aid for preventing a heart attack or even something helpful to take—after calling 911—when you suspect you are having a heart attack.

2. Be cautious of promotions that try to elicit an emotional reaction rather than present clear information that helps you make an informed decision about the product. Marketing strategies play upon our emotions to get us interested in buying a product. Promoters of questionable health products prey upon the emotions of the vulnerable and the desperate. People are asked if they are tired of fad diets, then are presented with yet another. Outrageous claims scare people into thinking their water, or food additives, or the air in their homes is poisoning them. And once the ad has you feeling scared, you're ready to try anything that claims to protect you.

Guilt is another emotion that's effective in a sales pitch. Here's a quote from the booklet we mentioned that was distributed through the mail: "Let me be blunt: Cancer, heart disease, stroke, and the other major killers now fall into the category of 'diseases for dummies.'" The implication is that if you get any of these diseases, it's your own fault! If only you had bought these products earlier!

3. When only anecdotal or testimonial evidence is used to support claims of a product's effectiveness, beware. Quotes from numerous satisfied customers, even satisfied doctors and nurses, adorn these Websites, these ads on TV and radio and in magazines and newspapers. When a celebrity endorses a product, that's meant to convey even stronger evidence that the product actually works even though the celebrity is no more qualified to speak about the product than you are.

4. Even the quacks and frauds will claim to have scientific evidence supporting their therapies. Watch out for the following:

- Few or no references given to original research studies.
- Studies done by only one researcher.
- Studies done at obscure, unknown institutions.
- Studies reported in small or virtually unknown journals.
- Studies reported decades ago.
- Studies that have not been repeated.
- Funding of research by someone with a financial or professional stake in the results.

By the time you have finished reading this book we hope you will know why these are important considerations. However, it may be difficult to find some of the studies and takes some training to be able to evaluate them. That's one of the reasons why we have searched out and summarized the original research on the therapies we evaluate in the second half of the book. If the promotional material only says "studies have shown," there may be important reasons why they are not making it easy to evaluate the original research.

5. Is the information about the therapy or product being provided by a professional lacking in the proper credentials? The essence of quackery is someone without adequate training giving medical advice. Do the therapists or experts have an alphabet soup of unfamiliar credentials after their names?

6. Are technical words used without a clear definition? "Energy" is one of those words. "John had more energy after just three treatments." A good night's sleep can give anyone more energy.

7. Would a treatment require you to abandon any well-established scientific laws or principles? This is often subtle in quackery, blatant with fraud. For example, psychic surgery requires you to believe that a hand, without first cutting an opening, can enter the human body, perform whatever surgery is necessary to remove tumors or organs, then be withdrawn, all with no marks, no obvious place where the flesh was separated. Since it violates so many scientific laws, it may be fraudulent. If it actually works, then it most likely involves supernatural forces. Christians should then have a host of spiritual concerns.

8. Do proponents claim that research was so flawless ("airtight") that there is no need for further testing? A different outcome is not possible? No area of medicine is 100 percent certain. Nor does it always work for all patients.

9. Is the treatment said to be effective for a wide variety of unrelated physiological problems? If something really does work, it usually has a limited effect—a specific action on a specific part of the body. If a treatment or product is said to cure everything, chances are it cures nothing (though it may be a powerful placebo).

10. Is the product a quick and easy fix for a complicated and frustrating condition? A "favorite" is called Exercise in a Bottle to help people lose weight and boost athletic performance. It appeals to our desire to find easy answers, avoid the difficult lifestyle changes needed to lose weight and get fit. But the idea that you can get the benefits of exercise by taking a pill is ridiculous.

11. Does the proponent of the therapy claim to be criticized unfairly? Portrayed as a martyr, does he or she claim to be crucified by the government, the medical establishment, or some other organization with a stake in keeping you unaware of the breakthrough? A physician claims his license to practice medicine was revoked in order to silence him. Check the facts. The real reason for the license revocation may have been due to quackery that was endangering the health and lives of patients. He may have been censured in the public interest, not against it.

12. When challenged, do defenders attack the critic instead of responding to the challenge? Proponents of a therapy with sufficient evidence to back up their claims do not need to attack the challenger.

13. Are persecution and conspiracy theories used to attack challengers? This goes back to the idea that somehow the medical and pharmaceutical establishments are protecting their lucrative territory.

14. Is the formal training needed to give the therapy offered only at obscure private institutions instead of accredited professional schools? Can anyone, with payment of a sizable tuition or fee, become a practitioner after only a few hours or days?

15. Do proponents use expertise in other areas to lend weight to their claims in medicine? Find out if the "expert" has any training in medicine or a related health care field.

16. Is a therapy encouraged simply because it's been used for centuries by some natives in a remote region? It might simply mean that those people have nothing else to use. If the best texts on the subject are decades or centuries old, you'll probably find that many of the old ideas were discredited long ago. Medicine evolves—just think about all we have discovered about nutrition in the last few decades. Continued use adds to our knowledge, uncovers side effects, fine-tunes dosage, and brings change.

17. Do proponents use statements that are basically true but unrelated to the therapy? Promoters of energy-based therapies like Therapeutic Touch and Reiki often mention the value of massage and touch. Both massage and touch are valuable and helpful, but irrelevant here because energy-based therapies are said to work through some nonphysical energy that does not require touch.

18. When asked to demonstrate a therapy or document proof of claims, does the proponent blame any failure on skepticism or outright nonbelief of observers? For example, a physician who uses applied kinesiology stated in a training video that his therapy doesn't work well when skeptical relatives of patients are present. He recommended that practitioners allow only "believers" in applied kinesiology to be present during their sessions. We acknowledge the role of psychological factors in healing, but an effective therapy should work whether the person believes or not.

19. When someone expresses skepticism about a therapy, does the proponent say an explanation of how the therapy works is too difficult for most to understand, or that only the "enlightened" can understand? Do they add that there are lots of things we have to accept without fully understanding them? Do they claim that research will prove the therapy is effective as soon as some is conducted? In legal arenas, ignorance of the law is no defense. In science, a lack of data never supports a conclusion.

20. Does the proponent disguise the truth with vague and misleading statements? A statement such as, "This therapy has been thoroughly tested by seven leading medical research facilities" may fail to add that the tests showed the product is worthless. The "research facilities" should be legitimate, independent organizations whose findings are made available for independent review. See our entry on pyruvate for a good example (pages 412–15)

21. Does the product you're considering require advance payment? You may never receive what you bought or get your money back.

22. Does the advertisement promise a "money-back guarantee"? Fraudulent businesses will have closed shop and moved on before you have a chance to complain.

23. Is the therapy available only in other countries? Foreign countries can have legitimate clinics, but they can also have fraudulent ones. Some countries have very lax regulations. Physicians may not be required to have the same credentials as you would expect in the United States. Before traveling, contact the local health authority where the clinic is located.

24. Watch out for conflicts of interest. Health care providers who recommend and sell products may not be as objective about the product as you would hope. You need to be as cautious about doctors and nurses selling magnets and herbs as you do an acupuncturist selling vitamins. This holds true for both conventional and alternative medicine. If practitioners tell you they have discovered a great new product, then try to sell it to you, you need a second opinion from someone who does not stand to gain financially from the sale.

25. Is the term "natural" the main advantage of the remedy? Do promoters claim that the product is safer because it's natural? Natural does not necessarily mean safe. Nature contains many poisons that are fatal (like certain mushrooms), highly irritating (think about poison ivy), or cause allergic reactions (like pollen or even milk, for some people). If something natural has the potential to heal, it also has the potential to hurt.

A popular "quack-buster" is Stephen Barrett, M.D., a nationally renowned author, editor, and consumer advocate. An expert in medical communications, he is medical editor of Prometheus Books and consulting editor of *Nutrition Forum*, a newsletter emphasizing the exposure of fads, fallacies, and quackery. He has published forty-seven books, including *The Health Robbers: A Close Look at Quackery in America.* He is a board member of the National Council for Reliable Health Information, a Scientific Advisor to the American Council on Science and Health, and a Fellow of the Committee for the Scientific Investigation of Claims of the Paranormal (CSICOP).

Dr. Barrett usually is not spoken of in glowing terms by most practitioners of alternative medicine. They claim he is not licensed to practice medicine (without mentioning that while practicing medicine he was licensed to do so). Many believe he is closed to new ideas, a crusader out to preserve the antiquated ways of conventional medicine.

We feel he gets closer to the truth than most of them do—at least on scientific grounds. His Website, www.quackwatch.com, is usually a good one for discovering the latest research on this or that health fad.

The Gurus

What we have said so far applies primarily to evaluating products and advertisements. We must also look at how to evaluate the claims of the writers who popularize the ideas behind the alternative medicine movement. For many, these are the "gurus" of the movement, the men and women whose latest books are scooped off the shelves by their followers. We will examine two of the most famous alternative medicine gurus who support their ideas and claims with extensive media campaigns that sell a specific approach to wellness.

DEEPAK CHOPRA, M.D.

The popular Deepak Chopra, M.D., has become one of the most prolific and popular authors in alternative medicine. His numerous books include some best-sellers, and all have enticing titles: *Creating Health*, *Quantum Healing*, *Perfect Health*, and *Ageless Body, Timeless Mind*.[2] More recently, he has focused on promoting the religious and spiritual views that underlie his approach to health.[3]

Chopra was trained as a physician in India, and in 1970 moved to the United States where he focused on endocrinology (the study of the hormones that regulate much of the body). In 1985 he was appointed chief of staff at what is now called Boston Regional Medical Center.

While Chopra had achieved much success in medicine, he became disillusioned with modern Western medicine. All he did as a doctor, he has said, was write prescriptions to alleviate symptoms: "Medical training doesn't equip doctors to help patients make changes that will have a significant impact on their health."[4]

Chopra read about Transcendental Meditation (TM) and put it into practice (see Meditation, page 246). Within weeks he had stopped smoking and drinking whiskey. He started reading about the medicine of his native India, called "Ayurveda" (see Ayurvedic Medicine, page 155). He returned to India to rediscover his "roots" and was soon involved with Maharishi Mahesh Yogi, the man who introduced TM to the West. Maharishi asked Chopra to start a company with him called Maharishi Ayur-Veda Products International, Inc. Together they distributed herbal remedies, teas, oils, and other Ayurvedic products (the hyphen allowed them to register Ayur-Veda as a trademark). Shortly after this Chopra resigned his hospital position to direct an Ayur-Veda health clinic in Lancaster, Massachusetts, which soon attracted the rich and the famous. With all this success Maharishi, in 1989, bestowed upon Chopra the title "Dhanvantari (Lord of Immortality), the keeper of perfect health for the world."[5]

During this time, Chopra started writing books that sold widely. A charismatic and extremely persuasive speaker, he was soon on the best-sellers' lecture circuit (charging $25,000 per lecture[6]) and appearing on television.

In 1993, Chopra resigned from all involvement with the TM organization and started a clinic in California as part of Sharp Healthcare. With reported charges to clients of $4,000 a week, its focus was obviously on the rich and famous.[7] The California clinic abruptly closed in 1995, and Chopra has since focused on writing and speaking. After leaving the TM organization, the Maharishi removed all Chopra's materials from his clinics and deleted all references to Chopra from Ayur-Veda materials.[8]

Chopra's Philosophy

Chopra provides an important example of why Christians need to critically evaluate the spiritual claims made by some within alternative medicine. A complete analysis of these claims would take up our whole book. An excellent book on this topic, including a more detailed evaluation of Chopra's philosophy, has been written by a group of Christian physicians.[9]

Chopra's views on health and medicine appear to us to be based on his modernized version of Ayurveda and Hinduism mixed with some conventional medicine. For this reason, it is difficult to separate his views of health from his religious beliefs, so we will consider them together. He preaches that to be healthy, people first need enlightenment. Chopra states:

> We all need to be healed in the highest sense by making ourselves perfect in mind, body and spirit. The first step is to realize that this is even possible. To create health you need a new kind of knowledge based on a deeper concept of life. Although our package of skin and bones looks very convincing, it is a mask, an illusion, disguising our true self which has no limitations.[10]

Chopra's approach is that we need to realize we are both infinite and all-powerful. In his own words: "The truth is: I am here, but I am also everywhere else. That you are there, but you are also here because here is there, and there is everywhere, and everywhere is nowhere, specifically."[11] And again: "We all have the power to make reality."[12] Once we come to believe these things, according to Chopra, we can create the health we so deeply desire. For Chopra, mind has complete control over matter. "People can become happy simply by realizing that the source of change is inside themselves. The responsibility for all illness and all cure resides within us."[13]

We get ill, Chopra claims, when our mind and our consciousness are not aligned with what he calls the Universal Consciousness. "Sickness, disease is a self-correcting signal to realign the patterns that structure the whole."[14] In other words, we get sick when our thoughts distract us from the way things really are. "Our physiology is the physiology of nature."[15]

Chopra believes that the Universal Consciousness is all-powerful, all-knowing, perfect, and good. According to Chopra, we, too, are like this: perfect and all-knowing. If we are sick, it is because we don't believe what Chopra believes. If we did believe it, we would be aligned with the Universal Consciousness. We would be healthy if we believed that our true nature is one of perfection and complete goodness. Health will arise, he says, when we can affirm that "I know myself as the immeasurable potential of all that was, is and will be. . . . There is no other I than the entire universe. I am being and I am nowhere and everywhere at the same time. I am omnipresent, omniscient; I am the eternal spirit that animates everything in existence."[16] In other words, Chopra claims each of us is God.

Chopra says that to come to believe this about ourselves involves meditation and a return to Hinduism. Meditation is how we reestablish contact with our inner self, which is more closely aligned with the Universal Consciousness. Chopra disagrees with the Western view that meditation is just a mental activity. He states that "meditation is a spiritual practice."[17]

We agree, which is why we are very concerned about the type of meditation someone promotes. For Chopra, meditation allows people to "settle down to a silent state of awareness, beyond thought, to the experiential level of total unity with the universe. You experience the fact that you are part of the larger wholeness."[18] Assuming that the Universal Consciousness is loving and cares for us, we will sense guidance and direction when meditating. "You will tap into the cosmic mind, the voice that whispers to you non-verbally in the silent spaces between your thoughts. This is your inner intelligence and it is the ultimate and supreme genius that mirrors the wisdom of the universe. Trust this inner wisdom and all your dreams will come true."[19]

Part of what makes Chopra's system so attractive is his declaration that the fulfillment of our dreams for health, wealth, and happiness are legitimate. In fact, our purpose in life is to be satisfied. He declares that when we live according to his Seven Spirituals Laws, "we experience the ecstasy and exultation of our own spirit, which is the ultimate goal of all goals."[20] To help people attain this goal, Chopra developed a special treatment for his clinics, called the "Pizzichilli treatment."[21] This involves two technicians massaging and bathing a naked patient in warm sesame oil for two hours. We find it hard to determine whether this practice is a therapy or self-indulgence!

Meditation is central to Chopra's approach to health, but he also recommends other products and practices. Ayurvedic remedies are herbal, but given to stimulate and balance life energy (or *prana*), which is described in more detail under "Energy Medicine" (see Energy Medicine, page 193). "In Ayurvedic terms, they stimulate the intelligence of the body, which is the ultimate and supreme genius mirroring the wisdom of the universe."[22] More traditional Ayurvedic approaches include the importance of detoxification, personality typing, pulse diagnosis, adequate rest and exercise, and attention to relationships. (See Ayurvedic Medicine, page 155.)

Deepak Chopra's immense popularity points to the high value many Americans place on personal comfort and pleasure. His system offers the universe—literally. Only the rich and famous can afford many aspects of his approach to health and healing. Yet their enthusiasm for his services makes the whole system more attractive to the masses. An editorial accompanying a *Newsweek* article on Chopra is well worth reading. In it, Wendy Kaminer points out that "gurus" like Chopra "always confirm our essential godliness. They lead by flattery. . . . Gurus often tell us exactly what we want to hear."[23]

Unfortunately, Chopra's approach to health contradicts the biblical approach. The Bible teaches that humans are not "little gods," and we are not, by nature, extensions of the Big God. The Bible's spiritual laws conflict drastically with Chopra's spiritual laws. Both cannot be right.

The Bible teaches that we humans are fallen human beings, creatures created by the One, True Creator. Romans 3:23 states that "all have sinned and fall short of the glory of God." Yes, we are extremely valuable to God, and have great potential. The psalmist thanks God for how he made humanity. "You made him a little lower than the heavenly beings and crowned him with glory and honor. You made him ruler over the works of your hands; you put everything under his feet" (Psalm 8:5–6). But our potential is not realized by listening to our inner selves and having our selfish dreams fulfilled. We need to listen to the Voice of God, which comes through his Word and his Holy Spirit. But this message is not as attractive to rebellious humans as a Pizzichilli massage. Nor is it an easy path to pursue.

In contrast, as Kaminer points out in her *Newsweek* editorial, Chopra and his fellow gurus ask very little. "The spiritual peace and enlightenment offered by pop gurus doesn't require a lifetime of discipline. It requires only that you suspend your critical judgment, attend their lectures and workshops and buy their books."[24]

While this may be more appealing, we question its long-term value and its spiritual veracity. Chopra's approach is sprinkled with enough good information about diet, sleep, and relationships that applying his ideas will bring some improvements to those who have not cared for their health.

However, when faced with serious illness and disease, his system appears to us to have little to offer. When pressed for scientific support for his remedies and therapies, Chopra admits, "I am not at all attached to the scientific worldview at the moment. I see myself as a bum on the street who has a lot of fun writing."[25] However, he doesn't forget to include his "M.D." on his books and continues to speak to an apparently adoring and growing choir of Americans committed to consumerism and postmodernism.

Chopra is like many other alternative medicine experts. We feel that his teaching must be rejected for the scientific and spiritual reasons we describe throughout our book. Chopra seems to truly believe in his methods, theories, and spiritual path. He feels that utilizing Ayurveda and other practices will result in the best possible health. He has achieved fame and, presumably, a significant degree of wealth from promoting his ideas. However, the discerning Christian seeking wellness needs to recognize that popularity, fame, and financial success do not prove that the possessor has an inside track on healthy living. Nor do they indicate a right relationship with God.

LARRY DOSSEY, M.D.

Chopra is not alone as a doctor-writer who has discovered "new answers." Others offer an approach with a seemingly Christian subtext. Larry Dossey is a physician who has come to public prominence through his books on prayer and healing: *Healing Words*, *Prayer Is Good Medicine*, and *Be Careful What You Pray For. . . You Just Might Get It.*[26] Raised in a fundamentalist Christian home in Texas, he drifted away from his religious upbringing into agnosticism.[27] However, as a physician, he was confronted by the way many of his patients relied on prayer. He undertook a spiritual journey that brought him into contact with Eastern religions. Here he claimed to find the universal aspects of all religions, and has come to view all world religions leading people in basically the same direction.

Dossey's Views on Health, Prayer, and God

Dossey proposes a view called "nonlocal medicine." According to this belief, each person does not have an individual mind confined to his or her own brain. Instead, Dossey believes that the minds of everyone are joined in one Universal Consciousness. This means that each person, through prayer or other distance healing (or hurting) method, such as telepathy, clairvoyance, or voodoo, can affect the mind of another. Dossey admits his view is not supported by scientific evidence, but this is because these anomalous, nonlocal events "seem to have no possibility, even in principle, of being explained in the local, physicalistic, reductionistic framework of" current science and medicine.[28]

For Dossey, then, "prayerfulness" is more important than "prayer." By prayerfulness he means "a sense of simply being attuned or aligned with 'something higher.' Prayer tends to follow instructions laid down by the great religious traditions; prayerfulness does not. It is a feeling of unity with the All, rather than with specific leaders, traditions, or holy books."[29] In many ways, Dossey understands the problems Christians sometimes have when they pray. He says we sometimes arrive at God's doorstep with a laundry list of expectations rather than with the humble attitude God calls on us to express. In *Healing Words*, Dossey writes:

> Intercessory prayer has a tendency to ask for definite outcomes, to structure the future, to "tell God what to do," such as taking the cancer away. Prayerfulness, on the other hand, is accepting without being passive, is grateful without giving up. It is more willing to stand in the mystery, to tolerate ambiguity and the unknown. It honors the rightness of whatever happens, even cancer.[30]

While Dossey's emphasis on the attitude for prayer seems on the surface to be biblically sound, his last sentence reveals where his theology differs from our view of orthodox Christianity. Dossey seems to us to have rejected the notion of a personal God whose loving will determines the outcomes of prayer. He claims this biblical view of prayer arises from a world view which "is now antiquated and incomplete" and constitutes a "uniquely 'pathological mythology.'" He acknowledges that his view of prayer is "far different" from the "old biblically based views of prayer" where requests were offered to a God distinct from humans.[31]

In Dossey's view, a Cosmic Consciousness directs all things. Interestingly, Dossey refers to this Consciousness as loving, trustworthy, caring, benevolent, wise, and something with which we can communicate. All these are personal attributes, yet Dossey never seems to admit this. Nor does he give us any reasons to explain why we should accept his description of Consciousness. Instead, we are left to take it on faith that the universe is loving, that cancer, for example, must be right.

In contrast, it seems to us that the biblical explanation is much more satisfying and reasonable. The Bible teaches that the universe (cosmos) is not loving, wise, and benevolent. The universe is not the way it should be, but one day it "will be liberated from its bondage to decay and brought into the glorious freedom of the children of God. We know that the whole creation has been groaning as in the pains of childbirth right up to the present time" (Romans 8:21–22). Cancer, pain, and suffering are not right; they are the tragic consequences of living in a fallen world. We do not have to, as Dossey has written, "honor the rightness of whatever happens, even cancer."[32] We can grieve the loss, suffering, and death that disease brings, decry the existence of such suffering, express our pain, and turn to the loving Creator of this world for comfort. He did not make the world to be this way, and he promises in his Word to one day restore it to how it ought to be. Because of this, God says we can have confidence that he will get us through the illness or disability we face.

Dossey ultimately seems to hold that prayer is a form of language, or energy. It is a way that minds have of interacting with one another. He refuses to believe that a personal God is needed to determine what outcomes will arise; the words need only be spoken, or the thoughts expressed.

We might want to have this type of powerful prayer that always works, but it raises the ominous possibility that our thoughts might also harm people. According to Dossey, even an inadvertent "God damn it!" thus becomes a dangerous weapon. This is the focus of Dossey's book on harmful prayer.[33] As such, he admits that his view of prayer has become a magical one. All those negative thoughts we think of others, or things we mumble under our breath, become expressions of the Cosmic Mind that impact the people against whom they are directed.

Dossey is to be admired for tackling such a controversial and unpleasant topic. Yet his conclusion is, to us, completely unsatisfactory and unscriptural. Given his belief in prayer as something like an energy, independent of our will or the will of God, he is forced to conclude that these negative thoughts do "hit" others. He uses stories about voodoo hexing as illustrations of this effect.

We therefore ask why people do not die when people maliciously or inadvertently tell them to "Drop dead." Dossey's answer is that humans "have evolved forms of protection against the negative thoughts of others—a kind of 'spiritual immune system' that is analogous to our immune system against infections."[34] As with most of Dossey's assertions, he has no evidence to back up his claims. He has to invent new theories to resolve problems in his old theories.

In contrast to this spiritual "word ping-pong," we can take comfort in the fact that our thoughts are not all-powerful. Dossey certainly raises good points about the impact of our attitudes toward others. People can often sense the negative attitudes and feelings we harbor toward them, which could be potentially harmful to them. This is not because of some energy that emanates from our mind to the Cosmic Mind and into the other person's mind. We harm them because these thoughts usually lead to actions. "For out of the heart come evil thoughts, murder, adultery, sexual immorality, theft, false testimony, slander" (Matthew 15:19).

At the very least, thinking negatively about others distracts us from focusing on how we might love and serve them. "Let us consider how we may spur one another on toward love and good deeds" (Hebrews 10:24). Instead, Paul urges us: "Whatever is true, whatever is noble, whatever is right, whatever is pure, whatever is lovely, whatever is admirable—if anything is excellent or praiseworthy—think about such things" (Philippians 4:8).

Our thoughts and words are filtered through the Mind of God. David prayed: "Search me, O God, and know my heart; test me and know my anxious thoughts" (Psalm 139:23; cf. Hebrews 4:12). God hears our requests but does not automatically act upon them in the way we feel is best. He determines what is most loving, most just, most needed in a situation. And he sees the totality of the other options, not just the limited view we have. That is why we cannot predict the outcome of prayer like we can the effects of an injection or X-ray. Prayer belongs in the spiritual realm, which is one occupied by many spiritual beings who are personal. Many of the methods of clinical research are designed to minimize the effects of personal will in therapies. Until we find some way to control the divine will, we will not be able to design an adequate study to completely and totally examine the effects or effectiveness of prayer (for more on prayer research, see Prayer for Healing, page 252).

Dossey's books on prayer have done much to stimulate discussion, research, and interest in prayer for healing. As such, his contributions are welcome. However, Christians cannot welcome his ideas with open arms. His beliefs about prayer, as he himself admits, are based on completely different views of reality, people, and God. His description of prayerfulness is quite insightful, but not as satisfying to us as the biblical perspective. Dossey's proposals suffer from a number of ironic twists. While rejecting the God of the Bible, he still wants to hold on to a "god" who has many of the attributes of God. There are obviously aspects of the biblical God that Dossey does not want to accept. But he fails to provide evidence for why we should accept those bits of Christianity he wants to hold on to. Nor does he show why we should accept the eclectic nature of his view of prayer. Christians who choose to be exposed to his teachings should read his books with a critical eye, realizing he makes some good points, but that his message is fundamentally at odds with the message of the Bible.

OTHER WRITERS ON HEALING

There are numerous other examples among the writers of wellness and spiritual healing books. Some are more like Chopra, with whom we find little to agree with. They use some good medical common sense to promote a form of spirituality that is completely alien to Christian spirituality. They often endorse a variety of other products that prove to be financially rewarding for them. Others are more like Dossey, who use their medical credentials to speak on spiritual issues. They take well-established Christian concepts, and completely redefine them. In either case, Christians need to evaluate all that is being said in light of biblical revelation and sound medical research.

All these writers, who adhere to an approach to healing far different from that with a biblical base, must be questioned in the same manner as we examine the therapies and herbal remedies. In some instances their work should be avoided because it requires the acceptance of religious ideas and values in opposition to those of orthodox Christianity. In other instances, they fall into the realm of medical uncertainty, fraud, or quackery. Either way, be as wary of the gurus as you are of quackery and fraud.

Reflect on the following passages and how they apply to your reading about health. We believe they call on us to actively engage our minds, to think critically and biblically, whenever our reading addresses spiritual issues. And, of course, we should also pray as we read on these issues.

Let no one deceive you with empty words, for because of such things God's wrath comes on those who are disobedient. Therefore do not be partners with them. For you were once darkness, but now you are light in the Lord. Live as children of light (for the fruit of the light consists in all goodness, righteousness and truth) and find out what pleases the Lord. Have nothing to do with the fruitless deeds of darkness, but rather expose them. For it is shameful even to mention what the disobedient do in secret. But everything exposed by the light becomes visible, for it is light that makes everything visible.

Ephesians 5:6–14

See to it that no one takes you captive through hollow and deceptive philosophy, which depends on human tradition and the basic principles of this world rather than on Christ. For in Christ all the fullness of the Deity lives in bodily form, and you have been given fullness in Christ, who is the head over every power and authority.

Colossians 2:8–10

Timothy, guard what has been entrusted to your care. Turn away from godless chatter and the opposing ideas of what is falsely called knowledge, which some have professed and in so doing have wandered from the faith.

1 Timothy 6:20–21

Use Common Sense

The spiritual teachings of the health gurus must be evaluated spiritually. Their health-related advice must be evaluated medically and scientifically. In the end, your decisions will often come down to using common sense. With all of its flaws and limitations, the scientific method remains the best way we have to figure out whether something works or not. A number of later chapters focus on how you can best use the results of these scientific studies. While scientists are never completely unbiased, they look to data and empirical evidence as the bottom line in discovering truth. Promotion of health-related products on any other basis must remain questionable.

Notes

1. David G. Williams, *Read This Or Die* (Rockville, Md.: Mountain Home Publishing, n.d.).

2. Deepak Chopra, *Creating Health: Beyond Prevention, Toward Perfection* (Boston: Houghton Mifflin, 1985); *Quantum Healing: Exploring the Frontiers of Mind/Body Medicine* (New York: Bantam, 1989); *Perfect Health: The Complete Mind/Body Guide* (New York: Harmony, 1990); *Ageless Body, Timeless Mind: The Quantum Alternative to Growing Old* (New York: Harmony, 1993).

3. Deepak Chopra, *Everyday Immortality: A Concise Course in Spiritual Transformation* (New York: Harmony, 1999); *How to Know God: The Soul's Journey into the Mystery of Mysteries* (New York: Harmony, 2000).

4. Deepak Chopra, quoted in Judith Graham, ed. *Current Biography Yearbook* (New York: H. W. Wilson, 1995): 91–96.

5. Andrew A. Skolnick, "Maharishi Ayur-Veda: Guru's Marketing Scheme Promises the World Eternal 'Perfect Health,'" *Journal of the American Medical Association*, 266, no. 13 (October 1991): 1741–50.

6. John Leland and Carla Power, "Deepak's Instant Karma," *Newsweek* (October 20, 1997), 52–58.

7. Elise Pettus, "The Mind-Body Problems," *New York* (August 14, 1995): 28–31, 95.

8. Pettus, "The Mind-Body Problems," 31.

9. Paul Reisser, Robert Belarde, and Dale Mabe, *Examining Alternative Medicine* (Downers Grove, Ill.: InterVarsity, 2001).

10. Deepak Chopra, *Journey Into Healing: Awakening the Wisdom Within You* (Random House Audio, 1995), audiocassette.

11. Deepak Chopra, *Ecaping the Prison of the Mind: A Journey from Here to Here* (San Rafael, Calif.: New World Library, 1992), audiocassette.

12. Chopra, *Journey Into Healing*.

13. Deepak Chopra, *Creating Health*, rev. ed. (Random House Audio Publishing, 1995), audio-cassette.

14. D. Scott Rogo, "The Healing Reality: An Interview with Deepak Chopra, M.D." in *New Techniques of Inner Healing* (New York: Paragon, 1992), 158.

15. Rogo, "The Healing Reality," 158.

16. Chopra, *Escaping the Prison of the Mind*.

17. Chopra, *Ageless Body, Timeless Mind*.

18. Rogo, "The Healing Reality," 161.

19. Chopra, *Journey Into Healing*.

20. Deepak Chopra, *The Seven Spiritual Laws of Success: A Practical Guide to the Fulfillment of Your Dreams* (San Rafael, Calif.: Amber-Allen, 1994), 93.

21. Pettus, "The Mind-Body Problems," 30.

22. Rogo, "The Healing Reality," 162.

23. Wendy Kaminer, "Why We Love Gurus," *Newsweek* (October 20, 1997), 60.

24. Kaminer, "Why We Love Gurus," 60.

25. Zina Moukheiber, "Lord of Immortality," *Forbes* 153, no. 8 (April 11, 1994): 132.

26. Larry Dossey, *Healing Words: The Power of Prayer and the Practice of Medicine* (New York: HarperSanFrancisco, 1993); *Prayer Is Good Medicine: How to Reap the Healing Benefits of Prayer* (New York: HarperSanFrancisco, 1996); *Be Careful What You Pray For...You Just Might Get It: What We Can Do About the Unintentional Effects of Our Thoughts, Prayers, and Wishes* (New York: HarperSanFrancisco, 1997).

27. Dossey, *Healing Words*, preface.

28. Ibid., 44.

29. Ibid., 24.

30. Ibid., 24.

31. Ibid., 7.

32. Ibid., 24.

33. Dossey, *Be Careful*.

34. Ibid., 8.

9

Taking a Closer Look at 'Christian' Therapies

They had gathered on the stage, nervously, prayerfully. One weary man, a self-employed laborer who had been working through the night to help a customer fix a flooded basement, was dressed in coveralls and boots. He had come without changing his clothing because there was no time. He needed this healing, needed it desperately. He was too young for Medicare, too poor for health insurance, and earned too much money to qualify for Medicaid. He had been experiencing difficulty urinating and suspected he had prostate trouble. Prostate cancer had eventually taken the lives of his grandfather, his uncle, and his father. The man had seen a doctor who had recommended periodic checks. But that was a few years ago. There was no money for that. The man was having enough trouble paying for food and shelter, and keeping his old truck in working order, the truck he needed to get from job to job. That's why he came to be healed by the preacher who claimed to have "the gift."

Near the man was a young woman, little more than a teenager, with a beautiful face, a torso that would have delighted an artist, and withered limbs that forced her to move slowly, painfully on crutches. Her physician had told her the defects with which she was born could not be altered. He advised her to consider her limited mobility, her upper body beauty, and her ability to work at a well-paid job as blessings from God.

The young woman understood that her doctor meant well. She knew he was speaking about the limits of medical knowledge. Still, she sought a second opinion, and she came forward when the evangelist announced that "Dr. Jesus will be healing tonight!"

There was an elderly woman with "the sugar"—diabetes. There was a man in a wheelchair, his head lolling slightly to the side, felled by a stroke that had left him weak, disabled. But his mind was still clear, and he was extremely frustrated. There were people with heart conditions, withered limbs. Some approached with uplifted hands. Some had tears in their eyes.

All were filled with hope. All were deeply believing Christians who felt the man about to lay hands on them, to slay them in the spirit, send them falling back, healed, into the arms of one of the "catchers," was a vehicle for God.

One by one they went down the healing line. One by one the television evangelist said a prayer, then struck each forehead with the palm of his hand. "Heal!" he proclaimed, and they, he said, were healed—provided they had adequate faith.

The evangelist, in his books on God, Christianity, and health, makes it clear what he means by "faith." When you go through his healing line, he explains, God heals you. It might take a limb a few days or weeks to return to normal. You might still have chest pains, shortness of breath, or other symptoms of your former problem, at least for a little while. But, he insists, you are healed.

The problem with the healing is with "doubters." He includes as "doubters" anyone who returns to a medical doctor after a "healing." The evangelist considers seeing a doctor after going through his healing line as proof that the person lacks faith. He warns that if those who have been healed consult a doctor, they will be punished with many times the number of problems for which they originally came to be healed.

Another television evangelist with a healing line also talks of God's ability to heal everyone and the need to have faith when accepting the healing. But, unlike the first man, the second speaks and writes about a "partnership" with the Lord. He talks about the diabetic who is healed by God, but must change his diet, increase his exercise, and see his physician to regularly check his health. God heals, the second evangelist stresses, in part through our cooperation in doing what is medically advisable.

Do 'Christian' Therapies Go Too Far in Their Claims?

It is hard to criticize a man or woman with a passion for the things of God. They are so certain, so joyous, we start thinking that all their pronouncements must be solidly based in Scripture.

Yet the truth is that the person of passion is also human. When celebrating our Lord, he or she can sometimes go too far in ascribing to God that which is of man. Such is often the case with what are being called "Christian alternative therapies."

The problem comes when someone who is alive with the Spirit, who has a passion for the Lord, enters the health field, offering ill-founded health advice with the same authority as the Word of God. Sometimes the therapy, recommended by a medical professional, appears to be a soundly reasoned program of healing or treatment. Other times the therapies, based on faulty views of the Bible, are recommended or even "preached" by sincere Christians who have little or no medical background or evidence to support them.

Christian therapies are frequently based on personal experience or the experience of individuals close to the proponent of the therapy. They were often discovered when someone benefited a lot from the therapy—someone improved or had a healing. Widespread promotion of the therapies sometimes begins with members of the clergy, lay theologians of note, or others with ready access to the media, especially Christian radio.

Rarely can anyone question that a healing did occur. There usually is no question that God's hand was involved in the healing. Yet the confusion is in the details. No one can say with certainty what caused the original healing. But you'd never know that from the way the therapy is promoted: it is presented as if this were God's answer to human ailments.

These Christian therapies are said to be biblically justified. Some fit into the theology of the particular denomination to which their proponents belong. They sound good. Unfortunately, some are not medically sound. Other remedies have an important role in health and healing, but that role is expanded well beyond what is scientifically supported. We sent away for an audiotape advertised as containing the Bible's recipe for healthy living. The tape presented some helpful information about the importance of vitamins, made many speculative claims about dietary supplements, and never once mentioned the Bible. The advertisement appeared to us to be no more than a marketing ploy to entice Christians into buying the company's products.

Christians are, and should be, concerned about their health. We want our book to help Christians choose alternative therapies wisely. We also believe that God sometimes grants a miracle of healing. When a Christian experiences healing, either directly from God or through a therapy, he or she may become convinced that others can similarly be healed. Some start to reflect on exactly what they did immediately prior to the healing. Had they just changed their diet? Had they just started praying a little differently? Had they just taken a dietary supplement? Had they started attending a new church? Motivated by a desire to help others, they search for those crucial steps that led to their healing. They hear others' experiences and develop a list of additional factors needed for healing. Soon they have formulated a new Christian therapy. Their experience, and the successes of others who have tried it, are the only proof they need that this new therapy really works. Besides, their intentions are only to share God's blessings, and the therapies are so "gentle" they couldn't harm anyone. Why should anyone be concerned?

We are concerned. It is one thing to rejoice with the person who has received renewed health. We cannot deny that someone has experienced a healing. But it is quite another matter to promote the therapy that developed out of that experience. Good intentions are not enough when making recommendations that affect people's health. And then labeling the therapy as "Christian," or "God's own," or "biblically supported" raises a host of other concerns.

What we suggest, in every case, is caution and wisdom. Let's examine one such therapy that goes by a variety of names.

The Genesis 1:29 Diet

Christian vegetarians point to the story of the Garden of Eden that seems to imply that Adam and Eve were meant to live in harmony with the animals, taking their food from what grows in the ground. The most-cited verse is Genesis 1:29: "Then God said, 'I give you every seed-bearing plant on the face of the whole earth and every tree that has fruit with seed in it. They will be yours for food.'"

Some scholars believe this verse can be correctly interpreted to mean that humanity, at least in the Garden of Eden, was designed to be vegetarian. From this belief stem several diet plans that are circulating in the church today, going by names such as "The Hallelujah Diet," "God's Original (or Optimal) Diet," "God's Ideal Diet," and "The Genesis 1:29 Diet." Their promoters claim that, since plant food was given to Adam and Eve, God still intends for people to eat only plant-based food.

But a significant amount of biblical teaching is difficult to square with this interpretation. You do not have to read very far in the Bible to find it. In Genesis 4 we learn that Abel was a keeper of livestock. In Genesis 9 God gave meat as food. In Genesis 18 Abraham served his angelic guests butter, milk, and meat—and they ate them. In Genesis 27 Jacob prepared venison for Isaac to receive his blessing. In Exodus 16 God sent quail, a bird, to the Israelites to feed them. In God's law, he lists clean and unclean animals and says of the clean animals, "Of all the animals that live on land, these are the ones you may eat" (Leviticus 11:2).

Furthermore, Jesus ate more than just plant foods (i.e., fish) and gave them to those he loved. One example is the well-known story of the loaves and the fish (Matthew 15:32–38). Another is the time after Jesus' resurrection when he appeared to the disciples and asked, "'Do you have anything here to eat?' They gave him a piece of broiled fish, and he took it and ate it in their presence" (Luke 24:41–43). Later, they all met on the beach. "Jesus said to them, 'Come and have breakfast.' None of the disciples dared ask him, 'Who are you?' They knew it was the Lord. Jesus came, took the bread and gave it to them, and did the same with the fish" (John 21:12–13).

Why would Jesus give his apostles fish to eat if he wanted everyone to be vegetarian? An apostolic council commanded the Gentile believers to abstain only from certain meats ("from the meat of strangled animals and from blood" Acts 15:20). And, in Romans 14:1, Paul states that dietary teaching is one of the "disputable matters."

Paul teaches that dietary regulations and dogmatism on disputed issues should not divide the Christian community:

> One man's faith allows him to eat everything, but another man, whose faith is weak, eats only vegetables. The man who eats everything must not look down on him who does not, and the man who does not eat everything must not condemn the man who does, for God has accepted him.
>
> Romans 14:2–3

The teaching of the Bible seems clear to us, that humans are not commanded to abstain from meat. Vegetarianism should not be promoted as required for Christians, either on its own or as part of a therapy. On the other hand, the typical Western diet is too high in animal products and saturated fat, too low in fruits and vegetables and fiber, and too high in processed food. Medical studies are virtually unanimous in agreeing that this type of diet causes and worsens a variety of diseases.

People would be wise to eat a more plant-rich diet. Yet a purely plant-based diet is not taught in Scripture and has some potential for harm. In fact, we now know that one of the vitamins essential for health—vitamin B_{12}—is lacking in all vegetarian diets (although vitamin B_{12} supplements are now available). In the past, vitamin B_{12} could only be obtained by eating at least some meat, as was certainly a part of the diet of Jesus and his disciples.

Some who still believe that "God's Ideal Diet" is vegetarian teach that God gave meat to humans in Genesis 9 (and thereafter in the Bible) to shorten their life span. We believe this is false teaching. For anyone wishing more detailed and balanced information on this topic, we recommend Dr. Michael Jacobson's book *The Word on Health*.[1]

We could give many other examples, but our point is not to attack one Christian therapy or another. Our point is to give a broad overview of concerns we have with promoting certain therapies as "Christian" or "biblical." We as Christians are blessed with God's biblical guidance and the direction of the Holy Spirit. We are blessed with many therapies, and the Bible and the Holy Spirit can guide us as we select the ones to pursue. But we should be very cautious about labeling any therapy as "Christian."

Some Pull a Therapy from Specific Bible Verses

Some Christians promote a therapy after finding one or more verses in the Bible that appear to support their perspective. Some proponents of herbal medicine claim the Bible specifically teaches that people should use herbs as medicine. They sometimes quote verses, and seem to usually use the King James Version (KJV). The following examples of verses come from a handout distributed by a visitor promoting herbal remedies at one of our churches:

> And to every beast of the earth, and to every fowl of the air, and to everything that creepeth upon the earth, wherein there is life, I have given every green herb for meat; and it was so.
>
> Genesis 1:30 KJV

> He causeth the grass to grow for the cattle, and herb for the service of man: that he may bring forth food out of the earth.
>
> Psalm 104:14 KJV

> And by the river upon the bank thereof, on this side and on that side, shall grow all trees for meat, . . . and the fruit thereof shall be for meat, and the leaf thereof for medicine.
>
> Ezekiel 47:12 KJV

Those who use these verses to promote herbal medicine seem to forget one of the primary principles of biblical interpretation: first seek to understand what the text meant to the original writer and audience, not to us today. Two Hebrew words are translated "herb" in the KJV and they both mean green plants or grass. Psalm 104:14 even states what the purpose of the "herbs" was: to serve as food. Just as grass feeds cattle, "herbs" or green plants feed humans (see also Psalm 37:2). This is poetry. English poetry uses rhyme. Hebrew poetry repeats the same thought in two ways.

When the King James Version was translated, the English word "herb" had a broader meaning than it does today. To take our modern usage of this word as a medicinal remedy, and read that meaning back into an English translation of the Bible, is to us inappropriate. Our belief is confirmed in more recent translations which replace the KJV "herb" with "green plants" or something similar. To us, these verses therefore have no bearing on whether Christians should or shouldn't use herbal remedies, or any other forms of medicine.

Ezekiel 47:12, however, does teach that trees can have leaves which bring healing. This interpretation has been noted throughout history without any disagreement. However, this verse gives no help in determining which herbs bring healing, which are poisonous, and how much should be used. This verse makes no statement on whether herbs or pharmaceutical drugs are preferable. In fact, it is questionable whether this verse has anything to do with the trees that grow on earth today. This section of the book of Ezekiel contains a series of prophecies about the future kingdom of God. Many scholars hold that this kingdom is yet to come, especially given the middle section of the verse, left out of the promotional literature we have seen. The following is the complete verse in the NIV:

Fruit trees of all kinds will grow on both banks of the river. Their leaves will not wither, nor will their fruit fail. Every month they will bear, because the water from the sanctuary flows to them. Their fruit will serve for food and their leaves for healing.

Ezekiel 47:12

Leaving out the middle of the verse hides the fact that these clearly are not typical trees. These trees bear fruit every month and have leaves that never wither. This makes the applicability of this verse to today's herbal remedies very questionable.

When investigating any claim that something is a Christian therapy, basic principles of biblical interpretation should be utilized. Before accepting any "Christian teaching," carefully compare it with what the Bible actually teaches. Try to discern the plain meaning of the text in its most recent scholarly translation. If verses are cited, read them in your own Bible. Read the passages around those verses to ensure that the interpretation fits the context. Detailed examination of claims may require learning about how the Bible should be translated and interpreted, a study that will bear a wealth of fruit for your spiritual vitality. It may well protect you from going astray from the clear teaching of the Bible. This type of study, practiced by the early believers in Berea, was commended and complimented by Luke when he wrote in Acts 17:11, "Now the Bereans were of more noble character than the Thessalonians, for they received the message with great eagerness and examined the Scriptures every day to see if what Paul said was true."

Use Caution on Any 'God-Ordained' Diet or Remedy

One version of the Genesis 1:29 Diet, called the Hallelujah Diet, exemplifies other concerns we have about many Christian alternative therapies. One of the more widely promoted Christian therapies at this writing, the Hallelujah Diet is no better or worse than others. The fervor of passionate Christians who feel they experienced a healing because of this Christian therapy is understandable. Their actions are based on faith and must be respected, but may still be critiqued (see Hallelujah Diet, page 202).

In brief, our concern is with anyone who puts the imprimatur of God on his or her advice, who puts a "Thus sayeth the Lord..." on a therapy recommendation. It is a bold statement to claim that one's advice is directly from God, or that one's therapy is God's ordained diet or remedy. At stake is God's credibility in the eyes of others, both those within the church and those outside the church. Consider the effect of when some Christians claim God's advice on diet is one thing, others claim his advice is something else, and still others claim he favors yet another diet.

Such divergent claims can discredit God before the world—especially when the Bible declares that Christians should not argue over dietary guidelines. Those who hear these contradictory views may well question the reliability of anything called "God's advice." Their doubts may even extend to questions of whether anyone knows God's instructions on salvation.

The Word of God does not give a clear statement of doctrine on many issues. What we get in such cases are biblical principles to apply to the issue. While we can still develop clear biblical positions on some issues not addressed in the Bible, we must remain tentative on other issues. Most Christian therapies appear to us to be in the latter category. They are not based on God's Word. They are based on someone's interpretation of the Word—someone's opinion. And in some cases we believe that person's opinion is wrong.

When scientific misinformation and confusion are promoted as part of a "Christian" therapy, Christianity can be further discredited. The proponents usually are not deliberately trying to mislead anyone. But they often have no medical training or experience. They are acting on a dramatic personal experience and what we feel is an incomplete understanding of Scripture. In addition to any discredit caused, Christians facing serious health problems who aren't aware of all the facts may actually be harmed by these therapies if they neglect effective treatment for their condition.

Teachings Are Not in Accordance with God's Word

Many Christians are accepting these therapies as biblical doctrine and fact. They are even using these teachings, which we believe to be unbiblical, to judge others in the body of Christ. Worse yet, the church is beginning to be divided over these "false" teachings—which, we suspect, is exactly what Satan would desire.

These types of therapies, promoted as Christian therapies, should be no surprise to wise, Bible-based Christians. God, in his Word, warns us about false prophets—those teachers or preachers who *appear* to be from God, whose advice *appears* to be from God, but whose instructions are *not* in accordance with God's Word.

We need to pay attention to his Word.

Be very careful, then, how you live—not as unwise but as wise, making the most of every opportunity, because the days are evil. Therefore do not be foolish, but understand what the Lord's will is.

Ephesians 5:15–17

Notes

1. Michael Jacobson, *The Word on Health: A Biblical and Medical Overview of How to Care for Your Body and Mind* (Chicago: Moody Press, 2000).

10

How Science Tests Therapies and Remedies

Science has developed a method of seeking truth about the physical world that requires objective, repeated, and repeatable testing of ideas. One of its goals is to provide conclusions that, as much as possible, are independent of people's prior beliefs and assumptions. The scientific method is meant to slice through the anecdotes and find truth. Anecdotal evidence, the stories people tell of how a particular therapy relieved their pain or cured their illness, is the starting point for scientific discovery, not the "proof." Success of a therapy can be checked by creating tests to see if the results are repeatable and consistent or due to chance.

Science values evidence over opinion. What distinguishes science from other branches of inquiry is the high priority placed on objective information, such as observable data and repeatable experiments. Ideally, theories arise from observations, then are changed or discarded when new data arrive that contradict or expand previous information.[1]

We are actually speaking of an ideal—scientists basing their conclusions on objectively demonstrated facts and observations. This is not to say that the users of the scientific method are always true to the ideals of the concept.

Problems arise when scientists ignore information that does not fit a prevalent theory. Science can be influenced by irrelevant or incorrect theories and the authority of those making pronouncements about some aspect of life. Some scientists don't recognize how influential their beliefs and assumptions are in forming the questions they ask and how they go about answering them. When scientists ignore their own assumptions, they can start with a conclusion and hunt for facts to support that conclusion. Some serious medical researchers are so convinced of the rightness of their theories they tailor their research to ensure they get the results they desire. Sometimes this is done subconsciously, but some scientists have been caught skewing their data in an attempt to convince others of their theory.

Researchers must be able to step back from their data and weigh all the relevant factors before they can honestly say their experiments support their theory or discover that their original belief was erroneous.

Unfortunately, even in medicine, some therapies have been vigorously defended or rejected because of how they lined up with prevailing theories, not because of how well they fit experimental data.

A good example of this is cinchona, an herbal treatment for malaria. Despite objective evidence of its effectiveness, seventeenth-century doctors rejected cinchona because it was first brought to Europe by Jesuit priests. The doctors' opposition was due to their bias against Catholicism and their adherence to flawed medical theories[2] (see page 119).

Even today, some proponents defend the use of therapies such as Therapeutic Touch and Bach flower remedies for many conditions for which no scientific evidence supports their effectiveness. These proponents insist these therapies are effective because of their belief in the existence of human life energies and the properties of the auras they believe people have.

Christians believe in miracles, and thus do not expect everything to be scientifically verifiable. But this can make Christians prone to accept reports of divine healing without examining the evidence surrounding the alleged or actual miracles.[3] We believe firmly that miracles have occurred and still do. But we do not believe that every claim of a miracle should be accepted without evaluation. Science provides an important way to determine if the person was truly healed. Science is completely compatible with belief in God and his healing miracles. In fact, the more a scientist discovers about life, the more his or her reverence for God can deepen through understanding God's creation.

Scientists Start with Specifics to Evaluate a Treatment

In order to evaluate a therapy, whether conventional or alternative, we need to be as specific as possible about what we are looking at. If we are looking at an herb's healing ability, it is best to know the active ingredient(s) within that herb—those compounds that cause healing. Ideally, we should know the quantity of the active ingredient, whether or not the amount is consistent from herb to herb (or bottle to bottle, company to company), and what other influences affect it, such as heat, light, and moisture. The soil in which the herb is grown, the amount of sunshine and rain, when it is harvested, how it is preserved, and how it is packaged all provide important information. If any of these vary from batch to batch, the effects of the herb on those who take it can vary significantly.

Anecdotal Evidence Should Be Only a Starting Point for Study

Sometimes, all we have is anecdotal evidence—stories of people who say they have been helped or harmed. But that evidence should be a starting point, and is never the "proof" of effectiveness. Anecdotal evidence of healing alone is not enough to come to any valid conclusion about what caused the healing. Focusing solely on positive results ignores the possibility that for some people, the therapy may do nothing or even prove dangerous. Focusing solely on negative results can result in rejection of what might actually be a new and important treatment for an illness.

With the exception of unsubstantiated opinion, anecdotal evidence is the least useful of the types of evidence available to judge medical therapies. Anecdotal evidence has supported the usefulness of many of the most unlikely and bizarre treatments in the world. However, anecdotal evidence generally does not take into account the many other things going on in a patient's life that have contributed to what happened.

For example, imagine a widow whose husband died two years ago. Each year, on the anniversary of his death, the widow becomes deeply depressed. Friends, not remembering the exact date, assume her depression is "chemical" and suggest she try an over-the-counter product advertised as being more effective and safer than any pharmaceutical.

The widow takes the product but about the same time decides to volunteer in a church outreach program. There she meets a widower who shares many of her interests and values in life. They go to church together. They go to lunch together. They begin dating. They both discover that you can move on and love someone new. The widow thanks God for the new life that has brought her joy. Her friends, seeing the dramatic improvement in her outlook, start recommending the over-the-counter product to others because of what they perceive it has done to help her.

But their observations do not match the reality of her healing. Their observations may be valuable—even accurate—however, their conclusion that the product erased the depression is false.

The importance of anecdotal evidence is in suggesting that something about a treatment may be effective. Hippocrates, the physician of ancient Greece whose oath is still revered, depended on anecdotal evidence to design his therapies for others. Thus, no less true in our day than his, if many people report being helped by a therapy, it may warrant further investigation. This is why, for example, the herbal remedy St. John's wort was and is being tested in several clinical trials. Anecdotal evidence overwhelmingly suggested it had value in treating mild depression. The scientific method is now confirming what was suspected. One of the recent studies, involving a small group of people with mild to moderate depression, found St. John's wort to be as effective as a popular pharmaceutical antidepressant.[4]

Proponents of alternative medicine and herbal medicine often claim that centuries of use of a therapy should count as valuable evidence of its efficacy. "Why else would people have kept using it?" they reason. Most scientists and physicians would agree that this does constitute valuable evidence. However, this "anecdotal" or "testimonial" evidence is of the least value when evaluating the effectiveness of any therapy.

Anecdotal evidence is a report about someone's experience when he or she tried a certain therapy or treatment. We all tell these stories. We tell what happened when we did or took something, especially when the product helped us. While these stories can be more interesting than a dry report of a scientific study, we must always remember the type of evidence each provides. Anecdotes tell us *what* we perceived happened but not necessarily what actually happened, and certainly not *why* it happened.

Anecdotes do play an important role in suggesting new ideas to be researched, but do not provide evidence of the effectiveness of a treatment. The National Center for Complementary and Alternative Medicine acknowledges that there is a hierarchy in the different types of evidence for therapies, with anecdotal at the bottom. The following table is adapted from the center's Five Year Strategic Plan.[5]

HIERARCHY OF EVIDENCE	TYPE OF RESEARCH
Highest	Large randomized clinical trial
	Small randomized clinical trial
	Uncontrolled trials
	Observational studies
	Case reports
Lowest	Anecdotes

Historical usage of a remedy is just another form of anecdotal evidence. It records *what* happened, not *why* it happened. In fact, there could have been many reasons why a remedy was used for centuries. People sometimes use a remedy because there is nothing else available. Or they may use a remedy because it is intricately interlinked with their culture and religion. Or, because the illness lasts only a short time, or comes and goes in cycles, they do not realize the relief they experience has nothing to do with the remedy.

Birth control at one time was believed to involve a woman avoiding particular sacred areas. A woman might be resting by the water of a sacred lake and feel her baby moving within her for the first time. Because the time between sexual intercourse and first awareness of a baby growing in the womb was so long, the connection between the two was not made. Thus birth control for that woman, and her culture, might mean avoiding the watery area.

Most people over the age of fifty remember being told that if they were burned while cooking, they should immediately cover the burn with butter. Years later emergency medical personnel are still trying to explain that grease not only doesn't work, it might delay the healing effect of proper treatment. Cold water (not ice), we now know, is the best therapy to use on a burn before seeing a physician or going to an emergency care center.

Many other examples exist. The longer a culture has used a therapy, the more likely it is to have some value. But that value may be minimal. The positive result may be nothing more than a placebo effect. Or it may be based on only a small number of reports of positive experiences, repeated over and over, with the negative experiences forgotten.

Early Testing Was Little More Than Careful Observation

As medical science began to develop in the sixteenth century, early experiments focused on careful observation. For example, a common treatment for poisonings in ancient times was the bezoar stone. Legend had it that these stones were the crystallized tears of a deer bitten by a snake (actually, they were gallstones). The legend was that when they were swallowed, they would stay in the stomach and absorb any poison taken by the person. A French surgeon, Ambroise Paré (1510–1590), conducted an observational experiment that would not be viewed as ethical today. Paré, better known for bringing respectability to medieval surgery at a time when it was a barber's side-trade, gave a bezoar stone to a palace cook who had been condemned to death for stealing. The cook was given mercuric chloride, a common poison, and subsequently died in agony, despite having been given the "antidote."[6] Clearly, the bezoar stone was useless.

Reporting the results of a treatment on a single patient still occurs today in what are called "case reports." These are more complete descriptions of the factors surrounding a patient's experience, but they remain limited by being a form of anecdotal evidence. If several case reports are published for a particular treatment, especially if the patients have similar conditions, someone is likely to initiate a more controlled study.

The Observational Study Compares Response to a Treatment

One of the earliest methods developed to compensate for the limitations of anecdotal evidence was the comparative, or observational, study. Anecdotes and case reports are descriptions of what has already happened. Observational studies are set up ahead of time to closely observe what happens as patients are treated in a certain way. When comparing people's responses to treatments, everyone tested should be in a similar environment. Observational studies allow doctors to control some of the factors influencing a treatment, and thus are the simplest of controlled studies.

One of the earliest controlled trials was carried out by James Lind (1716–1794), a Scottish physician in the British Navy. Scurvy was a major problem in the navies of the world at that time. One estimate claimed that scurvy took the lives of about 1 million British sailors between 1500 and 1800, more than all those who lost their lives at sea through warfare and accidents during the same period.[7]

Lind conducted an experiment in which two sailors were given a quart of apple cider a day, two more were given an elixir of vitriol (a copper-based tonic), two took two teaspoonfuls of vinegar three times daily, two drank half a pint of seawater a day, two were given an electuary (a sweet-tasting medicine made from cooking herbs), and two more were given two oranges and a lemon daily. By comparing the effects of different treatments on people in similar situations, Lind showed that citrus fruits not only cured scurvy but also could be used to prevent it. However, his story also demonstrates how long it takes for some new findings to be accepted. The British Navy did not add citrus fruits to sailors' rations until the year after Lind died, forty-eight years later.

Why was the British Navy so slow to make changes based on, what seems to us today, such clear-cut evidence? Why do some insist on using therapies that others claim are completely ineffective? While complete answers to these questions are complicated, at least two factors associated with this phenomenon are important to our discussion. One is the natural course of illness and disease. Many illnesses and pains will diminish or disappear on their own. Some estimates claim that people will recover from as much as 80 percent of all illnesses regardless of what treatments they use.[8] There is much common sense behind the saying that if you have a cold: "Take an antibiotic or an aspirin and it'll be gone in a week; do nothing and it'll be gone in seven days." Even illnesses as serious as cancer are known to inexplicably disappear, which is known medically as "spontaneous remission." Many chronic conditions fluctuate in their severity, so if a treatment is started when the condition is at its worst, it may appear that the treatment helped when in fact the condition merely improved on its own, only to return later.

Controlled Clinical Trials Help to Test Effectiveness

The second factor related to why people believe in therapies not supported by research is the placebo effect, which we discussed at length in chapter 2. The placebo effect is the combination of factors that give therapies beneficial effects, but which are not caused by any direct physiological action. The classic placebo is the sugar pill. Recognition of the placebo effect led scientists to realize that many remedies used throughout the history of medicine were placebos. Clinical research trials have developed in large part to figure out whether a therapy is beneficial in and of itself, or whether it works primarily by the placebo effect. Many people remain convinced that certain therapies help them, when in fact they are benefiting from the placebo effect.

The primary tool for discovering whether a treatment is effective in and of itself is the "controlled clinical trial." This research tool was not widely implemented until the middle of the twentieth century, even though its development began in the seventeenth century. Ironically, while conventional medicine emphasizes controlled clinical trials, this approach was developed with what would today be called alternative therapies.

A number of important events can help us track the development of controlled clinical trials and thereby help us understand the importance of the sort of evidence they provide. During the seventeenth and eighteenth centuries, developments in human anatomy and microbiology occurred which contradicted many of the assertions and theories of Galen, a Greco-Roman physician (A.D. 131–200).

For example, Galen held that ingested food was continuously converted into blood in the liver. The blood, according to Galen, then permeated all the tissues of the body, passing through the heart, where it mysteriously picked up the "vital spirit" which controlled all bodily functions.

William Harvey (1578–1657) dissected animals and discovered that blood circulates continuously around the body, pumped by the heart. Harvey emphasized the importance of observation in medicine, and was the first to use quantitative analysis. He calculated the volume of blood in the body, showing that this was incompatible with Galen's theories about blood.

Harvey feared what might happen to his livelihood if he published his controversial results. After they were published, he reflected, "But now the die is cast; my hope is in the love of truth and in the integrity of intelligence."[9] But Harvey's claims could be objectively demonstrated for all to see, which is an important feature of the scientific method. Harvey's discoveries weakened the influence of Galen's theory and opened the possibility that the ineffectiveness of popular remedies based on his theories might soon be demonstrated. Gradually, the influence of Galen on medical training began to wane.

Around the same time as Harvey was conducting his experiments, European explorers discovered the medicinal uses of cinchona bark *(Cinchona succirubra),* long known to Peruvian Indians. Jesuit missionaries returning from Peru introduced cinchona into Europe in 1638.[10] Malaria had been a common and devastating disease in Europe for centuries. In accordance with Galen's medical theories, different remedies were used for months to rid the body of the corrupting humors, all to no avail. In contrast, cinchona rapidly cured the protracted and intermittent fevers that accompany malaria.

Curiously, cinchona cured malarial fevers, but did not work on other types of fever, which demonstrated an important principle in validating cures. If a remedy has a specific action on a specific condition, it is likely to be due to an active ingredient in that remedy (which, for cinchona, was later shown to be quinine). Remedies said to cure a wide variety of unrelated conditions (called "panaceas") are more likely to be placebos, if they work at all.

The reaction of the medical establishment to cinchona reveals another important principle. In spite of its demonstrated efficacy, especially in curing Charles II of England and Louis XIV of France, many physicians of the day rejected its use. Following the Protestant Reformation, anything associated with the Roman Catholic Jesuits was frowned upon or dismissed by many non-Catholic physicians. In addition, ineffective, adulterated, and counterfeit cinchona products were being sold which were less effective and sometimes harmful. This reduced people's confidence in the authentic product's efficacy.

But the primary reason for the rejection of cinchona was that it did not fit in with the prevailing medical theory of the day. "The history of cinchona illustrates the way in which powerful a priori beliefs prevented intelligent and highly trained physicians from recognizing an effective treatment and led them to reject one of the most useful drugs in the history of medicine."[11] This tendency remains today among those who do not value the evidence of controlled trials.

Throughout the nineteenth century, more and more controlled studies were conducted, especially with controversial therapies like homeopathy and paranormal healing. Some people held on to the cures and remedies that had been popular for centuries. But there gradually arose a group of physicians who became known as the New School of Medicine. They pursued a form of medicine that would offer only what had been demonstrated to be effective—that which was based on the best evidence available. A leader of this group, William Osler (1849–1919), put it this way:

The characteristic of the New School is firm faith in a few good, well-tried drugs, little or none in the great mass of medicines still in general use.... The battle against poly-pharmacy, or the use of a large number of drugs (of the action of which we know little, yet we put them into bodies of the action of which we know less), has not been fought to a finish.... A new school of practitioners has arisen which cares nothing for homœopathy and less for so-called allopathy. It seeks to study, rationally and scientifically, the action of drugs, old and new. It is more concerned that a physician shall know how to apply the few great medicines which all have to use, such as quinine, iron, mercury, iodide of potassium, opium and digitalis, than that he should employ a multiplicity of remedies the action of which is extremely doubtful.[12]

Osler's commitment to science did not diminish his compassion for patients, an accusation often leveled against conventional medicine. In spite of his enthusiasm for scientific developments in medicine, he also noted: "Perhaps in no particular does nineteenth-century practice differ from that of the preceding centuries more than in the greater attention which is given to the personal comfort of the patient and to all the accessories comprised in the art of nursing."[13] He remained concerned for justice in health care, as when he stated: "There is no higher mission in this life than nursing God's poor."[14] A commitment to science and caring should always go hand-in-hand in health care.

Double-Blind Studies Control As Many Aspects As Possible

Early in the twentieth century, researchers realized the importance of controlling as many aspects of a trial as possible. A study of drugs being used to treat angina represented an important development.[15] The drugs were all xanthine alkaloids, a chemical group of which caffeine is the most familiar. Two other xanthines, theobromine and aminophylline, had been widely used since 1895 for the relief of angina pain. By 1932 almost every cardiac patient used them. However, one physician-researcher, Harry Gold, was skeptical of their efficacy and started an experiment where some patients got the drug and some got a lactose (or milk-sugar) pill. This was a "single-blind trial." The patients didn't know which pill they got, but the physicians evaluating them did.

After more than two years of treatments, Gold and his colleague, Kwit, noticed that patients were giving contradictory answers to questions about their pain levels. Upon closer review, they discovered that the physicians talking to patients would ask different questions depending on whether the patient was receiving the xanthines or the placebo. In effect, they were asking patients leading questions that were biasing the results and introducing errors. The researchers suspected the patients were answering questions according to what they thought the physicians wanted to hear, thus undermining the value of the study.

Gold and Kwit changed their methodology so that the physicians did not know whether they were giving their patients the placebo or the drug. This was the first example of a clinical trial using a placebo where neither the patients nor the physicians knew what was being given. This type of controlled study would later become known as a "double-blind study"—

the patient and the physician are both "blinded" to whether the patient was receiving the active or inactive intervention.

Kwit summarized the essence of this method: "Toward the end of the study we realized that the doctor must not know what he gives, the patient must not know what he receives, and the questioner must not know what was given."[16] With this new element of control introduced, the study went on to reveal that xanthines were no more effective at relieving angina pain than placebo, a finding confirmed by later studies.

Many other studies have shown that patients have an amazing ability to detect whether or not researchers expect to see them improve.[17] A more recent study of pain relief after tooth extraction used two placebo groups.[18] Researchers told one group of physicians that their patients would receive either a placebo or a pain enhancer (which blocks the body's natural pain-relieving mechanisms). A second group was told their patients would receive a placebo, pain enhancer, or pain reliever. All patients in the study actually received a placebo.

The patients in the first group reported increased pain to their physicians, while the patients in the second group reported reduced pain.

The only difference between the groups was what the physicians had been told. In the first group, the physicians believed their patients would not get a pain reliever. And those patients' pain, on average, got worse. In the second group, the physicians believed their patients had a one in three chance of getting a pain reliever. Those patients, on average, reported pain relief. Somehow the physicians' expectations influenced the patients' response to the treatment. When the physicians believed there was some chance the patients would benefit from the treatment, the patients benefited. When they knew there was no chance of benefit, no one benefited.

Studies like this show that researchers who know whether they are giving patients a placebo or the test treatment can bias the test results. Somehow they inadvertently or even subconsciously transmit their knowledge or expectations to the patients. This can occur in very subtle ways, through facial expressions, body movement, and tone of voice.[19] People differ in their ability to pick up on these cues, an ability which has even been demonstrated in animals. Hence, the best research must control researchers' expectations by keeping them unaware or "blinded" about which treatment they are giving. That is the essence of the double-blind clinical trial. Research over the years has confirmed that the double-blind controlled study is much more likely to give accurate results than the single-blind controlled study—and both are far superior to anecdotal reports.

Randomization in Research Improves Accuracy of Results

The first randomized clinical trial (RCT) was conducted with tuberculosis patients around the same time as Gold's research with angina patients. During the nineteenth century, tuberculosis led to one in every seven deaths. Many different remedies had been touted as cures, only to later find they made little difference. Then they would be replaced by yet another ineffective remedy. Up until the 1940s, standard treatment for tuberculosis in one lung was to deliberately collapse that lung; if both lungs were infected, bed rest was the only treatment.[20]

Sir Austin Bradford Hill is often referred to as the "father of clinical trials" because of his influence on clinical research. Hill contracted tuberculosis (during World War I) and was one of the fortunate to survive. He was seriously ill for five years, making it impossible for him to attend medical school. His love of medicine led him to study statistics, which he applied to medical questions as an epidemiologist working in public health. Epidemiology is the study of how frequently diseases occur in a population, and the factors that contribute to increasing or decreasing that frequency.

Hill remained interested in studying tuberculosis, and was a member of the British Medical Research Council when a new drug, streptomycin, was reported to be effective against tuberculosis. The council designed a clinical trial for streptomycin that incorporated Hill's expertise in statistics.[21] Researchers at this time were becoming aware that if the individuals in the placebo group were not very similar to those receiving the test treatment, the results could be biased.[22] For example, if by chance one group contained mostly younger people and another mostly older people, different results might be due to the age differences, not the treatment. These other factors (like age, gender, and economic status) are known as "confounding variables." The best way to avoid such differences is to randomly assign people to the groups, and use statistical methods to check whether the groups are similar in all known and relevant ways.

Today these random assignments are made based on computer-generated random allocation tables. Then, researchers have no way of knowing which patients will end up in which group. This can be done best by having someone who does not even see the patient determine the group assignment, and not tell the researcher until after the study is completed. Research that is not properly randomized has, on average, been found to overestimate the treatment's benefit by 41 percent.[23]

Hill's streptomycin study emphasized the importance of assigning people to different groups in random ways. In this study, one group received streptomycin injections and bed rest, and the other group received bed rest alone. The study would have been stronger if the second group had received a placebo (injections containing no active drug). However, other considerations sometimes have to outweigh the scientific issues. Streptomycin was given in four intramuscular injections daily for six months. These injections are painful. To give this number of painful placebo injections was viewed as inappropriate. The researchers recognized that the scientific value of a placebo was overridden by the ethical issue of avoiding needless patient pain and discomfort.

Obviously, the patients knew whether they were in the treatment group or the placebo group. The researchers compensated for this by blinding the radiologists who read patients' chest X-rays and the physicians who evaluated the patients clinically. The results showed that the streptomycin group had less than half the death rate of the placebo group and almost double the rate of improvement. Thus, the study provided important evidence for the efficacy of an early antibiotic.

The Impact of World War II on the Modern Era of Drug Testing

World War II impacted the development of clinical trials in a number of ways. Infectious diseases such as malaria and typhoid were major killers in regions where soldiers were being sent to fight. Cinchona had been almost exclusively available from Indonesia, which was occupied by Japanese forces in 1942, thereby cutting off cinchona supplies.[24] Nonfatal wounds often became infected and then caused death. Penicillin and sulfonamide, discovered prior to the war and shown to dramatically reduce wound infections, were available in only small amounts. Their large-scale production thus became a priority. A major push to find and manufacture effective antibiotics was launched, resulting in many new and powerful drugs—streptomycin, Aureomycin®, and chloramphenicol. The production and sale of these new drugs was surprisingly profitable for their manufacturers. Therefore, after the war, pharmaceutical companies widened their scope of interest to find or develop drugs for other diseases.

Along with this impetus to find new drugs came the need to test them. Most people are surprised to learn that very few of the drugs that are developed by pharmaceutical companies actually make it to commercial production. In a twenty-year search for antimalarial drugs alone, 300,000 chemicals were tested on animals, of which only twelve were found useful and safe enough to try with humans.[25] Fewer made it onto the market. During World War II, the need to develop reliable ways to evaluate effectiveness was very pressing. This applied not only to drugs but also to other items important to the war effort, such as food, clothing, shelter, and vehicles.[26] From this effort came scientists trained in comparing the effectiveness of similar products using the most objective methods possible.

Further impetus for conducting controlled clinical trials came from legislative pressure. In the late 1950s, a new drug was introduced in Europe as a mild sedative. Since large doses appeared to result in little harm, it was viewed as safe and recommended for morning sickness caused by pregnancy, high blood pressure, and migraines.[27] In 1961, reports surfaced of deformities among babies born to women who had taken this drug when they were pregnant. The drug, thalidomide, was quickly taken off the market throughout the world, but not before about 8,000 children were born deformed, often with missing limbs. These deformities appeared in about 20 percent of the pregnant women who had taken thalidomide.

Thalidomide had never been approved for sale in the United States, but not because anyone suspected it could harm unborn children. Drug manufacturers were required to show that their products were safe before receiving permission from the Food & Drug Administration (FDA) to market them in the United States. Because some animals given thalidomide suffered nerve damage (technically called "peripheral neuropathy"), the FDA kept the drug off the market. During clinical trials in the U.S., thalidomide was given to some pregnant women, resulting in seventeen children being born with the characteristic deformities.

Many believed the FDA regulations averted a much larger tragedy. As a result, even stricter regulations were introduced. A bill passed by Congress in 1962 added the requirement that manufacturers submit "adequate and well controlled experiments by experts qualified by scientific training and experience to evaluate the effectiveness of the drug involved."[28] Gradually the precise nature of these experiments was defined. Since the early 1980s, FDA approval of new drugs has effectively required the use of randomized, placebo-controlled, double-blind clinical trials.

Incidentally, in July 1998 the FDA approved marketing of thalidomide for a rare skin disease associated with Hansen's disease, the technical term for leprosy.[29] There is clear evidence that it effectively treats this condition, but those taking it are required to agree to strict contraceptive measures.

Some fear thalidomide will be used for other conditions for which it is not approved. Thalidomide is anecdotally reported to be beneficial for a wide variety of conditions such as mouth ulcers associated with HIV, rheumatoid arthritis, diabetes, and some cancers. Many fear that if thalidomide is promoted on the basis of this anecdotal evidence, some unborn children will again become victims, and end up either deformed or aborted.

The most reliable evidence for effectiveness comes from properly designed and conducted randomized, double-blind, controlled clinical trials. These have been defined as "any planned therapeutic, diagnostic, or preventive study involving humans comparing concurrently one intervention (drug, device, or procedure) to another intervention (placebo), or no intervention, to determine their relative safety and efficacy."[30] Appropriate statistical comparisons between the two groups (the treatment group and the placebo group) are at the core. These groups should be as similar as possible in every way, other than the therapy being evaluated.

While we have focused on the role of a placebo control, other controls are sometimes used, such as a "no-treatment" control group. A no-treatment control group will show whether the natural course of the illness is similar to the changes occurring with the treatment. The test treatment can also be compared to the current standard treatment. Even if a new therapy is effective and safe, it is important to learn whether it has any advantage or disadvantage compared to what is already being used.

The Power of the Placebo Must Be Understood

The role of the placebo effect is probably the most important aspect to control in clinical trials. Studying its effect is complicated by the fact that it varies between people and procedures. It is often reported that the placebo effect can account for a third of the improvements found with any therapy. In fact, if the measured placebo effect is too small, it will cast doubt on the validity of the study. The claim that about one-third of all patients will improve via the placebo effect is based upon an influential 1955 article.[31] But the author found that 35 percent was the *average* placebo effect. It can be much larger.

For example, angina was sometimes treated surgically in the 1950s. A double-blind study compared patients who received this surgery to a group who received only a skin incision (the ethics of these types of studies are seriously questioned and debated today, but that is another issue). Over half of those who received the placebo surgery reported significant improvements, approximately the same proportion as those who received the actual surgery.[32] Another study shortly after this one reported that every patient getting the placebo surgery showed significant improvements. This surgery was soon abandoned, but remains an important symbol of the importance of the placebo effect.

Placebos are more effective in treating certain types of disorders. They work best with pain, nausea, phobias, depression, and anxiety.[33] Disorders related to blood pressure and bronchial airways also respond well to placebo therapy. However, placebos do not appear to work as well in acute situations (like a heart attack) or in degenerative diseases.

It is critically important for the reader to understand that the conditions in which placebos work well are, for the most part, the same conditions for which alternative therapies are commonly used. We also point out that studies have shown that people pursuing alternative medicine tend to be more anxious than the general population.[34] Some commentators describe them as "the worried well" who monitor their bodies carefully and "spend more on all forms of health care, even though most are fairly healthy."[35] This heightened anxiety is relevant here because anxiety is one of the conditions most strongly affected by placebos.[36] A positive interaction between patients and health care professionals can strongly influence the placebo effect, which is why we place such importance on this interpersonal aspect of alternative therapies.

How Researchers Judge the Clinical Significance of a Treatment

Results of clinical trials must eventually be evaluated. Every patient does not respond in the same way or to the same extent. If treatment results are not drastically different from the placebo, how different do they need to be before we can be sure the therapy is useful? In other words, how do you tell which differences are significant?

Differences between two groups could be due to chance, or they could be due to the treatment really being better. Sometimes reports of studies will state that the treatment was beneficial, but not at a statistically significant level. That means there is a higher probability that the positive results were due to chance, and we cannot place much confidence in the effectiveness of the therapy. In those cases, it is important not to make definite statements about the treatment based on that study, other than saying that the results for the two groups are not statistically different and that a larger study might be warranted.

In clinical research, the more patients enrolled, the more reliable the results. The fewer the patients, the less reliable the study and the more likely that any differences are due to chance.

Alternative Therapies Are Believed Safe Simply Because They're Old

The "scientific method" is quite different from the traditional justification for alternative therapies. Alternative therapies are usually regarded as safe and effective because they have been used for decades or centuries and the preponderance of anecdotal evidence says they work. Sometimes this reasoning is accurate, and scientific testing is able to demonstrate that the therapy is effective and may even go on to uncover why the therapy works. Other times, even scientific claims about the anecdotes turn out to be inaccurate.

We have seen this most recently when studying the eating habits of various Western nations. Traditional French cuisine was always rich in sauces full of ingredients that contribute to heart disease. Yet the French had a lower rate of heart disease than Americans eating meals just as rich in fat. This observation became known as the "French paradox." Epidemiologists examined many reports from different countries trying to figure out what protected the French. This research led to speculation that drinking a glass of wine with dinner might somehow protect people from heart disease.[37] It sounded like scientific validation of the age-old practice of drinking wine!

The protective quality of various grapes, both fermented and unfermented, due to certain active ingredients (called antioxidants) became a topic of serious experimentation that continues to this day. However, what was not raised in the publicity surrounding the heart issue was something just as important. The French who consume wine regularly do have a lower incidence of deaths from heart problems than Americans with a similar diet, but the French have a higher incidence of death due to alcohol-related causes.[38] The French are not somehow magically protected from alcohol abuse just because their consumption of wine is both routine and ritualized at meals. Yet there were Americans who decided that they should increase their alcohol intake based on the French experience. One commentator recently quipped, "Eat like the French, die like the French." To avoid the extra alcohol, others recommend taking supplements of grape seed extract (see Antioxidants, page 298).

The lesson to be learned here is that scientific studies are not all alike. Epidemiological studies are more similar to anecdotal reports than they are to randomized, clinical trials. Epidemiologists survey people, asking them lots of questions about lifestyle issues, such as their diet. These studies can identify correlations: that those who drink wine moderately have less heart disease. But this does not prove causation: that heart disease is prevented by moderate wine consumption. This would require a controlled study in which one group added wine to their diet and another did not. The scientific evidence does not yet support adding wine to one's diet. Doing so prematurely could even lead to the alcohol-related problems found in France.

Willow bark offers another interesting case. Willow bark has been used for centuries as a natural remedy for headache and joint inflammation. During the nineteenth century, scientists decided to investigate whether willow bark worked by the placebo effect or actually contained some active ingredient that did relieve pain. Scientists found that willow bark contains salicylic acid, which does relieve pain. However, it is very irritating to the stomach. To make it less irritating, they chemically converted it to acetylsalicylic acid—what we know today as aspirin. In this way, an herb with a long tradition led to a scientifically verifiable medication.

Some now promote the use of willow bark as a "natural alternative" to pharmaceutical aspirin. They cite the scientific evidence supporting the safety and effectiveness of aspirin as support for willow bark. It is easy to assume that one is as effective as the other. But the first step in testing this claim would be to measure the amount of the active ingredient in each. Aspirin is manufactured to standard specifications. Two regular-strength aspirin tablets each contain the same amount of the active ingredient, so you can expect the same results. They may be positive (easing a headache or reducing joint inflammation) or negative (stomach irritation) or both. Results will be consistent.

With willow bark, you cannot have the same expectation. Even though willow bark has a long history of use, aspirin has the scientific support. The amount of active ingredient in the particular sample will vary depending on where the willow bark was obtained, when it was harvested, and how it was packaged. If the bark is then used to prepare a tea, many other variables will be introduced, such as the amount used, the temperature of the water, and how long the bark was soaked. The active ingredient may be similar to aspirin (and similar does not mean identical), but the quantity and quality may be very different. (See Willow Bark, page 457.)

These are some of the reasons why we believe everyone should learn how to evaluate the various medical claims made about all sorts of therapies. Only then will you be able to figure out what is most likely to be effective for you, using products that are proven to be reliable, safe, and effective. Without that knowledge, we as a society risk the continued and unnecessary expenditure of billions of dollars per year for harmful or ineffective medical therapies.

Reviewing the Literature Is Vital But Time-Consuming

With the widespread use of clinical trials today, physicians now have a new problem: the shear volume of information available. There are about 22,000 medical publications of a serial nature, about 16,000 of which are journals.[39] Over two million medical articles are published every year. If placed on top of one another, these articles would make a pillar over 150 feet high.[40] Many of these medical articles contain reports of clinical trials. But even with this amount of written information, only about half of the clinical studies conducted are ever published in written form, the rest being reported orally at meetings or not accepted for publication.[41]

All this information has to be condensed and combined into a usable form for busy practitioners. For this purpose, systematic reviews are done. Reviewers search for all the studies conducted on a certain therapy or drug, and summarize their findings in some way. The most common way of doing this is called a "narrative review." The reviewer, usually an expert in the field, selects the important studies on a treatment and writes an essay on the strengths and weaknesses of each. The reviewer comes to some conclusion about all the evidence and its implications for clinical practice. These reviews provide concise summaries from someone very familiar with the details of that research.

While narrative reviews are very useful, they have an important limitation. Most reviewers are likely to have some preconceived idea about the research, and there is a natural tendency for this bias to come through in the conclusions. This is especially the case if the reviewer has done some of the research on the therapy. Reviewers must work hard to be as objective as possible. A number of safeguards are now put in place by publishers to help minimize this sort of bias.

A famous case of this involved the usefulness of vitamin C for treating the common cold. Linus Pauling (1901–1994) was a biochemist who won two Nobel prizes, one in 1954 for chemistry and in the other in 1963 for peace. He reviewed the available research on vitamin C and the common cold, publishing two books on his findings. He concluded, from the research done by others, that high doses of vitamin C would both prevent colds and, if you have a cold, decrease its severity and duration, adding, "Catching a cold and letting it run its course is a sign that you are not taking enough vitamin C."[42]

Pauling referred to thirty studies in his review. However, he did not state how he found them or how exhaustively he looked. He rated some studies as being of high quality and some poor, but nowhere explained how he made those evaluations. He did not state if he "blinded" himself to the findings of the studies when evaluating their quality. The best way to review a study is to evaluate its quality without looking at the results. In other words, a reviewer who thinks vitamin C helps with colds will have to fight against a tendency to judge studies supportive of this conclusion as being of higher quality. In Pauling's review, most studies supported his conclusion, and those that didn't he labeled as "unfortunately flawed" without explaining why.

Years later, a researcher was preparing to conduct another clinical trial on vitamin C and the common cold, and he reexamined Pauling's data.[43] He searched exhaustively for all previous studies and found sixty-one. He had decided ahead of time what would constitute high quality and low quality in a study. He then covered up the results section of each study while grading how well the study was conducted. Only then did he look at their conclusions.

On a scale of 0 to 12 (with 12 being the best), only 15 of the 61 studies scored 7 or more points. Based on the results of the best 15 studies, this reviewer concluded: "Vitamin C, even in gram quantities per day, cannot prevent a cold. On the other hand, if you already have a cold, a megadose of, say 1 g vitamin C may slightly decrease the duration and severity of your cold (perhaps by 10%)."[44]

This more rigorous and objective form of review is called a "systematic review." This conclusion, not Pauling's, has been consistently supported, which is why large doses of vitamin C are still not recommended by conventional medicine to prevent or cure colds.[45]

In spite of safeguards, no review can be absolutely objective since no human reviewer can be completely unbiased. Since decisions have to be made on what constitutes high and low quality, and what score counts for inclusion among the "best studies," any review will be somewhat biased. However, the more explicit the review, the easier it is to determine how objectively it was done.

Unfortunately, media reports of therapies tend to use the most unreliable and unobjective methods of "reviewing" therapies. Far too often, people who market alternative therapies try to promote or sell those therapies by using either media reports or poorly performed medical studies. For example, media reports or promotional materials stating, "studies have found…"

or "the latest evidence shows . . ." tell us nothing about the overall quality and significance of the research.

In fact, these reports can be completely misleading as they can selectively pick the studies that support only the conclusion the author wants to promote. It takes a lot more time and work to do a comprehensive review of the literature. When making decisions about therapies, though, these are the sorts of reviews we should rely on.

A newer method of reviewing research, called a "meta-analysis," has been developed to eliminate even more bias. This is a statistical method of combining the results of several trials that have given unclear or conflicting results. Most clinical trials with alternative therapies tend to be very small and are often poorly controlled. The theory behind the meta-analysis is that instead of running another large, expensive trial with hundreds of patients, the results of numerous small trials can be combined to give statistically significant results.

However, a meta-analysis is only as good as the quality of the original studies. In other words, if the studies included in a meta-analysis are of poor quality, then the meta-analysis will be of poor quality. All the studies combined in a meta-analysis must be very similar for the conclusion to be valid, and this is not always possible. A chain of evidence made up of weak links will not be made stronger by adding more weak links.

The best meta-analyses start by grading, as objectively as possible, all discoverable studies—whether published or not. Most of the nonpublished studies are those that show no difference between treatments. In addition, data is often available from ongoing studies that have not yet been published. So, many researchers who perform meta-analyses will seek to find quality data that is both published and unpublished. Then, the statistical evaluation should be performed on only the best studies that are most similar. However, objective and ethical researchers will disclose the studies that they excluded and the reasons for their exclusion.

Even Scientific Methods for Testing Remedies Have Weaknesses

Overall, conventional medicine has developed methods of reliably determining whether treatments work or not. The randomized double-blind clinical trial has made important contributions to conventional medicine's ability to determine safety and effectiveness. However, these methods are not without problems.[46] Probably the biggest problems arise when studies are thought to be controlled studies when in fact they are not. Much training is needed to properly conduct clinical trials. Such training may not be available to some researchers and is ignored by others. Hence, some studies that have significant methodological flaws get published by inexperienced or unscrupulous researchers. Studies of that type, especially with controversial therapies, make evaluations of the therapies even more complicated.

In spite of this, randomized, double-blind, controlled clinical trials remain the gold standard of clinical research. Even with their limitations, they provide the best evidence for discovering the truth about any particular treatment. The author of an article on clinical trials in the prestigious journal *Science* concluded: "Even the sharpest critics of the way clinical trials are currently conducted, however, would not advocate that they not be done, for one simple reason: There's no better alternative."[47]

The only alternative would be a return to the type of medicine where everyone tries and promotes whatever he or she likes, with no scientific evidence to back up claims. We recognize that there is a certain amount of trial and error in medicine. There are limitations to diagnosis and prognosis. Every patient is different and responds somewhat differently to the same therapy.

But conventional medicine has developed a reliable means of determining what works and what doesn't. Health care providers and patients should provide or accept only those therapies that are based on the best scientific evidence. That way we can restrict ourselves to using only reliable, safe, and effective treatments. We would encourage our readers not to ask of physicians, "What do you think of this or that therapy?", but rather, "What is the evidence supporting this or that therapy?" Why? Because the therapy, if chosen, will be applied to one of the most valuable possessions on earth:

> *Do you not know that your body is a temple of the Holy Spirit, who is in you, whom you have received from God? You are not your own; you were bought at a price. Therefore honor God with your body.*

1 Corinthians 6:19–20

Notes

1. For example, quantum theory appeared to contradict much of classical physics. Yet the results of many experiments showed that its predictions were correct. It was also eventually shown that quantum and classical physics did not contradict one another, but that classical physics fits within quantum theory. Classical physics describes large objects best, while quantum physics describes submicroscopic objects best. When science works well, the data speak for themselves, regardless of who did the experiment. The data (if accurate and reliable) may require changes in current theories. Unfortunately, this is not always how science has been practiced. For example, Galileo's discoveries were rejected for years because the scientific community at that time was strongly influenced by Catholic Church beliefs.

2. Leonard J. Bruce-Chwatt, "Cinchona and Its Alkaloids: 350 Years," *New York State Journal of Medicine* 88, no. 6 (June 1988): 318–22.

3. Ernest Lucas and Peter May, "The Significance of Jesus' Healing Ministry," in *Christian Healing: What Can We Believe?* ed. Ernest Lucas (London: Lynx, 1997), 85–108.

4. Ronald Brenner, Vadim Azbel, Subramoniam Madhusoodanan, and Monica Pawlowska, "Comparison of an Extract of Hypericum (LI 160) and Sertraline in the Treatment of Depression: A Double-Blind, Randomized Pilot Study," *Clinical Therapeutics* 22, no. 4 (April 2000): 411–19.

5. National Center for Complementary and Alternative Medicine, *Draft Five Year Strategic Plan.* Accessed at http://nccam.nih.gov/ on April 10, 2001.

6. Anonymous, "Charitable Chirurgion," *MD* 4 (May 1960): 188–93.

7. Sherman M. Mellinkoff, "James Lind's Legacy to Clinical Medicine," *Western Journal of Medicine* 162, no. 4 (April 1995): 367–69.

8. Arthur K. Shapiro and Elaine Shapiro, *The Powerful Placebo: From Ancient Priest to Modern Physician* (Baltimore and London: Johns Hopkins University Press, 1997), 51, 134.

9. M. E. Silverman, "William Harvey and the Discovery of the Circulation of Blood," *Clinical Cardiology* 8, no. 4 (April 1985): 244–46.

10. Bruce-Chwatt, "Cinchona and Its Alkaloids," 318–22.

11. Shapiro and Shapiro, *Powerful Placebo*, 22.

12. William Osler, "Medicine in the Nineteenth Century," in *Aequanimitas: With Other Addresses to Medical Students, Nurses and Practitioners of Medicine*, 3d ed. (Philadelphia: Blakiston, 1932), 254–55.

13. Osler, "Medicine in the Nineteenth Century," 257.

14. William Osler, "Nurse and Patient," in *Aequanimitas: With Other Addresses to Medical Students, Nurses and Practitioners of Medicine*, 3d ed. (Philadelphia: Blakiston, 1932), 158.

15. Harry Gold, Nathaniel T. Kwit, and Harold Otto, "The Xanthines (Theobromine and Aminophylline) in the Treatment of Cardiac Pain," *Journal of the American Medical Association* 108, no. 26 (June 1937): 2173–79.

16. Kwit, quoted in Shapiro and Shapiro, *Powerful Placebo*, 142.

17. Robert Rosenthal, *Experimenter Effects in Behavioral Research* (New York: Irvington, 1976).

18. Richard H. Gracely, Ronald Dubner, William R. Deeter, and Patricia J. Wolskee, "Clinicians' Expectations Influence Placebo Analgesia," *Lancet* 1, no. 8419 (January 1985): 43.

19. Rosenthal, *Experimenter Effects*, 281–302.

20. Flávio D. Fuchs, Michael J. Klag, and Paul K. Whelton, "The Classics: A Tribute to the Fiftieth Anniversary of the Randomized Clinical Trial," *Journal of Clinical Epidemiology* 53, no. 4 (April 2000): 335–42.

21. Medical Research Council, "Streptomycin Treatment of Pulmonary Tuberculosis," *British Medical Journal* 2 (October 1948): 769–82.

22. Theodore H. Greiner, Harry Gold, McKeen Cattel, Janet Travell, Hyman Bakst, Seymour H. Rinzler, Zachery H. Benjamin, Leon J. Warshaw, Audrie L. Bobb, Nathaniel T. Kwit, Walter Modell, Harold H. Rothendler, and Charles R. Messeloff, "A Method for the Evaluation of the Effects of Drugs on Cardiac Pain in Patients with Angina of Effort: A Study of Khellin (Visammin)," *American Journal of Medicine* 9 (August 1950): 143–55.

23. Kenneth F. Schulz, Iain Chalmers, Richard J. Hayes, and Douglas G. Altman, "Empirical Evidence of Bias: Dimensions of Methodological Quality Associated with Estimates of Treatment Effects in Controlled Trials," *Journal of the American Medical Association* 273, no. 5 (February 1995).

24. Bruce-Chwatt, "Cinchona and its Alkaloids," 318–22.

25. Ibid.

26. Shapiro and Shapiro, *The Powerful Placebo*, 158.

27. George J. Annas and Sherman Elias, "Thalidomide and the *Titanic*: Reconstructing the Technology Tragedies of the Twentieth Century," *American Journal of Public Health* 89, no. 1 (January 1999): 98–101.

28. Kefauver-Harris Amendment to the Food and Drug Act (1962), quoted in Shapiro and Shapiro, *Powerful Placebo*, 172.

29. Annas and Elias, "Thalidomide."

30. Kay Dickersin, Roberta Scherer, and Carol Lefebvre, "Identifying Relevant Studies for Systematic Reviews," in *Systematic Reviews*, ed. Iain Chalmers and Douglas G. Altman (London: BMJ Publishing Group, 1995), 19.

31. Henry K. Beecher, "The Powerful Placebo," *Journal of the American Medical Association* 159, no. 17 (December 1955): 1602–6.

32. Leonard A. Cobb, George I. Thomas, David H. Dillard, K. Alvin Merendino, and Robert A. Bruce, "An Evaluation of Internal-Mammary-Artery Ligation by a Double-Blind Technic," *New England Journal of Medicine* 260, no. 22 (May 1959): 1115–18.

33. Vernon M. S. Oh, "The Placebo Effect: Can We Use It Better?" *BMJ* 309 (July 1994): 69–70.

34. John A. Astin, "Why Patients Use Alternative Medicine: Results of a National Study," *Journal of the American Medical Association* 279, no. 19 (May 1998): 1548–53.

35. Paul H. Ray, "The Emerging Culture," *American Demographics* (February 1997), 7.

36. Judith A. Turner, Richard A. Deyo, John D. Loeser, Michael Von Korff, and Wilbert E. Fordyce, "The Importance of Placebo Effects in Pain Treatment and Research," *Journal of the American Medical Association* 271, no. 20 (May 1994): 1609–14.

37. E. N. Frankel, J. Kanner, J. B. German, E. Parks, and J. E. Kinsella, "Inhibition of Oxidation of Human Low-Density Lipoprotein by Phenolic Substances in Red Wine," *Lancet* 341 (February 1993): 454–57.

38. Malcolm Law and Nicholas Wald, "Why Heart Disease Mortality Is Low in France: The Time Lag Explanation," *BMJ* 318 (May 1999): 1471–76. This article sparked considerable controversy from numerous authors, whose comments are found in *BMJ* 318 (May 1999): 1476–80; *BMJ* 319 (July 1999): 255–56; *BMJ* 320 (January 2000): 249–50.

39. Dickersin, Scherer, and Lefebvre, "Identifying Relevant Studies," 17–36.

40. Cynthia D. Mulrow, "Rationale for Systematic Reviews," in *Systematic Reviews*, ed. Iain Chalmers and Douglas G. Altman (London: BMJ Publishing Group, 1995), 1.

41. Dickersin, Scherer, and Lefebvre, "Identifying Relevant Studies," 17–36.

42. Linus Pauling, *How to Live Longer and Feel Better* (New York: W. H. Freeman, 1986), 122; see also *Vitamin C and the Common Cold* (San Francisco: W. H. Freeman, 1970).

43. Paul Knipschild, "Some Examples of Systematic Reviews," in *Systematic Reviews*, ed. Iain Chalmers and Douglas G. Altman (London: BMJ Publishing Group, 1995), 9–16.

44. Knipschild, "Some Examples of Systematic Reviews," 11–12.

45. Institute of Medicine, *Dietary Reference Intakes for Vitamin C, Vitamin E, Selenium, and Carotenoids* (Washington, D.C.: National Academy Press, 2000), 126–27.

46. Rachel Nowak, "Problems in Clinical Trials Go Far Beyond Misconduct," *Science* 264 (June 1994): 1538–41.

47. Nowak, "Problems in Clinical Trials," 1541.

Part Four

POPULAR ALTERNATIVE THERAPIES, HERBAL REMEDIES, VITAMINS, AND DIETARY SUPPLEMENTS

11

How to Use the Rest of This Book

To help you make better choices, the alternative therapies, herbal remedies, vitamins, and dietary supplements listed alphabetically in this section are presented in as concise a manner as possible. We wanted to give you the most useful information in the least space.

You will learn the origins of each, learn explanations of the beliefs about how and why they "work" as well as the scientific information, if any, that supports or refutes the various claims made about each. In addition, you will learn whether there are aspects of these therapies that may be dangerous physically, mentally, or spiritually, and see that some are counter to biblical teaching. We have also rated the evidence using a standard and easy-to-understand research scale for each therapy, remedy, and supplement (see key below).

Unfortunately, finding reliable products in the field of alternative medicine is fraught with problems and dangers. Often the only approach available is one of trial and error.

We believe that eventually there will be standards for herbs and other natural products, similar to those for pharmaceuticals. Currently, the only guidance for product quality comes from some independent agencies. For example, products that claim to be produced to *The United States Pharmacopoeia* (USP) standards of quality, purity, and potency (and carry the USP symbol on their label) are supposed to be laboratory tested and theoretically should be— but are not necessarily—of higher quality than products not meeting this standard. *The United States Pharmacopoeia* is an independent pharmacy organization, not a government agency. A commercial company doing something similar makes its conclusions available by subscribing to its Website (*www.consumerlab.com*).

Until national standards are in place, recognize the dangers and use caution. If you decide to use a particular product, first try to find a brand that has been certified by an independent testing laboratory or another country's regulatory agency (such as Commission E in Germany). If neither is available, then try to find a brand that seems to work well for you and stay with that brand.

How We Rated the Evidence

Evidence for Using Therapies

If the evidence shows a therapy has benefit, we rated the *evidence* (not the benefit) using the following criteria based on how much evidence, and the type of evidence, supports the therapy:

✔✔✔✔ Multiple randomized, controlled trials demonstrate the efficacy and safety of this therapy.

✔✔✔ At least one randomized, controlled trial or nonrandomized trial supports the use of this therapy.

✔✔ Nonrandomized series or numerous case reports in the peer-reviewed medical literature support the use of this therapy.

✔ Anecdotal evidence in humans exists to support the use of this therapy.

EVIDENCE AGAINST USING THERAPIES

If the evidence shows no benefit, the potential for harm, or actual harm, we rated the *evidence* (not the potential for harm) using the following criteria:

✗✗✗✗ Multiple randomized, controlled trials demonstrate the lack of benefit or potential for harm with this therapy.

✗✗✗ At least one randomized, controlled trial or nonrandomized trial supports the lack of benefit or potential for harm with this therapy.

✗✗ Nonrandomized series or numerous case reports in the peer-reviewed medical literature show the lack of benefit or potential for harm with this therapy.

✗ Anecdotal evidence in humans exists to show the lack of benefit or potential for harm with this therapy.

THE KEY: READER GUIDE

Since the evidence for any particular therapy can include evidence that not only supports its benefits but also shows its potential for harm, we have compiled a single guide that we hope will be useful. This rating is our "best estimate" of the benefit or harm of any particular therapy for any particular indication. Others could (and often do) look at the same evidence and derive different conclusions:

☺☺☺☺ 75%–100% confidence that the therapy is potentially beneficial

☺☺☺ 50%–74% confidence that the therapy is potentially beneficial

☺☺ 25%–49% confidence that the therapy is potentially beneficial

☺ 0%–24% confidence that the therapy is potentially beneficial

☹ 0%–24% confidence that the therapy is of no benefit or potentially harmful

☹☹ 25%–49% confidence that the therapy is of no benefit or potentially harmful

☹☹☹ 50%–74% confidence that the therapy is of no benefit or potentially harmful

☹☹☹☹ 75%–100% confidence that the therapy is of no benefit or potentially harmful

Categories of Therapies

Each therapy or herbal remedy also is categorized to define how it can be viewed according to our present knowledge. Some fit in several categories. The categories are:

CATEGORY	CATEGORY NAME
1	Conventional Therapies
2	Complementary Therapies
3	Scientifically Unproven Therapies
4	Scientifically Questionable Therapies
5	Energy Medicine
6	Quackery or Fraud

1. CONVENTIONAL THERAPIES

Conventional therapies are those we associate most closely with medical physicians, hospitals, and the modern Western health care system. Conventional medicine focuses on the use of pharmaceuticals, surgery, technology, and physical devices to prevent, diagnose, and cure disease. These are the therapies either practiced routinely by Western-trained physicians or taught in nearly all medical schools.

2. COMPLEMENTARY THERAPIES

Complementary therapies are the therapies either not practiced routinely by Western-trained physicians or not taught (or incompletely taught) in most medical schools. However, these therapies are increasingly being integrated into conventional therapy. They are not primarily designed to cure illness, but focus instead on promoting health and preventing illness. Some of the more popular complementary therapies include nutrition, exercise, stress reduction, marriage and parenting classes, support groups, massage, prayer, and spirituality. Common sense and mounting evidence from studies show that many of these therapies are important for healthy lifestyles and the prevention of illness. For this reason, some view many of these therapies as part of conventional health care, not alternative medicine.

Because complementary therapies include spirituality in general, and even a number of spiritual practices, there is concern that complementary therapies are really "New Age therapies." At times these therapies can be infused with New Age ideas, but this is not always the case. Many of the ideas behind these complementary therapies are not New Age concepts. Complementary therapies provide the opportunity to be fully healthy in ways that surgery and medication alone may not achieve.

Christians should affirm the need to provide biblically appropriate complementary therapies: those that have either been scientifically validated as being effective or are taught in the Bible. In fact, Christians should be leading the way in providing them. Meeting people's spiritual, relational, and community needs is central to the mission of the church.

3. Scientifically Unproven Therapies

Scientifically unproven therapies are usually, but not always, based on established scientific principles. However, these therapies have not gone through even the most basic testing required for scientific demonstration of effectiveness and safety.

Despite this lack of testing, these therapies need not be rejected outright. Uncertainty about their claims should be admitted, but this does not mean they should be completely avoided until proven to be effective. We advise waiting until there is evidence that the therapy is safe. But sometimes it may be appropriate to try a therapy that shows some evidence of effectiveness if there is no evidence of it causing harm and its cost is reasonable. However, you must remember that anything that affects your body chemistry can prove dangerous. Herbal products, including those marketed as dietary supplements, are drugs. They can be harmful or even fatal. They can interact with other medicines and even foods you are taking, including prescription medications or a variety of over-the-counter products, such as aspirin.

Consider therapies that are scientifically unproven as holding hope for the future. Approach them with caution.

4. Scientifically Questionable Therapies

Scientifically questionable therapies are those that have little or no scientific evidence to back up their claims. They also are based on theories or principles that contradict widely held scientific beliefs. This category can include therapies that have been proven ineffective or even harmful.

For example, we categorize homeopathy as not only unproven but as scientifically questionable because of the theory upon which it is based. Homeopathic remedies are made by repeatedly diluting and shaking various herbal and mineral ingredients. Homeopathy claims that increasing the dilution increases the strength of the solution's effect. This contradicts the scientific finding that the more dilute a drug's concentration, the weaker its effect on the body. Homeopathic dilutions are continued, in some cases, to the point where every molecule of the original "active" ingredient has been diluted out of the solution. In other words, none of the starting material is left in the final solution, and yet homeopaths claim these have the strongest effects.

We remain very skeptical of scientifically questionable therapies. However, if good quality evidence shows that a therapy of this type is effective, we would have to examine that evidence carefully. The proposed explanation for why something works may be wrong, yet the therapy itself may have some usefulness via some unknown mechanism. However, until that evidence is available, we would not recommend using scientifically questionable therapies.

5. Energy Medicine

Energy medicine takes us into an area of alternative medicine that is highly problematic for Christians and believers of other faiths, especially monotheistic religions. Energy medicine is a general term for a collection of diverse practices based on what are called "life energy," or spiritual, principles. Many of these practices are based on a nonphysical life energy, or force, also called *prana, chi, ki, ka,* or *orgone.* According to these perspectives, the basic substance of the human body is not matter, but energy and information. This life energy is nonphysical and universal, animating and sustaining all living things. The energy of each person is a localization of infinite fields of energy that pervade the universe. This energy enters the human body through what are called *chakras*. True health, these practitioners say, results from a balanced flow of this energy through the body and unblocked exchange of this energy with one's environment. Imbalances or blockages in the flow lead to physical symptoms that we recognize as illness, aging, and death.

Belief in this life force is not just on the fringes of alternative medicine. It underlies the vast array of energy medicine, which includes Therapeutic Touch, Reiki, reflexology, Deepak Chopra's Ayurvedic medicine, Larry Dossey's healing words, and many other therapies.

Some practitioners claim that acupuncture, chiropractic, herbal medicine, and homeopathy also work by influencing this energy. Some proponents even claim, "No matter what therapies a traditional healer depends upon, he or she essentially is treating the life force itself."[1]

Since this energy is said to be nonphysical, most teach that no instruments can detect or measure it. Instead, we are told, humans must train themselves to become more sensitive to it. Meditation, or centering, is needed to enter a state of consciousness where you can detect this energy. In this state, trained practitioners claim they not only sense the energy field, or aura, around a person but also see it in a variety of colors and shapes. They claim that illness can be detected, and health restored, once imbalances or blockages in the field are detected because the fundamental essence of who we are is in our energy fields, not our bodies.

These beliefs are integral to what are called "vitalistic" belief systems, which traditionally included Eastern mystical religions, New Age belief systems, and occult religions. Yet these beliefs are growing in acceptance even among health care professionals and Christians. Clearly these therapies require theological evaluation even more than scientific analysis because they are based on principles that go beyond the natural world and into the spiritual world. While some proponents claim this energy is nonspiritual—just another natural energy that we do not yet understand—the burden is on them to show that it is not spiritual. As Christians, we are called to test all spirits, and thereby all spiritual teaching and claims. The standard is clearly described in 1 John 4:1–3:

> *Dear friends, do not believe every spirit, but test the spirits to see whether they are from God, because many false prophets have gone out into the world. This is how you can recognize the Spirit of God: Every spirit that acknowledges that Jesus Christ has come in the flesh is from God, but every spirit that does not acknowledge Jesus is not from God. This is the spirit of the antichrist, which you have heard is coming and even now is already in the world.*

6. QUACKERY OR FRAUD

False claims, unproven products, and products known to be ineffective rob the public of money, trust, and, frequently, their health. The sad truth is that some individuals will intentionally deceive others about a treatment's efficacy just to make money. That's fraud.

Almost as bad are the therapies touted by people who truly believe they are of value even though they are not. That's quackery.

See chapter 8, "The Gurus: Fraud, Quackery, or Wisdom?" for examples of both and the warning signs you should be aware of in order to protect yourself from falling for these.

Picking a Therapist

In addition to knowing about a therapy, discernment must be exercised when choosing the practitioner who will provide the therapy. The same therapy can be practiced in different ways. For example, a Christian chiropractor could treat you holistically, in a biblical sense, based on the best scientific evidence available for your condition, including referring you to a conventional physician when needed. Another chiropractor, who claims to be able to treat all of your ailments, may manipulate your aura, introduce you to Eastern meditation, and sell you dietary supplements. Both are practicing what they call "holistic health care," but their approach is different, and what their patients receive is very different.

Another complication arises when practitioners mix different therapies. You may think you are receiving only a massage when in fact the practitioner is mixing massage with Therapeutic Touch and color therapy.

Because of these differences in the way therapies are administered, it's important to investigate each practitioner and what they believe. Take your time. Ask questions of the practitioner and staff. Seek the advice of others.

Consider carefully not only the therapy but also the character and world view of those offering the treatment. Medical literature now gives health care providers guidance on discussing issues of spirituality with patients. One such tool uses the mnemonic SPIRIT to remind physicians of the types of questions they might ask patients.[2] Patients could use the same types of questions to gather information on a therapist's spiritual views.

S for spiritual belief system. Ask therapists to describe their belief system.

P for personal spirituality. Ask what they believe personally, and how important spirituality is for them.

I for integration into a spiritual community. Ask if they are involved in a spiritual group, formally or informally.

R for rituals and restrictions. Ask if they include any spiritual rituals in their therapies, or if their beliefs restrict them from offering certain therapies.

I for implications for medical care. Most importantly, ask how their spiritual beliefs impact the care and therapies they offer.

T for terminal care (probably the least relevant here). Ask about how their beliefs impact the care they offer when patients reach the end of their lives.

Taking such a "spiritual history" on a therapist will alert you to potential spiritual conflicts—before they become an issue. It can help you avoid those therapists who want to draw you away from faith in Jesus Christ and convert you to their religious beliefs. Remember, attractive remedies may sometimes be nothing more than lures to draw us into deception. Reflect on the following Scriptures:

> *The Spirit clearly says that in later times some will abandon the faith and follow deceiving spirits and things taught by demons.*
>
> 1 Timothy 4:1

> *For the time will come when men will not put up with sound doctrine. Instead, to suit their own desires, they will gather around them a great number of teachers to say what their itching ears want to hear. They will turn their ears away from the truth and turn aside to myths.*
>
> 2 Timothy 4:3–4

Notes

1. Deborah Cowens, *A Gift for Healing: How to Use Therapeutic Touch* (New York: Crown Trade Paperbacks, 1996), 20.

2. Todd A. Maugans, "The SPIRITual History," *Archives of Family Medicine* 5 (January 1996): 11–16.

12

Popular Alternative Therapies

How We Rated the Evidence

For a complete explanation, see chapter 11.

EVIDENCE FOR USING THERAPIES

If the evidence shows a therapy has benefit, we rated the *evidence* (not the benefit) using the following criteria based on how much evidence, and the type of evidence, supports the therapy:

✔✔✔✔   Multiple randomized, controlled trials demonstrate the efficacy and safety of this therapy.

✔✔✔   At least one randomized, controlled trial or nonrandomized trial supports the use of this therapy.

✔✔   Nonrandomized series or numerous case reports in the peer-reviewed medical literature support the use of this therapy.

✔   Anecdotal evidence in humans exists to support the use of this therapy.

EVIDENCE AGAINST USING THERAPIES

If the evidence shows no benefit, the potential for harm, or actual harm, we rated the *evidence* (not the potential for harm) using the following criteria:

✘✘✘✘   Multiple randomized, controlled trials demonstrate the lack of benefit or potential for harm with this therapy.

✘✘✘   At least one randomized, controlled trial or nonrandomized trial supports the lack of benefit or potential for harm with this therapy.

✘✘   Nonrandomized series or numerous case reports in the peer-reviewed medical literature show the lack of benefit or potential for harm with this therapy.

✘   Anecdotal evidence in humans exists to show the lack of benefit or potential for harm with this therapy.

THE KEY: READER GUIDE

Since the evidence for any particular therapy can include evidence that not only supports its benefits but also shows its potential for harm, we have compiled a single guide that we hope will be useful. This rating is our "best estimate" of the benefit or harm of any particular therapy for any particular indication. Others could (and often do) look at the same evidence and derive different conclusions:

☺☺☺☺ 75%–100% confidence that the therapy is potentially beneficial

☺☺☺ 50%–74% confidence that the therapy is potentially beneficial

☺☺ 25%–49% confidence that the therapy is potentially beneficial

☺ 0%–24% confidence that the therapy is potentially beneficial

☹ 0%–24% confidence that the therapy is of no benefit or potentially harmful

☹☹ 25%–49% confidence that the therapy is of no benefit or potentially harmful

☹☹☹ 50%–74% confidence that the therapy is of no benefit or potentially harmful

☹☹☹☹ 75%–100% confidence that the therapy is of no benefit or potentially harmful

ACUPRESSURE

What It Is

Traditional Chinese medicine appears to have much in common with the contemporary concept of holism. More than 2000 years ago, traditional Chinese physicians began stressing moderation in all things and the importance of being in harmony, both with one's body and with nature. They stressed wellness, in part because they received money only if patients stayed healthy.

The broad theory of traditional Chinese medicine is a belief that all life has *yin* and *yang*, two parts that must be in balance. The organs of the body are further divided into two parts—the *zang* and the *fu*. *Yin* organs are for storage. *Yang* organs are for elimination. A few parts of the body, such as the brain and blood vessels, have both *yin* and *yang* functions.

Traditional Chinese medicine teaches that within our bodies is life energy known as *qi* (pronounced CHEE and often spelled "*chi*"). *Chi* provides protection from illness. *Chi* is a mix of inherited energy, passed from parents to children at the time of conception, and energy derived from the food and air that sustain us throughout life.

Chi is transported by a system of meridians throughout the body that link the skin to the *zang* and *fu* organs. Within this belief system, the concepts of both acupressure and acupuncture evolved. As long as *chi* is flowing through the meridians, you are said to be in good health. Disease occurs when the flow is interrupted.

In diagnosing an ailment, a traditional Chinese doctor listens to the patient's breathing, coughing, and voice. The doctor smells the patient's body to see if there are any pungent or foul odors, both of which they believe can indicate disease. The doctor may study the patient's tongue, believing that different sections of the tongue reveal what is happening with different organs of the body. The doctor also studies the patient's spirit, complexion, and overall appearance. With touch, the doctor checks the pulse in three different places along each wrist. Practitioners believe they can detect almost thirty different qualities in the pulse, each of which can indicate an imbalance to be corrected.

Acupressure practitioners work with "acupoints" on the body. A practitioner diagnoses where and how the flow of *chi* has been stopped, then puts pressure on the appropriate acupoints to remove blockage of the energy channel. This returns the body to balance and restores health.

Claims

Acupressure is most commonly believed to reduce nausea and vomiting with pressure on an acupoint on the wrist (called "P6," or "Inner Gate"). Some companies market a do-it-yourself acupressure device with small metal or wooden balls positioned on a strap in such a way that when the device is strapped around the wrist, a ball will press on P6. These are sold in stores catering to boaters, air travelers, and others who suffer from motion sickness.

Another acupoint between the thumb and index finger (called "Meeting of the Valleys") is believed to help digestion. Acupressure is also believed to relieve pain, particularly headaches, back pain, and migraines.

Some claim acupressure can treat and cure just about every illness and disease. A form of acupressure called "One Touch Healing" claims to offer "joyous health and freedom from illness for the rest of your life." Once you buy their book, "you can say goodbye to dangerous drugs, expensive treatments and tasteless special diets." Many testimonials are given of people being cured of heart failure, asthma, arthritis, hearing loss, and many other diseases. According to their promotional material, "Not only does new One Touch Healing let you cure the worst illnesses safely and permanently, it can even work to reverse the aging process." Such extravagant claims can mislead and deceive people.

Study Findings

Research on acupressure has focused primarily on the relief of headaches, nausea, and vomiting. Several studies involved wristbands to apply pressure on the P6 acupoint to relieve morning sickness. Most of the studies (✔✔✔) found that acupressure was effective in relieving morning sickness, but some found no benefits. Studies (✔✔✔) on headaches also had mixed results.

Objective studies have not demonstrated the existence of the acupoint and meridian system. Though there are charts mapping this invisible system, they are only guides. Traditional Chinese medicine teaches that acupressure points vary from person to person. Western scientists question the validity of the entire concept.

Conventional medicine recognizes that acupressure works for some people some of the time, especially for headaches and the nausea and vomiting of pregnancy. The question is whether this is because it acts the way traditional Chinese medicine teaches, or by some poorly understood but scientifically verifiable mechanism, or simply via the placebo effect.

Cautions

Although most treatments are gentle, and acupressure is without serious side effects, some types of acupressure are applied with enough pressure to cause minor aches and pains that continue hours after the procedure has been completed.

Of greater concern is the belief system accompanying the therapy. Belief in the concept of life energy and its manipulation is fundamental to Eastern religions. Certain acupressure teachers expose practitioners to these ideas and may want to convert patients to their beliefs. Some practitioners call upon spiritual powers to assist in diagnosis and treatment, exposing patients to occult concepts and powers. For that reason, Christians must use careful discernment when choosing a practitioner.

Recommendations

Therapists give acupressure treatments in sessions that may take as long as an hour and may continue over several weeks, affording ample opportunity to expose clients to the religious ideas underlying *chi* therapies. Considering the modest results found in research on acupressure done by therapists, there seems little value to exposing yourself to this therapy. If you do try it, great care should be taken to ensure no occult spiritual powers are called upon during treatment. Another option would be to choose a conventional therapist—a physical therapist or physician—who could teach you to perform acupressure on yourself. Patients who do acupressure on themselves may be able to get some relief from certain forms of headaches or from the nausea and vomiting in pregnancy. The over-the-counter acupressure wristband can be used without any exposure to Eastern religious beliefs. Although results are mixed, if it works for you, great.

Treatment Categories

Complementary Therapy

Morning sickness	☺☺☺☺
Nausea and vomiting	☺☺☺
Headaches	☺☺☺

Scientifically Unproven
    All other uses

Scientifically Questionable
    All other uses

Energy Medicine
    As used by some practitioners

Further Reading

Cassileth, Barrie R., *The Alternative Medicine Handbook* (New York: W. W. Norton, 1998), 209–12.

Woodham, Anne, and David Peters, *Encyclopedia of Healing Therapies* (London and New York: Dorling Kindersley, 1997), 95.

ACUPUNCTURE

What It Is

Acupuncture is a therapy that evolved from the same concepts in acupressure as part of traditional Chinese medicine. Traditionally, acupuncture is usually used in combination with other therapies. Fine needles are inserted into the skin just far enough so they don't fall out—a procedure that usually is painless. Both acupuncture and acupressure are based on the idea of the body having an invisible life energy force known as *chi* (pronounced CHEE) that is said to travel through invisible pathways known as meridians. The proper flow of *chi* helps all parts of the body adjust to various stresses, keeping the organs in balance (see Acupressure for a discussion of *yin* and *yang, zang* and *fu*).

Alteration or blockage of the normal flow of *chi* causes imbalances in the body that can cause disease. Traditional Chinese medicine practitioners believe acupuncture restores the proper flow of *chi*.

The earliest surviving Chinese medical texts show 365 acupuncture points; contemporary charts show as many as 2000. Each point is on a meridian that affects particular organs.

Originally a single needle was inserted at each point believed to be appropriate for restoring proper flow of *chi* based on the patient's symptoms. Today, many needles will be inserted.

Small variations are sometimes added to the acupuncture procedure. The needles can be twirled after insertion into the skin to increase the stimulation. Electro-acupuncture sends tiny electric charges through the needles for added stimulation. Laser acupuncture uses lasers instead of needles. In a more traditional variation called "moxibustion," the ends of the needles protruding from the skin are heated with burning cones of the herb mugwort. The needles are not allowed to get hot enough to burn the patient. Mugwort leaves are known to have an antibiotic effect. However, in moxibustion, mugwort is believed to help restore the flow of *chi,* whether the cone is burned to heat acupuncture needles or the leaves are used alone.

Modern interest in acupuncture was sparked during President Richard Nixon's visit to China in 1972. A reporter on the trip underwent emergency surgery for acute appendicitis and later received acupuncture for pain. News accounts of the procedure led to widespread interest in acupuncture.

But the news stories led to a misconception: that for centuries acupuncture was the standard anesthetic for surgery in China. While Western medicine has long considered surgery a tool of healing, traditional Chinese medicine, until very recently, rarely used surgery. Acupuncture is used as an anesthetic in the operating room, but its use is almost always in conjunction with traditional forms of anesthesia. The combination is believed to *reduce* the amount of conventional anesthetic needed, not eliminate the need.

Western medical scientists, not convinced of the existence of *chi* or meridians, have developed alternative theories about how acupuncture might work. One theory is that the needles release naturally occurring hormones called "endorphins" that regulate pain perception. Endorphin release reduces pain during childbirth. Athletes commonly experience the effect of endorphins when they run long distances. If acupuncture needles stimulate the release of these hormones, pain will be reduced.

Another theory is based on the observation that pain in one area of the body can be reduced when another area is irritated. Still other scientists say that acupuncture creates nothing more than a placebo effect.

Claims

Acupuncture is most commonly believed to reduce pain, both acute pain such as with surgery, and chronic pain. Anecdotal accounts report the use of acupuncture to control asthma, reduce nausea and vomiting, reduce weight, treat chronic sinus and allergy symptoms, and help people give up addictive behaviors, such as cigarette smoking.

Study Findings

In November 1997, a panel at the National Institutes of Health (NIH) released a review of research on acupuncture. Of the more than 2000 studies, few were determined to be high-quality clinical studies. Although the popular press generally reported the panel's findings as positive, the report actually concluded there was little evidence to support most of the claims. Good-quality evidence (✔✔✔) on the effectiveness of acupuncture was found for the reduction of nausea and vomiting after chemotherapy or surgery, and for relief of dental pain. Numerous studies (✘✘✘) have shown that acupuncture alone is not effective in controlling asthma or for weight reduction. Studies (✘✘✘) also showed it was not effective in stopping smoking.

Another report released by the British Medical Association in June 2000 came to almost identical conclusions, but reported new evidence concerning the effectiveness of acupuncture with chronic pain. A number of controlled studies have been conducted for treating low back pain, but the results have been variable. A meta-analysis of the four highest quality back pain studies indicated there was no difference between real and sham acupuncture. When lower-quality studies were included, a 1998 review concluded it was somewhat effective, but a 1999 (✘✘✘) review concluded it could not be recommended as a regular treatment. Studies with recurrent headaches and migraines (✔✔✔) have similarly shown some improvements, but with inconsistent results. Given the great variability in the origins of and responses to pain, some people's pain may respond well to acupuncture while others' pain does not.

Cautions

Acupuncture should not be used in the hope of curing an illness. It should not be used instead of proven effective therapies. At the most, it may relieve some symptoms and perceptions of illness. However, be aware that, although infrequent, infections have developed from the use of unsterile acupuncture needles. In a couple of cases (✘✘), death resulted from needles puncturing a patient's lung.

Recommendations

Despite its limited effectiveness, acupuncture's low cost and relative safety can make it a viable option for some conditions, such as pain relief in the situations specified by the NIH panel.

Use great caution when choosing a therapist, whether conventional or alternative. Verify that the therapist has had adequate training. Acupuncturists who are physicians may have had little training in acupuncture. Those who adhere to acupuncture's roots in traditional Chinese medicine and religion may try to convert patients to their Eastern world view, although this is not the case with every practitioner. Others may call upon spiritual powers to assist in treatments, thus exposing people to occult influences.

Treatment Categories

Complementary Therapy

Nausea and vomiting after chemotherapy or surgery	☺☺☺☺
Dental pain	☺☺☺☺
Headaches	☺☺
Back pain	☹☹

Scientifically Unproven

Asthma	☹☹☹
Weight reduction	☹☹☹☹
Smoking cessation	☹☹☹

Scientifically Questionable
All other uses

Energy Medicine
As used by some practitioners

Further Reading

British Medical Association, *Acupuncture: Efficacy, Safety and Practice* (Amsterdam: Harwood Academic, 2000).

National Institutes of Health, Consensus Development on Acupuncture, "Acupuncture," *Journal of the American Medical Association* 280, no. 17 (November 1998): 1518–24.

APPLIED KINESIOLOGY

What It Is

In 1964 chiropractor George Goodheart noted that weakness in certain muscles could be corrected by massaging seemingly unrelated muscles. His work was initially based on work done about twenty years earlier at Johns Hopkins University. That research concerned the evaluation of disability through a series of noninvasive muscle tests. Goodheart's work went much further, developing the idea that muscle dysfunction could be used to identify specific problems with glands and organs.

Within the theory of applied kinesiology, overall health is seen as involving a complex interaction among structural, chemical, and mental components, all requiring many different therapies. For example, the structural health of the body requires such therapies as conventional dentistry as well as chiropractic and acupuncture. Chemical health is treated through herbal remedies, homeopathy, and conventional medicine. And mental health is achieved through relaxation, energy medicine, and Bach flower remedies. According to applied kinesiology, the various muscle groups are connected to the body's vital organs and systems through interconnected "energy circuits" similar in concept to the meridians found in traditional Chinese medicine (see Acupressure, page 144).

The treatments recommended may involve any of those listed above, or other alternative therapies. One specific therapy involves gently massaging "pressure points" on the patient's scalp or body. These are usually located far from the affected muscles. The massage is believed to improve blood, lymph, and life energy flow to the related muscles.

To diagnose a problem, the strength of relatively large muscles is tested. For example, patients are asked to hold their arms out straight. Practitioners place their fingers on patients' arms and apply firm but gentle pressure. If a patient resists this pressure and the resistance feels normal to the practitioner, the systems related to the arm muscle are considered normal. If the muscle feels weak or sags under pressure, that's the sign of a problem. Further tests are carried out on other muscles to pinpoint the problem. Muscle weakness is said to be caused by life energy imbalances, physical problems, dietary deficiencies, and allergies.

Claims

Practitioners claim to be able to diagnose and treat most ailments, in particular chronic problems such as asthma related to allergies and environmental toxicity. To test for allergies, first muscle strength is tested in the usual way. Then a solution of a food, chemical, bacteria, etc., is placed on the patient's stomach, lips, or tongue, and the same muscle is retested. If the muscle seems as strong when retested, the patient is not allergic to the substance. If the muscle is weaker, the patient has an allergy to the substance. This type of muscle testing is also used to detect deficiencies in nutrients, vitamins, or minerals.

Study Findings

In our opinion, there is no compelling scientific evidence that applied kinesiology works for diagnosing or treating health problems. It's not that there have been no successes. Rather, this is not a true science. All practitioners do not apply the ideas in the same way. Different practitioners even reach different conclusions on the same patient. Outcomes vary depending on the amount of pressure applied, the angle at which pressure is exerted, and whether the patient or the practitioner pushes first. Practitioners have tried to develop instruments to standardize the muscle-testing method, but at this writing there has been no success. Even if such instruments were developed, additional time would be needed for testing to develop consistent replicated standards of diagnosis and treatment.

Cautions

While applied kinesiology may cause little harm, it could lead someone to postpone pursuing more conventional and effective diagnosis and treatment.

Particular caution should be exercised concerning the beliefs accompanying this practice. Practitioners who are strong advocates of life energy ideas may try to draw people into the New Age world view. This is particularly the case with Touch for Health, an offshoot of applied kinesiology developed by John Thie, a chiropractor and colleague of Dr. Goodheart. This popularized version, which has been significantly influenced by New Age beliefs, focuses on the need to balance "energy" in the body.

Recommendations

There is little or no reliable evidence that applied kinesiology does anything more than provide reassurance to those who have not been able to find relief through conventional medicine. As such, when it offers comfort, it probably works through a complicated placebo effect. The specific treatments involved are often not necessary and could waste valuable time and money. Given this, and the close connections between some of its many variants and New Age ideology, there seems to be no valid reason for Christians to use this practice.

Treatment Categories

Scientifically Questionable
    For any indication   ☹☹☹

Energy Medicine

Quackery or Fraud
    In the hands of some practitioners

Further Reading

Woodham, Anne, and David Peters, *Encyclopedia of Healing Therapies* (London and New York: Dorling Kindersley, 1997), 196–97.

A R O M A T H E R A P Y

What It Is

It might be said that the concept behind aromatherapy dates back thousands of years. Everyone knows the experience of encountering the aroma of a favorite food as it is being cooked for dinner, only to suddenly become hungry. We instantly remember the last time we ate that particular meal and the pleasure we experienced. We are anxious to repeat those feelings and look forward to when the food will be ready.

A woman wears a special perfume only when she plans an intimate rendezvous with her husband. The moment he becomes aware of the scent, he is aroused, anticipating the physical pleasure of his beloved.

Soldiers talk about the smell of death lingering in their nostrils. If they come upon a dead animal by the side of the road, the odor may instantly flash them back to emotions they had in a war zone many years earlier. They may become frightened, sad, or angry, all responses inappropriate for the moment, but quite normal when they were in the midst of combat.

Then there are the aromas of special places—the mix of hay, manure, and sweat we knew from a time spent happily caring for a horse on a grandparent's farm; the rose garden in which we played as children; the salty air of the seashore we visited on our honeymoon. Perfume companies experiment with scents to find ways to sell fragrances that will revive personal aromatic pleasures of long ago.

The universal way an aroma can affect people seems to be acknowledged in the Bible. Exodus 29:18 describes the aroma of sacrificial offerings: "Then burn the entire ram on the altar. It is a burnt offering to the LORD, a pleasing aroma, an offering made to the LORD by fire."

Aromatherapy is the systematic use of essential oils to attempt to improve people's well-being. Plants contain many constituents, including compounds that are not water soluble. These can be extracted from the plants using other oils (like castor oil or olive oil), by pressing on the plants, or by using heat distillation of the oil. Many of the essential oils produced in this manner have pleasant aromas. They are then diluted with other oils, like sunflower oil or sweet almond oil, and the resulting mix is usually massaged into the skin by an aromatherapist.

A variation of this practice involves the heating of the oils at home in order to fill a room with a scent. Oils may also be added to baths.

Claims

Aromatherapy adds a relaxing element to a lingering bath or a massage. Rooms with aromatic scents appropriate to the person using them are believed to create a calmer atmosphere and relieve stress. For these reasons, aromatherapy is used by some as an adjunct to analgesics for people with a variety of painful conditions.

Various specific claims are made for particular aromatherapy oils, much like the claims for herbal remedies. Each essential oil contains compounds particular to the plant from which it was obtained. For example, eucalyptus oil is said to treat infections. Rose oil is used to regulate menstruation. And lavender oil is said to promote the healing of burns and wounds as well as having a calming effect.

Study Findings

While the use of essential oils dates back centuries, little research has been done on their therapeutic uses. Certainly, smells can elicit memories and emotions that can influence people's thoughts and feelings (✔✔). Most people can relate to feeling at ease (or uncomfortable) walking into a room with an aroma associated with either a comfortable (or disturbing) memory. Aromatherapy accompanied by a massage and involving an interaction with a caring provider will relieve stress (✔✔✔). Someone who is seriously ill is likely to feel better for the experience, but such feelings are not cures for illness. A small number of preliminary studies (✔✔✔) have found that people experience some relief from pain during aromatherapy. Oils used in these studies come from herbs with pain-relieving or anti-inflammatory reputations, such as chamomile, marigold, or willow.

Claims that certain essential oils can cure or prevent illnesses or diseases have little evidence to support them. Most of these claims have not been tested, and research into therapeutic aromatherapy (or aromatology) is only beginning. Early results (✔✔) have shown that certain aromas influence brain activity of areas affecting sexual arousal or appetite. Whether this will lead to products which, for example, help people attempting to diet remains to be seen.

Cautions

When used as recommended, aromatherapy oils are generally safe and soothing for most people. However, these are plant products to which some people can have allergic reactions.

Other potential hazards may arise because these oils are very concentrated. They should never be taken internally. Some ingredients are absorbed through the skin during proper use, so large amounts could lead to potentially troublesome side effects. A number of oils (particularly from pennyroyal, parsley seed, and juniper) have reputations for causing abortions and thus should not be used during pregnancy. Children should be massaged with only small quantities of oils that have already been well diluted.

Recommendations

Aromatherapy provides a pleasant (though not always inexpensive) means of relaxing. No evidence supports claims the oils prevent or cure any illnesses. As with all forms of natural products, care should be taken to use reputable brands. Higher price tags do not necessarily mean higher quality. Some products have been adulterated with cheaper, synthetic oils. Essential oils are highly concentrated extracts of plants that can cause problems if taken internally. The oils should be kept out of the reach of young children.

Treatment Categories

Complementary Therapy
Relaxation, stress, or anxiety ☺☺☺☺
Pain ☺☺

Scientifically Unproven
Most specific healing uses

Scientifically Questionable
To cure or treat diseases

Quackery or Fraud
In the hands of some practitioners

Further Reading

Buckle, Jane, "Use of Aromatherapy as a Complementary Treatment for Chronic Pain," *Alternative Therapies in Health & Medicine* 5, no. 5 (September 1999): 42–51.

Cassileth, Barrie R., *The Alternative Medicine Handbook* (New York: W. W. Norton, 1998), 258–62.

Woodham, Anne, and David Peters, *Encyclopedia of Healing Therapies* (London and New York: Dorling Kindersley, 1997), 62–65.

AYURVEDIC MEDICINE

What It Is

Ayurveda is the traditional medicine of India. The word means "knowledge of life," and thus refers to a whole approach to living, incorporating medical, philosophical, and religious beliefs. It is thus very difficult to separate those parts of Ayurveda that deal with one's health from the religious components.

The central belief of Ayurveda seems compatible with contemporary Western medical thought: that health involves balance among physical, mental, spiritual, and environmental elements. If we don't look too closely at what this means for the practitioner, it would seem to be comfortably compatible with Christian beliefs. The best-known proponent of Ayurvedic medicine in the United States, Deepak Chopra M.D., has furthered this idea. This best-selling author and physician was for many years a part of the Transcendental Meditation (TM) organization, until they parted ways in 1993.

In its traditional form, Ayurvedic medicine teaches that life is sustained by the nonphysical life energy called *"prana."* Health exists when the body has a balanced flow of *prana,* a concept very similar to the *chi* of traditional Chinese medicine. When the flow of *prana* is blocked or out of balance, people get ill, age, and die.

Energy balance, Ayurvedic practitioners believe, is not just internal. Such balance is also needed among people and their environments, a concept they say is based on a belief in the unity and interconnectedness of the universe.

According to Ayurveda, at conception each person is given a unique combination of what are called the three *doshas—vata, pitta,* and *kapha.* Since no two people have the same *dosha* combination, a practitioner must do an individualized typing and diagnosis to ensure the proper *dosha* balance for the patient. The diagnosis is made by examining the tongue, breathing patterns, and the pulse in ways that are believed to reveal information about *prana.* Prescriptions for restoring energy balance are also individualized.

Given that Ayurvedic medicine is actually a world view, the practices recommended to balance *prana* and the *doshas* encompass every dimension of life. Meditation (of the Transcendental Meditation variety in the West) is viewed as essential for reducing stress and inducing altered states of consciousness. These changes are said to allow people to attain insight into their health and spirituality.

Ayurvedic practitioners use numerous products and practices to improve people's health. These include *rasayanas* (herbal supplements), gemstones, *panchakarmas* (purification procedures), and *yagyas* (religious ceremonies to solicit the aid of Hindu deities).

Removal of toxins from the body is also important in Ayurvedic medicine. Negative thoughts, foods, and habits lead to the accumulation of *ama*, a negative form of energy. Purification practices include bloodletting with leaches, vomiting, laxatives, sinus cleansing, and enemas. Chopra's version of Ayurveda includes the Pizzichilli treatment, where two "technicians" massage and bathe a naked patient who reclines in a warm sesame oil bath for two hours. Formerly reserved for "the pleasure of the kings," this is viewed as more appealing to Western customers than purging and bloodletting.

Claims

Ayurvedic medicine is a holistic approach to health and life. In its traditional setting, practitioners advise people on their diet, exercise, health, work, choice of spouse, sex life, personal habits, and religious beliefs. It emphasizes prevention of disease, but also claims to be able to cure any and every disease. Interestingly, while increasing numbers of Westerners turn to Ayurvedic medicine, many Ayurvedic practitioners in India are increasingly adding conventional therapies to their practices.

Study Findings

Some Ayurvedic herbal remedies have been subjected to research and appear to have some efficacy. However, many thousands of preparations are recommended which have never been scientifically investigated. At the 1987 annual meeting of the Society for Economic Botany, a number of presentations were made on Ayurvedic remedies that are still cited as evidence that these products have scientific support. One of the organizers of the meeting said this was little more than a publicity stunt. "While the submitted abstracts seemed reasonable, what they presented had little to do with their abstracts. In one presentation, they couldn't even provide the scientific names of the medicinal plants they claimed to have tested. The other presentation was a pitch for the Maharishi's meditation techniques—hardly appropriate for a botany meeting."

No rigorous, scientific evidence supports the claim that Ayurvedic remedies can cure serious diseases, a point apparently acknowledged in India, where 75 percent of the preparations recommended by Ayurvedic practitioners were modern pharmaceutical drugs. The lifestyle changes recommended as part of Ayurveda's holistic approach to health may be beneficial if they are based on sound dietary, stress-reduction, and relational principles.

Cautions

Certain parts of Ayurvedic medicine may be beneficial for disease prevention and promotion of a healthy lifestyle. However, much of it remains unproven, and aspects of Ayurveda such as the purification methods may have serious side effects for some patients. In pursuing Ayurvedic medicine exclusively, people with serious illnesses may neglect more effective conventional treatment.

Another problem concerns the quality and authenticity of products sold as Ayurvedic remedies. Authorities in India question whether commercial Ayurvedic preparations even conform to ancient Ayurvedic texts. Vaidya Balendu Prakash, chair of the advisory board on Ayurvedic medicine to the Ministry of Health in India, stated recently in the British journal *Lancet,* "The majority of Ayurvedic formulations on the market are either spurious, adulterated, or misbranded."

Of equal concern should be the intimate association between Ayurvedic medicine and Hinduism, along with its New Age variations including the Transcendental Meditation movement. The holistic approach of Ayurvedic medicine means that practitioners are interested in all aspects of a patient's life, including religious beliefs, and will often suggest changes in those beliefs. While someone can obtain surgery or a drug from a physician without any questions about their belief system, this is not possible with an Ayurvedic practitioner.

Recommendations

While certain aspects of Ayurvedic medicine may be beneficial, Christians should be extremely cautious and view it with a critical mind. It should not be pursued to the neglect of conventional medicine, especially for serious illnesses. Those parts of the Ayurvedic system that are beneficial (like some of its dietary and relaxation advice) can be put into practice without involving oneself in Ayurvedic medicine. There appears to be no good reason why Christians should pursue Ayurvedic medicine.

Treatment Categories

Complementary Therapies
　　Certain aspects only　　　　　　　　☺☺

Scientifically Unproven
　　Most aspects of this therapy

Scientifically Questionable
　　Most indications

Energy Medicine

Further Reading

Cassileth, Barrie, "Ayurveda," (New York: W. W. Norton, 1998), 22–27.

Kumar, Sanjay, "Indian Herbal Remedies Come Under Attack," *Lancet* 351 (April 1998): 1190.

O'Mathúna, Dónal, "Postmodern Impact: Health Care," in *The Death of Truth*, ed. Dennis McCallum (Minneapolis: Bethany House, 1996), 58–84.

BIOFEEDBACK

What It Is

One of the simplest ways to understand biofeedback is to think about how you drive a car, especially a stick shift. You probably don't even notice all the different things you do. You certainly don't have to tell your foot when to move from the accelerator to the brake. You change gears without watching your speedometer to decide when it's time to shift. All of the looking, listening, and moving of your arms and legs occur pretty much automatically.

Now think back to when you were learning to drive. Did you watch the speedometer to know when to shift gears? Listen to the sound of the engine? Did you look down when you moved the gearshift lever from one position to another? Was it awkward to parallel park? Back up?

You learned to drive with the help of feedback from the various dials and sounds in your car. You learned to process the input automatically. You no longer need to consciously think about these things.

Biofeedback offers you the same sort of help as you learn to "operate" your body. Think of your body for a moment. You have been working under intense pressure, leaning over your desk with terrible posture. Your nerves are on edge, your jaw is set as you race toward the deadline imposed by your boss—the slave driver. Finally, you go home. Your back aches, your neck aches. You have a headache. You want to relax, but your mind is so focused on your work and your hostility toward your supervisor, relaxing is impossible.

Enter the biofeedback machine. One device or another, such as an electromyography (EMG) instrument, is attached to your body by a biofeedback therapist. The machine can either measure the electrical activity of your muscles, the temperature of the skin, or the dampness of the skin. An indicator of how tense you are might be a sound that rises or lowers in pitch, a dial with a needle that moves, or it could be some other auditory or visual device.

Just as you used to watch your car's speedometer, or actively listened to the engine, you now watch or listen to the biofeedback machine. Just as you learned to drive a car, you can learn to control your skin temperature, heart rate, brain wave patterns, and many other functions once thought to be beyond conscious control. You would use the biofeedback machine to help you relax your muscles.

Sometimes the instrument is as simple as a handheld thermometer that displays your skin's temperature as you focus on warming your hand, an approach that could help improve your circulation.

No matter what the device, biofeedback is to be used only as a short-term aid. People learn to consciously make the desired changes in their bodies without needing a machine to tell them how well they are doing. The machine is an aid for a few sessions, not something needed for months or years.

Claims

The most common use for biofeedback is in learning to relax and reduce or eliminate pain. For example, when you are anxious, a number of physiological changes occur that are measurable—tensed muscles, colder hands, and raised heart rate and blood pressure. Biofeedback instruments help you learn to consciously alter all these factors and let you know what progress you are making in learning to relax, to reduce stress.

Biofeedback also is reported to help relieve migraine and tension headaches, and to help control incontinence and hypertension.

Study Findings

Numerous studies (✔✔✔) have shown that biofeedback can give most people control over functions they could not previously control. It has been shown to reduce blood pressure and relieve tension and anxiety. One study (✔✔✔) supports its use to restore continence. However, its effectiveness varies with different physiological conditions, and does not appear to work at all for some people.

Controlled studies (✔✔✔) have shown that for tension headaches, biofeedback is about as effective as relaxation training alone. Results with migraine and hand-temperature biofeedback have been less encouraging, although some studies (✔✔✔) do show it can be as effective in preventing migraines as relaxation training alone or even as the use of the drug propranolol.

Back pain is a symptom that occurs with a complex variety of problems, and, as such, the success of biofeedback has not been consistent (✔✔✔✔). This is to be expected. For some people, learning to relax works best with approaches that combine several techniques, such as biofeedback, hypnosis, and progressive muscular relaxation.

In some instances, such as heart disease, the biofeedback is used to reduce one or more elements that put you at risk, such as blood pressure (✔✔✔). However, whether or not this actually impacts your chances of developing heart disease, or the severity of the problem if it develops, remains less clear.

Cautions

Biofeedback instruments have not been reported to cause any harm, nor do they have side effects. Someone already using conventional medicine to control a condition (such as high blood pressure) should consult his or her physician before trying biofeedback, or any other alternative therapy, so that the conventional therapies can be appropriately adjusted if necessary. Do not stop medications or make other significant changes before starting biofeedback.

Recommendations

Biofeedback is an approach that has been shown to work for some people, allowing them to consciously control their symptoms and thus reduce or eliminate medications or other therapies. Those with chronic pain who have had little relief from other therapies may find it worth trying, though realizing it does not work for everyone.

As a method of relaxation, biofeedback is devoid of the need to alter one's consciousness or adopt non-Christian beliefs. As such, it is an alternative that is becoming more and more conventional.

Treatment Categories

Complementary Therapy

Reduce blood pressure	☺☺☺☺
Relieve tension and anxiety	☺☺☺☺
Restore continence	☺☺
Tension or migraine headaches	☺☺☺
Back pain	☺☺

Scientifically Unproven

For most other indications or to cure any illness

Further Reading

Cassileth, Barrie R., *The Alternative Medicine Handbook* (New York: W. W. Norton, 1998), 117–21.

Jessup, Barton A., and Xochitl Gallegos, "Relaxation and Biofeedback," in *Textbook of Pain,* ed. Patrick D. Wall and Ronald Melzack, 3d ed. (Edinburgh, U.K.: Churchill Livingstone, 1994).

CHELATION THERAPY

What It Is

The concept behind chelation therapy has made it one of the most talked about forms of alternative medicine for an aging population. As far back as 1948, it was in regular use by physicians in the U.S. Navy for treatment of lead poisoning. A chemical, most commonly ethylene diamine tetra-acetic acid (EDTA), is injected into the bloodstream. The EDTA molecules act like claws (the Greek word for claw is *chele*), engulfing other molecules. The injected substance traps the lead and other minerals, such as calcium, magnesium, and iron, and removes them from the body by way of the kidneys.

The early Navy experiments used injected EDTA to remove lead from poisoned seamen. It also used the liquid as a cleaning agent to remove calcium that had built up and was clogging pipes and boilers. Calcium plaque routinely builds up when someone suffers from atherosclerosis, so Dr. Norman Clarke Sr., in Detroit's Providence Hospital, theorized that EDTA chelation could be used to treat heart conditions and began experiments in the late 1950s.

Today EDTA is used in some areas as an alternative therapy for arteriosclerosis, despite the FDA recommendation that, "because of the potentially lethal side effects, [EDTA] should not be used for the treatment of generalized arteriosclerosis." Elevated cholesterol levels lead to a buildup of thick, hard plaque in arteries that can cut off blood circulation and lead to angina, peripheral arterial disease, heart attack, or stroke. Chelation therapists claim that people with higher blood levels of calcium may have an increased risk of developing atherosclerosis because EDTA pulls calcium out of plaques and cleans out a person's arteries.

Claims

Intravenous and oral EDTA chelation therapies are primarily used today to treat coronary heart disease and peripheral arterial disease. They are said to be economical, effective alternatives to coronary bypass surgery and angioplasty, and effective therapies for cleaning blocked arteries in the legs. However, some chelation therapists also claim they are effective in treating thyroid disorders, multiple sclerosis, cancer, Alzheimer's disease, and many other disorders. Adequate explanations for how they might act in these other disorders have not been proposed.

A variation of intravenous EDTA chelation therapy is called "oral chelation." Various substances are taken by mouth to reduce serum cholesterol and to treat problems such as heavy metal (nickel, mercury, etc.) toxicity. Among the suggested substances for oral chelation have been vitamin C, zinc, garlic, and certain amino acids. The concept is based only on anecdotal reports (✔).

Study Findings

When EDTA was first used for lead poisoning in the 1950s, patients who also had angina reported (✔) relief from their symptoms. Angina is chest pain resulting from inadequate blood supply to the heart muscle, often due to clogged coronary arteries. In the following years, many reports (✔✔) were published indicating that chelation therapy helped people with coronary heart disease. However, most of these were reports on small groups of patients where no controls were used to see if it was really the EDTA causing the improvements. A 1990 controlled study (✔✔✔), though with only ten people, reported benefits from chelation, which led to a number of larger, controlled studies. All of these, including a large randomized study, have found neither short-term nor long-term benefits from the therapy (✘✘✘✘). A 1997 review of the best of these studies (✘✘✘) concluded that use of chelation therapy for atherosclerosis "should now be considered obsolete." Another concluded chelation therapy "must be regarded as ethically unsound practice."

Not only have the results in patients been unsuccessful, but also the proposed rationale for how it might work has been shown to be scientifically implausible. One month of chelation therapy could remove no more than 1 percent of all the calcium in plaque. As quickly as it would be removed, more calcium released from the bones would replace it. Plus, calcium makes up only a tiny fraction of what is in plaque. Cholesterol and fibrous tissue are much more abundant, and there is no reason to believe that these are removed by EDTA. This is a good example of an alternative therapy based on ideas that appear scientifically sound, but upon closer examination are revealed to be implausible.

Cautions

Chelation therapy has potentially serious side effects. Dangerously low levels of blood calcium can result (blood calcium is more easily accessible than the calcium in plaque). These low levels could lead to tetany (muscle spasms). Severe kidney damage and even death have resulted from using EDTA in lead poisoning. These risks are justified only because of the bigger dangers of heavy metal poisoning. The American Heart Association and various physician organizations have reported many negative effects from the therapy and are against its use for atherosclerosis. Proponents say that some of the dangers have come from the amount of EDTA used, and that reducing the amount of EDTA reduces the risks. Intravenous infusions take three to four hours, usually requiring forty or more treatments over a couple of months. Chelation therapy is very expensive, costing between $3,000 and $10,000. This type of therapy—we believe for the right reasons—is virtually never covered by medical insurance.

Recommendations

Intravenous chelation therapy should only be used in cases of heavy metal poisoning where objective tests validate the presence of toxic levels of specific metals. The risks for other uses of intravenous chelation or any use of oral chelation are not warranted in light of the lack of evidence for the therapy's effectiveness. The significant amount of evidence against its effectiveness in heart disease raises serious ethical questions concerning the motives of those continuing to provide this therapy. The therapy is very expensive; it can be very lucrative for providers.

Treatment Categories

Conventional Therapy
  Heavy metal poisoning   ☺☺☺☺

Scientifically Questionable
  For any other use, particularly coronary artery disease,
    angina, and peripheral vascular disease   ☹☹☹☹

Fraud or Quackery
  In the hands of some practitioners

Further Reading

Sampson, Wallace, "The Pharmacology of Chelation Therapy," *Scientific Review of Alternative Medicine* 1, no. 1 (Fall/Winter 1997): 23–25.

Sorrentino, Matthew, "EDTA Chelation Therapy Not Recommended for Peripheral Vascular Atherosclerotic Disease," *Physician's Guide to Alternative Medicine*, ed. Marc S. Micozzi (Atlanta, Ga.: American Health Consulting, 1999), 127–29.

CHIROPRACTIC

What It Is

Daniel David Palmer was a self-taught healer at a time—the 1890s—when science had yet to have serious impact on medicine. The country doctor rode his horse and buggy from home to home, giving patients more loving comfort than meaningful treatment. Patent medicine remained popular, most of it so filled with alcohol that heavy users could forget their discomfort as long as there was another dose in the bottle. Many people used a new cola drink for a fast pickup, not realizing that one ingredient was cocaine (which has been removed and has *not* been used for about a hundred years). Bayer, the German pharmaceutical company, was just starting to market two products that would become well known in the twentieth century: one was aspirin—the other was heroin!

Palmer was a grocery store owner who had learned magnetic healing and mysticism. He also had the good sense to distrust much of contemporary medicine, and was determined to find a way to heal others without using drugs. The idea of spinal manipulation for the treatment of illness was not a new one when Palmer was doing his reading and research. It had been used in one form or another for centuries. What Palmer did was develop a series of manipulative procedures to bring health to muscles, nerves, and organs that had gotten out of alignment. And he named these procedures for the Greek words *cheirios* and *prakticos,* which translate to "done by hand," or "manipulation." Palmer called his method "chiropractic."

The start of chiropractic goes back to deaf janitor Harvey Lillard in Davenport, Iowa. Lillard was said to have been in good health until one day, when he was doing heavy labor, he felt something go wrong with his back. He was instantly deaf and remained that way for the next seventeen years until he encountered Palmer.

Lillard, so the story goes, had a lump on his back that Palmer determined to be a displaced vertebra. He applied pressure according to his carefully conceived theory, and the vertebra slipped back into place. Immediately the janitor could hear.

The frequent retelling of this story has left many details very sketchy. It is uncertain how the janitor became a patient of Palmer (he was not a doctor). Nor is it clear why he would allow the grocery store owner to manipulate his spine. What matters is that this story became the basis for Palmer's theories, theories he claimed to prove, at least to himself, with a second patient whose heart condition was eased through similar manipulation. His techniques are now called the Palmer Method of chiropractic.

The history of chiropractic is filled with divisiveness over what problems it relieves best and precisely how manipulations bring relief. Today the Palmer concept stresses that alignment of the spine assures good health. Misalignments, called "subluxations," interfere with the body's natural ability to heal itself and thus need to be corrected by spinal manipulation.

Palmer used the term "subluxation" in a metaphysical way. In his view, subluxations interfered with the flow through the body of Innate Intelligence (or spark or life or spirit). This energy was therefore a form of life energy, as used in Eastern medical systems. His son, Bartlett Joshua Palmer, claimed that subluxations were the cause of all disease. This led to a split between those loyal to both Palmers and chiropractors who sought a scientific basis for chiropractic. In the view of those seeking scientific explanations, subluxations are displaced vertebrae that somehow disrupt the flow of nerve impulses through the spine. These somehow cause pain and physical illness. However, the nature, location, and very existence of subluxations remains disputed, even by chiropractors.

Chiropractors typically use X rays and their hands to determine where manipulation is needed. One form of manipulation is done quickly, using hand thrusts involving different amounts of force. The manipulation causes adjustments that usually are accompanied by a distinctive cracking noise. Another form of manipulation involves slower gentle movements. With both, relief may be immediate, may require a number of visits, or may come after an initial period of increased discomfort.

Claims

The claims made vary, depending on which version of chiropractic a therapist uses. Some chiropractors treat only those conditions appropriate to their training. They strive to support as many clinical decisions as possible with rigorous chiropractic studies that have revealed clear benefits. Other chiropractors claim they can cure almost any disease and seek to practice as the equivalent of primary care physicians. These chiropractors point out that their training involves significant numbers of science-based courses, which they claim gives them extensive medical knowledge. Most fall in between, particularly when their scope of practice includes diagnosis of common ailments. Many chiropractors also function in the capacity of naturopaths—practitioners who resist the use of medicinal drugs and surgery, and emphasize natural approaches to healing. Chiropractors are recognized by the D.C. after their name, which stands for Doctor of Chiropractic.

Study Findings

Hundreds of studies have been conducted with chiropractic, leading to more than fifty reviews of the research. Unfortunately, many of the studies had significant methodological flaws that make using their results difficult. In spite of this, there is substantial evidence (✔✔✔) that chiropractic manipulations bring relief of acute (less than six weeks) lower back pain.

When compared to treatment by primary care physicians or physical therapists (✔✔✔), little differences were noted in effectiveness or speed of recovery, although patients reported being more satisfied with chiropractors. The evidence (✔✔) for chiropractic use in neck and shoulder pain is much less convincing. There is no compelling medical evidence (✘✘✘) that it is effective for other conditions such as asthma and allergies. Reports (✘✘) are similar for cancer.

Cautions

Chiropractic manipulation is not without side effects. A 1996 review (✘✘) in the *Journal of Family Practice* identified 165 accidents, including twenty-nine deaths, from chiropractic manipulations. Serious injuries and deaths are much more likely with neck manipulations because of the stress placed on the arteries at the top of the spine while the head is rotated. Manipulations of the lower spine are much safer. About 12 percent of patients reported mild adverse effects. While this risk is not very high if the treatment is effective, it becomes highly problematic if manipulation is done for conditions for which it has not been shown to be beneficial.

Chiropractors who adhere to Palmer's metaphysical roots are willing to promote or practice life energy therapies and even teach courses in New Age philosophy.

Recommendations

Chiropractors differ in their scientific foundations and spiritual beliefs. Some openly promote other New Age and shamanistic approaches to health and healing. Other chiropractors take a very scientific approach to their profession, and practice according to evidence-based guidelines. The Christian Chiropractic Association is to be highly commended for separating New Age beliefs and practices from the scientifically based practice of chiropractic.

Chiropractic can be a legitimate intervention, bringing welcome relief for specific muscular and skeletal conditions. Although many chiropractors claim it is also more cost-effective than conventional medicine, economic studies have found the opposite. Individual visits to chiropractors cost less, but more visits usually are recommended, and treatment is often continued for longer periods. A 1995 study in the *New England Journal of Medicine* found that different treatment approaches for back pain were equally effective. However, primary care physicians offered the least expensive regimen, with chiropractic care being the most expensive option, costing even more than orthopedic surgery.

Treatment Categories

Conventional Therapy
    Acute low back pain   ☺☺☺☺
    Some other musculoskeletal conditions   ☺☺☺

Scientifically Unproven
    Medical diseases or preventive medicine   ☹☹☹☹

Energy Medicine
    In the hands of certain practitioners

Quackery or Fraud
    In the hands of a few practitioners

Further Reading

Assendelft, Willem J. J., Lex M. Bouter, and Paul G. Knipschild, "Complications of Spinal Manipulation: A Comprehensive Review of the Literature," *Journal of Family Practice* 42, no. 5 (May 1996): 475–80.

Ernst, E., and W. J. J. Assendelft, "Chiropractic for Low Back Pain," *British Medical Journal* 317 (July 1998): 160.

Ofman, Joshua J., "Chiropractic Spinal Manipulation for Treatment of Acute Low Back Pain," *Alternative Medicine Alert* 1, no. 4 (April 1998): 45–46.

COLONICS

What It Is

Enemas (irrigation of the colon) are used medically for constipation and prior to colon operations or procedures. Colonic hydrotherapy (colonics or detoxification) is usually practiced outside of conventional medicine. Colon therapy in one form or another is actually many centuries old. Even in the early 1900s, the American Medical Association criticized colonic irrigation when used to allegedly remove toxins and enhance health. Scientific knowledge about these procedures has increased with the years, yet the treatments are still criticized.

Since the time of ancient Egypt, different theories have arisen tracing the origins of all human disease to feces. Those who advocate colonic hydrotherapy offer one of two theories on why patients should utilize it. The first theory, which has its roots in Darwin's concept of evolution, considers colonic hydrotherapy necessary to counter what is known as "ptosis." This term simply means that an organ has moved downward from its usual position. According to this theory, as humans evolved from four-legged to two-legged animals, gravity in the standing position pulled the abdominal cavity in a different direction. This pressure, so the theory contends, produced a drop, or ptosis, in the intestines that caused stress bands that narrowed the intestines, slowing passage of the contents. Treatment included massage to help move bowel contents along, and colonic irrigation to loosen the contents.

The second and related theory, championed by French physician Charles-Jacques Bouchard (1837–1915), is "autointoxication." Just when microorganisms were being identified as the cause of some diseases (leading to the germ theory of disease), Bouchard proposed that slower movement of waste through the colon would give microorganisms time to decompose that material. That would lead to the production of toxins, which could then be absorbed back into the body, causing disease and illness. This reabsorption leads to the body poisoning itself, which is what Bouchard and others called "autointoxication." He wrote, "Man is in this way constantly living under the chance of being poisoned; he is always working toward his own destruction; he makes continual attempts at suicide by intoxication."

Nobel Prize winner Eli Metchnikoff also promoted autointoxication and, later in his life, proposed a link between autointoxication and aging. His name and his Nobel Prize were widely used to promote the theory.

The most famous practitioner of colon therapy was Dr. John Harvey Kellogg of Battle Creek, Michigan, the man who would become most known for his breakfast cereals. The doctor was convinced that, by using colonic therapy, he had saved almost 40,000 sufferers of gastrointestinal illness from surgery. He claimed that only twenty of his patients had to undergo the knife.

Dr. Kellogg practiced in the early twentieth century, and by 1920 colon therapy had become quite popular. Many people utilized the colonic irrigation machines in doctors' offices. Some of the wealthy, such as heiress Doris Duke, who could afford to take advantage of the new concept in health, became addicted to the use of colonics and enemas.

Colonics are performed by inserting a soft tube into the rectum. The tube is connected to a machine that gently pumps liquid into the colon. FDA-approved colonic machines usually come with filters to remove bacteria from the infusion liquid. Although enemas are not true colonics, they can be included here. Enemas empty only the end of the colon.

Claims

Enemas have been used since ancient times. Ancient Egyptian, Babylonian, Greek, Roman, Chinese, and Ayurvedic physicians believed that agents in human feces caused disease. Enemas, which were believed to rid the body of toxins, became very popular in the eighteenth century. Mineral oil enemas, called "lavages," were used because it seemed the ideal way to eliminate feces while lubricating the colon.

More recently, colonics have been said to treat or cure arthritis, fatigue, depression, anxiety, headache, seizures, alcoholism, allergies, asthma, colitis, hypertension, parasites, skin disorders, fevers, and ulcerative colitis.

Study Findings

Unfortunately, there are no well-performed, controlled medical studies to support or refute this type of therapy. Some doctors feel that patients who feel better after colonics are only responding to a placebo effect induced by their belief that colonics are helpful.

Cautions

Reports show (✗✗) that colonic irrigation has been associated with at least one outbreak of amoebiasis (an infection caused by a tiny one-celled organism called an "amoeba" that can be spread by the use of improperly cleaned colonic equipment contaminated with fecal material). Other types of colon infections have been caused by colonics. Two deaths associated with coffee enemas have also been reported (✗✗). Some doctors worry that colonics might change the normal bacteria in the colon, but this has never been reported. Other unproven concerns include the loss of intestinal muscle tone and normal defecation reflex, water intoxication, electrolyte disturbances, and perforation of the colon. People with any intestinal problem or illness should consult a physician before undergoing colonics.

Recommendations

We could find no studies that prove or disprove that colonics enhance health. No medical evidence supports the use of colonics other than for constipation and pre- or postoperative reasons (✔✔✔). Adverse effects appear to be relatively infrequent. There is no scientific basis for using or recommending colonics for general health.

Treatment Categories

Conventional Therapy
Constipation (certain types)   ☺☺☺☺
Preparation for certain types of surgery ☺☺☺☺

Scientifically Questionable
Detoxification or other indications   ☹☹☹

Quackery or Fraud
In the hands of some practitioners

Further Reading

Ernst, E., "Colonic Irrigation and the Theory of Autointoxication: A Triumph of Ignorance Over Science," *Journal of Clinical Gastroenterology* 24 (1997): 196–98.

Sullivan-Fowler, Micaela, "Doubtful Theories, Drastic Therapies: Autointoxication and Faddism in the Late Nineteenth and Early Twentieth Centuries," *Journal of the History of Medicine and Allied Sciences* 50 (July 1995): 364–90.

CRANIOSACRAL THERAPY

What It Is

Craniosacral therapy was developed in the 1970s by osteopathic physician John Upledger as a variation of an older therapy called "cranial osteopathy." Although arising out of an osteopathic approach, craniosacral therapy is not typically viewed as a part of conventional osteopathic medicine.

Cranial osteopathy, on which craniosacral therapy is based, evolved from two controversial ideas. The first is the belief that the bones of the cranium (the part of the skull surrounding the brain) can be moved relative to one another. This is true with babies because movement of the bones is necessary for a normal birth. However, these bones are naturally fused during childhood, or at least held in place by very dense connective tissue, and therefore are no longer movable to any significant degree in older children, teenagers, or adults.

The second controversy deals with cerebrospinal fluid and the idea of cranial rhythmic impulse (CRI). Cerebrospinal fluid brings nutrients and protection to the brain and the spine. Cranial osteopaths claim they can detect pulsation in this fluid by holding the head in their hands. They claim they can restore CRI to normal by using pressure to adjust the relative positions of the cranial bones.

Craniosacral therapy also focuses on the soft tissues (various membranes and connective tissues) around the skull and spine, while cranial osteopathy focuses on the bones. The goal of both therapies is the same: restoration of an even, rhythmic CRI in the cerebrospinal fluid. Therapy is believed to improve the function of the central nervous system, the immune system, and other systems. Craniosacral therapists apply a gentle and subtle pressure to the head and sacrum (base of the spine) to manipulate the membranes said to control CRI.

Claims

The CRI is believed to influence the connective tissues that surround all the major organs and muscles of the body. Craniosacral therapy is used primarily to relieve chronic aches and pains throughout the body, but especially muscle problems and arthritis. It is also believed to relieve stress, lift depression, correct learning disabilities, and to assist in a patient's recovery from brain and head injuries, as well as stroke and meningitis. Therapists claim to be especially successful with children because their cranial bones are not yet fused.

Study Findings

There are many anecdotal reports (✔) of dramatic recoveries from chronic, persistent problems, especially through the Upledger Institute in Florida. However, a 1999 review of research literature found very few studies of the therapy. It remains controversial to claim that the bones of the cranium can be moved in adults. A number of controlled studies found that craniosacral therapists did not agree on the values of the craniosacral rhythms they detected or on the effects of one another's manipulations (✘✘✘).

Cautions

Craniosacral therapy appears to be very gentle, much more so than cranial osteopathy. There appears to be little danger from craniosacral therapy so long as serious problems are not missed when conventional care is avoided. While children appear to be more suited to these therapies, great caution should be exercised by anyone attempting to manipulate a child's growing bones. Cranial osteopathy is offered by osteopathic physicians, but craniosacral therapy can be offered by anyone who has completed a course in the therapy. CRI practitioners may have little medical training and are not qualified to diagnose medical problems.

Recommendations

There is little evidence that this therapy does anything more than help people relax. Many experts claim that simply lying down will produce greater changes in the pressure of the cerebrospinal fluid than any manipulation of the bones or membranes of the head.

Treatment Categories

Scientifically Unproven
For any indication

Scientifically Questionable

Quackery or Fraud
In the hands of some

Further Reading

Green, C., C. W. Martin, K. Bassett, and A. Kazanjian, "A Systematic Review of Craniosacral Therapy: Biological Plausibility, Assessment Reliability and Clinical Effectiveness," *Complementary Therapies in Medicine* 7, no. 4 (December 1999): 201–7.

Rogers, J. S., and P. L. Witt, "The Controversy of Cranial Bone Motion," *Journal of Orthopedic Sports and Physical Therapy* 26, no. 2 (August 1997): 95–103.

DIET AND NUTRITION

What It Is

Why discuss diet and nutrition—which conventional medicine has always recognized as important—in a book on alternative medicine?

Many surveys reporting on the popularity of alternative medicine include nutrition as an alternative therapy, sometimes with emphasis on dietary supplements to provide critical nutrients. In our opinion, these nutrients are best obtained through a healthy, balanced diet, though there are exceptions, including certain illnesses that make it necessary for some people to take specific nutritional supplements.

With the increased attention on dietary supplements, there is concern that some people might ignore good eating habits, trusting instead in supplements to meet their needs. Others may already be eating a healthy diet, getting everything they need, but add supplements since everyone else seems to be taking them. Or, for example, news reports that antioxidants in vegetables have health benefits might prompt some to begin taking dietary supplements containing these antioxidants rather than doing what would be cheaper and better: eat more vegetables.

Since dietary supplements are often inconsistent in their quality, you are better able to assure yourself the nutrition your body needs by eating a proper diet. And it's cheaper than relying on supplements.

The following information includes some of the most significant principles to keep in mind as you plan and cook meals. We will not focus here on specific dietary supplements (see chapter 13, "Herbal Remedies, Vitamins, and Dietary Supplements").

GUIDELINES FOR A HEALTHY DIET

Eat 50 to 60 percent "good" or complex carbohydrates, 20 to 25 percent "good" fat, and 20 to 25 percent protein. This should provide sufficient energy for everyday activities and the variety of compounds needed by the body to prevent many forms of illness and to replenish and repair tissues. The most widely recognized and scientifically supported set of guidelines for a healthy diet is the Food Guide Pyramid produced by the U.S. Department of Agriculture.

How much and when you eat may be as important as what you eat. If you eat more calories than you use in daily activities, you will gain weight. This extra weight will have negative effects on your health no matter what percentage comes from breads, meats, or

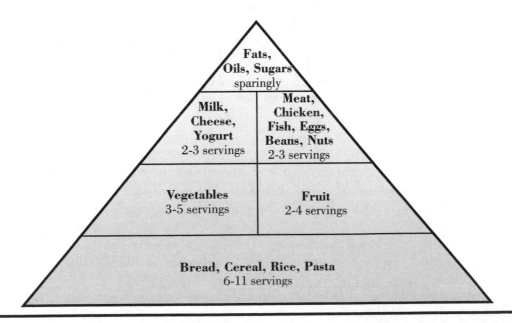

vegetables. Figure out what your "ideal" weight range is, given your height, sex, and other relevant factors. Ideal weight is often based on the appearance of underweight models, which is not healthy. The most recent research points to determining ideal body weight by measuring body mass index (BMI). A BMI of 19 to 25 is considered ideal body weight.

Based on your current weight and activity level, figure out how many calories you need to eat each day to either maintain your weight or move gradually toward your ideal weight range. Divide the number of calories you need each day among the recommended food groups. There are many excellent nutrition books available to help you with these calculations. One is *The American Dietetic Association's Complete Food & Nutrition Guide* by Robert Larson Duyff (Minneapolis, Minn.: Chronimed Publishing, 1998). Another by Frances Sizer and Eleanor Whitney, having an extensive list of calorie contents of many foods, is their eighth edition of *Nutrition: Concepts and Controversies* (Belmont, Calif.: Wadsworth/Thompson Learning, 2000).

THE RECOMMENDED FOOD GROUPS

Breads, cereals, rice, and pasta

Carbohydrates (sugars) in the breads and cereals group are an important, easy, and inexpensive food, in spite of all the current interest in losing weight with low-carbohydrate

BMI	18	19	20	21	22	23	24	25	26	27	28	29	30	31	32
Height	Body Weight (pounds)														
4'10"	86	91	96	100	105	110	115	119	124	129	134	138	143	148	15:
4'11"	89	94	99	104	109	114	119	124	128	133	138	143	148	153	58
5'0"	92	97	102	107	112	118	123	128	133	138	143	148	153	158	6:
5'1"	95	100	106	111	116	122	127	132	137	143	148	153	158	164	69
5'2"	98	104	109	115	120	126	131	136	142	147	153	158	164	169	75
5'3"	102	107	113	118	124	130	135	141	146	152	158	163	169	175	180
5'4"	105	110	116	122	128	134	140	145	151	157	163	169	174	180	186
5'5"	108	114	120	126	132	138	144	150	156	162	168	174	180	186	92
5'6"	112	118	124	130	136	142	148	155	161	167	173	179	186	192	98
5'7"	115	121	127	134	140	146	153	159	166	172	178	185	191	198	204
5'8"	118	125	131	138	144	151	158	164	171	177	184	190	197	203	210
5'9"	122	128	135	142	149	155	162	169	176	182	189	196	203	209	216
5'10"	126	132	139	146	153	160	167	174	181	188	195	202	209	216	22
5'11"	129	136	143	150	157	165	172	179	186	193	200	208	215	222	29
6'0"	132	140	147	154	162	169	177	184	191	199	206	213	221	228	235
6'1"	136	144	151	159	166	174	182	189	197	204	212	219	227	235	24:
6'2"	141	148	155	163	171	179	186	194	202	210	218	225	233	241	249
Underweight	Healthy Weight						Overweight						Obese		

Find your height along the left-hand side and look across the row until you find the number closest to your weight.
The number at the top of that column gives you your BMI.

diets (see Diets and Dieting, page 181). Bread, particularly bread made with stone-ground whole grains (complex, or "good," carbohydrates), was important in biblical times and remains the basic food for three-quarters of the people living in the Middle East. God nourished the Israelites for forty years in the wilderness with bread made from manna (Exodus 16:4). Bread was made from both wheat and barley grains (2 Samuel 17:28), although rye is mentioned occasionally (Isaiah 28:25). The importance of bread in the Jewish diet is reflected in Jesus' statement, "For the bread of God is he who comes down from heaven and gives life to the world" (John 6:33). He went on to proclaim: "I am the bread of life. He who comes to me will never go hungry, and he who believes in me will never be thirsty" (John 6:35).

Bread is an important food because of how many nutrients it contains. In addition to carbohydrates, bread contains protein, vitamins, minerals, and fiber. Grains are also valuable because of what they lack. Foods made from grains tend to be relatively low in fat, which is not the case with many protein foods. Stone-ground whole-grain bread is vastly more nutritious than highly processed (white) bread, even when white bread has been enriched, because the processing removes nutrients and fiber. Most fast-food and bakery-produced breadlike foods, such as donuts, pastries, and sweets, should be kept to a minimum because of their high content of "bad" fats and high calorie count. They represent "bad" carbohydrates, as do most simple sugars, or "sweets."

Fruits and vegetables

Many recent studies have documented the extensive health benefits of eating several servings a day of fruits and vegetables. But plant products are also mentioned throughout the Bible. They have been the primary source of nutrition throughout most of human history, and remain so for most of the world's population. In biblical times, grain, wine, and olive oil were the three main foods, with the wine and olive oil coming from fruits (Deuteronomy 7:13; Nehemiah 5:11; Hosea 2:8). Vegetables and fruits are commonly mentioned as part of the diet during biblical times. Some of the vegetables mentioned include lentils (Genesis 25:34), beans (2 Samuel 17:28), leeks, onions, and cucumber (Numbers 11:5). Fruit eaten include figs (Deuteronomy 8:8; Luke 13:6), apples (Proverbs 25:11), melons (Numbers 11:5), and, of course, grapes (Numbers 6:3; Matthew 7:16).

Plant foods contain nutritious complex ("good") carbohydrates, are high in fiber, low in fat, and are healthy sources of other substances (called *phytochemicals*) that include vitamins, antioxidants, and other plant products. An article by Johanna Lampe at the Cancer Prevention Research Program summarizes the numerous ways phytochemicals have health-promoting benefits. They have been shown to act as antioxidants, stimulate the immune system, lower cholesterol, improve many hormones, and assist the body's detoxification systems. While in some cases we know which individual phytochemical has which specific effect, the mixture of compounds found in food seems to work better than the individual components taken as supplements.

Fruits make a great snack and many are best eaten unpeeled, after thorough washing, as the skins are high in fiber. Most vegetables are best eaten uncooked, or lightly steamed, as prolonged cooking destroys many of the nutrients. However, some vegetables seem to have improved health benefits when cooked. Tomatoes are one example.

Dairy products

Dairy products are felt by many, but not all, experts to be an important primary source of nutrients and vitamins, containing proteins, carbohydrates, and fats. The Old Testament frequently describes the Promised Land as "a land flowing with milk and honey" (Exodus 3:8). The abundance of milk was often used as a metaphor for God's provision (Isaiah 55:1; see also Deuteronomy 32:14; Proverbs 27:27; Isaiah 7:22).

The dairy group includes milk, cheese, yogurt, sour cream, cottage cheese, and many other products. Milk products contain vitamins A, C, E, some of the B vitamins, and minerals like calcium and magnesium.

But the milk of today is not necessarily the milk of the Bible. Most milk is homogenized and pasteurized, which has led to debate over the benefits of processed milk. Processing prevents the transmission of many infections and makes it possible to reduce the fat content, but it also can damage some nutrients. Because of these concerns, some avoid all milk products, claiming a biblically based prohibition (see Christian Therapies, page 106, and the Hallelujah Diet, page 202). However, Abraham and the angels ate curds (or butter) and drank milk (Genesis 18:8), milk was recognized as important for healthy teeth (Genesis 49:12), and the Israelites kept milk available to drink (Judges 4:19).

Dairy products can contain significant amounts of fat, so low-fat or no-fat milk products usually are preferable for adults. Because of hormones and antibiotics given to cows in commercial diary operations, some turn to "organic" dairy products to avoid this type of exposure. Others use goat or soy milk, trying to gain the benefits of the protein without the possible detriments of commercial cow's milk.

Meat, poultry, and fish

Another food group recommended is a major source of protein. Various types of meat, poultry, and fish contain significant amounts of protein and numerous vitamins and nutrients. Meat varies in the type and proportion of saturated (or "bad") fat it contains. Expensive cuts of beef contain about 20 percent saturated fat, whereas up to half of some types of ground beef can be fat. Animal fat tends to be primarily saturated fat, which is not as healthy as the unsaturated fat found to a greater extent in plants and fish. The Bible seems to indicate that meat was eaten only on occasion, except for the rich who could afford to eat it regularly (Genesis 18:6–8; 27:3–4; 1 Samuel 2:13–15). Fish was an important part of the diet during the time of Jesus.

The Old Testament law was very specific about which meat was clean or unclean (Leviticus 11; Deuteronomy 14). These laws demonstrate that vegetarianism is not obligatory for Christians, although some may choose such a diet (see Hallelujah Diet, page 202). Vegetarians who avoid meat and dairy products must be careful to obtain sufficient protein elsewhere, and supplement their diet with certain nutrients and vitamins, especially vitamin B_{12} (see Hallelujah Diet, page 202). Sufficient protein can also be obtained relatively easily from dry beans, nuts, and soy protein, which also are sources of other important nutrients.

Fats, oils, and sweets

The small tip of the Food Pyramid represents the importance of reducing the amount of fats and sweets in the diet. The American Heart Association recommends that fats make up no more than 30 percent of the diet. Some, such as Pritikin and Ornish, suggest this should be as low as 10 percent. In contrast, the proportion of fat in the average American diet increased steadily during the twentieth century, at times approaching 50 percent. To reduce the amount of fat, the types of foods and the way food is prepared must change. For example, fried food has more fat than the same food cooked any other way. Instead of flavoring dishes with cream sauces or butter, use herbs and spices. When cooking with eggs, don't use the yolks. Remove the skin and fat from poultry. Eat less.

All fat is not alike. There are "good" fats and "bad" fats. The "bad" ones are saturated fats, hydrogenated fats, and the trans-fatty acids (TFAs). Most margarine, baked goods, and fast-foods have high levels of hydrogenated fats and TFAs. Food labels indicate (under ingredients) whether hydrogenated fats are in the food, but TFAs are not indicated on these government-required labels.

The "good," or "healthy," fats include the omega-9 fatty acids (contained in olive oil) and the omega-3 fatty acids (contained in cold-water fish oils [cod, salmon, halibut, swordfish, etc.] and virtually all types of nuts). These "good" fats appear to have many health benefits, and a diet deficient in the "good" fats is actually associated with some poor health outcomes. What is called the "Mediterranean Diet" is very low in the "bad" fats and has up to 25 percent "good" fat—especially olive oil. The healthiest of the olive oils appear to be "cold-pressed, extra virgin" olive oil, which can be used instead of butter (some call it "Italian butter") and in salad dressings. However, cooking has to be done in "regular" olive oil, as the regular olive oil has a higher smoke point than extra-virgin olive oil.

Water

Not listed in the Food Guide Pyramid is water, a vital component of our diet. At birth, the body was three-fourths water. This decreases as we age, but water remains the single most common substance in our bodies. We need water to transport nutrients around the body and remove wastes. Water plays a central role in regulating body temperature. Most chemical reactions that allow life to continue occur within a liquid environment. Water is one of the starting materials required for some reactions our cells carry out, including breaking down all of the major food groups.

To provide the body with enough water, most healthy adults need to drink at least eight to ten 8 oz. glasses of water a day. Some experts recommend that we drink even more water. A common rule-of-thumb is to take your weight in pounds, divide it in half, and drink that number of ounces of water every day. A 150-pound person should drink about 75 ounces of water per day, more than two quarts.

Most parts of the United States have a plentiful supply of clean, safe water. In other parts of the world, people live or die depending on whether their water supply is maintained. In biblical times, an abundant supply of drinking water was another reminder of God's loving provision. "For the LORD your God is bringing you into a good land—a land with streams and pools of water, with springs flowing in the valleys and hills" (Deuteronomy 8:7; see also Isaiah 41:17–20). Jesus used the importance of water for physical life as a metaphor for the spiritual life he offered: "Jesus stood and said in a loud voice, 'If anyone is thirsty, let him come to me and drink. Whoever believes in me, as the Scripture has said, streams of living water will flow from within him.' By this he meant the Spirit, whom those who believed in him were to receive" (John 7:37–39; see also John 4:10–14).

The rise in purchases of bottled water has prompted a number of city water departments to check the quality of their tap water against the quality of the mineral and spring water available at a much higher cost. In most instances, the quality of the tap water was higher—especially water purified using an ionization process as opposed to a filtration process. In fact, some studies have shown that as much as 50 percent of the bottled water samples tested had excessive amounts of viruses, bacteria, or other impurities. Water from a "natural spring" does not guarantee quality. There are health food purists who say the only water to drink is steam distilled. Certainly a safe alternative, but in most large cities, steam distilled water is, in our opinion, a needless expense.

Water is so readily available for most of us that we are not content with "just" water. We have become used to beverages with taste—with caffeine or sugar to keep us going. Sugar is a source of needless calories, and caffeine, a diuretic, causes the body to eliminate fluids. While some people need diuretic drugs, for most of us caffeine works against the body's need to remain hydrated. Dehydration can lead to much more than just being thirsty. It can cause headaches, intestinal problems, and even be a factor in more serious illnesses. Learning to increase your intake of pure water and to decrease your intake of other beverages seems to be a healthy choice.

When ill, it is especially important to drink lots of water. That's one of the reasons you'll see so many people in a hospital hooked up to an IV bag. Remember to also adjust your water intake based on weather and your activity level. Those exercising in warm weather should drink two to four extra glasses of water in the hour before exercising, a glass of water every thirty minutes during exercise (if practical), and afterwards, three glasses of water for every pound of weight lost during exercise (that was mostly water loss through sweating). That's a lot of water, but it has been shown to improve exercise performance and may also lead to a better overall feeling of well-being.

Study Findings

The dietary recommendations given in the Food Pyramid and discussed above are widely accepted by different professional organizations. In April 2000, the *Journal of the American Medical Association* reported findings (✔✔) that women who ate more of the recommended foods had lower death rates during the three years of the study. The survey asked more than 40,000 women (average age 61) whether they ate certain foods at least once a week. Twenty-three of these foods (like apples, dried beans, baked fish, high-fiber cereal, 2 percent milk) are on the Food Pyramid. Based on how many recommended foods they ate at least once a week, the women were divided into four groups. Each group contained roughly one-quarter of the women. After making allowances for age differences and other relevant factors, the group with the highest scores (14 to 23 out of 23) had a 30 percent lower death rate than the group with the lowest scores (0–8), a statistically significant difference.

Other epidemiological studies (✔✔) have had similar positive findings. For example, women who daily ate food from only two of the recommended food groups had a 40 percent higher risk of death than women who daily ate from five different food groups. In another study, men with healthier diets had a 13 percent lower risk of death. These studies are somewhat limited because there might be something else about people who eat according to the recommended guidelines that reduces their risk of death.

However, in a randomized controlled study (✔✔✔), people who started eating according to these dietary recommendations had significantly lower blood pressure within eight weeks, regardless of whether they started with normal or high blood pressure. Clearly, eating according to the Food Guide Pyramid can quickly produce changes known to be more conducive for good health.

Most of the positive research findings have come from epidemiological studies. These large surveys are designed to measure different factors that might give some clues as to what aspects of people's lifestyles make an impact on their health. Winston Craig, a professor of nutrition, reported that out of 156 of these types of studies (✔✔), 82 percent found that increased fruit and vegetable consumption significantly protected people against a wide variety of cancers. Those who ate the most fruits and vegetables had roughly half the risk of getting cancer, especially those cancers that involve epithelial cells found in the lung, cervix, stomach, and colon. Similar types of effects have been found in relation to cardiovascular disease. A 1999 study (✔✔) found that men and women who ate five to six servings of fruits and vegetables per day had a 31 percent lower risk of stroke compared to those who ate one serving per day.

The limits of epidemiological studies have recently led to some controlled clinical studies of the effects of making dietary changes. Unfortunately, two such trials reported in the April 2000 *New England Journal of Medicine* (✖✖✖) did not produce the results researchers had hoped to achieve. Both were randomized controlled trials of patients after removal of colorectal polyps, which can be an early sign of colon and rectal cancer. One group in each study was given intensive counseling and assigned a high-fiber diet believed to prevent colorectal polyps.

While the test group in the first study was assigned the low-fat, high-fiber diet, the control group was given a brochure on healthy eating, but no further nutritional counseling. Both groups were examined four years later to see if polyps had recurred. Both had the same rate of recurrence (40 percent).

In the second study, the two groups were assigned to add either 13.5 grams or 2 grams of wheat-bran fiber to their daily diet. After three years, the polyp recurrence rate was 47 percent in the high-fiber group (13.5 grams) and 51 percent in the low-fiber group (2 grams), which is not a statistically significant difference (the difference can be explained by random chance). While these results were disappointing, they do not necessarily mean that diet plays no role in the development of colorectal cancer. For one thing, both studies were of fairly short duration, and these cancers can take many years to develop.

Researching the health effects of dietary intervention is frustrated by its complexities. Benefits noticed in an epidemiological study may have more to do with general lifestyle than any one food. Mary Serdula, a physician-researcher at the Center for Disease Control and Prevention, has shown that studies (✔✔) demonstrating health benefits from eating more fruits and vegetables also found that those who ate more of these foods tended to exercise more, and those who ate fewer tended to exercise less, smoke more, and drink heavily.

Many people, despite news reports on the importance of diet for overall health, do not follow the recommended dietary guidelines. Professor Winston Craig reviewed a survey which found that the average American eats only one and one-half servings of vegetables per day, and less than one serving per day of fruit. On the day the survey was taken, almost half the people said they had eaten no fruit. Only about one-third of Americans eat the recommended servings of grains, and only one-quarter consume the recommended number of dairy products.

Modern research is confirming the age-old wisdom underlying the saying, "An apple a day keeps the doctor away." Yet in spite of both ancient wisdom and modern research, unhealthy eating habits are proving to be hard to break.

Cautions

Remember the proper role of diet and nutrition. Evidence for claims that certain diets cure people of serious illnesses, such as cancer, is weak or nonexistent. Although we are discovering that a healthy, balanced diet can play a role in preventing certain illnesses, this does not mean that a particular diet can cure someone of a disease unless the disease is due to a dietary deficiency or another factor related to food.

An important example of the latter involves milk. Some people become less able to tolerate milk as they get older, due to a particular type of sugar in milk, called "lactose," which requires an enzyme called "lactase" to be digested. People whose ancestors came from northern and western Europe continue to produce lactase as they get older and usually have no problem with milk. But people of any other ethnic origin tend to produce less lactase as they age. This gives rise to a condition called "lactose intolerance," which leads to various intestinal problems and pain whenever milk is consumed. This condition is easily treated by reducing (or eliminating) milk products in the diet, or by taking supplements of lactase. These are now readily available (one example is Lactaid®), to be taken whenever milk products are consumed.

Milk can also be the source of other problems. Milk is one of the most common sources of food allergies, best treated by avoiding milk products altogether. A more serious problem, called "galactosemia," occurs in a small number of newborn babies. The heel-prick blood test done on all newborns checks for the presence of this genetic condition (and others). When lactose is digested, it makes another sugar called "galactose," which must then be converted into glucose before being used in the body. If the enzyme for this conversion is not present, galactose builds up in the blood and can lead to brain damage. A baby with this condition must avoid all milk sugar.

If you suspect that an illness is linked to food, get advice from a professional trained in nutrition. You should be aware that anyone can call themselves a nutritionist. There is no generally accepted standard for training or certifying nutritionists. However, registered dietitians are nationally certified. In most cases, a registered dietitian should be consulted.

Recommendations

A balanced diet that meets the recommendations of the Food Guide Pyramid can go a long way toward maintaining good health and reducing the risk of a number of chronic diseases. More and more research is finding that we can make significant improvements in our health, and our long-term outlook, by adhering to these guidelines. Most people are not successful in completely overhauling their diet in one swipe. Plan instead to make small, consistent steps toward your goal. Studies have found that even small dietary changes lead to some health improvements. Remember that these changes are primarily beneficial in the prevention of disease, not its treatment.

Treatment Categories

Conventional Therapy
Reducing risk of cardiovascular diseases,
cancer, and other chronic diseases ☺☺☺☺

Complementary Therapy
Reducing risk of many other chronic diseases ☺☺☺
Improving general well-being ☺☺☺☺

Scientifically Unproven
   Curing diseases

Quackery or Fraud
   Certain "miracle" foods and diets

Further Reading

Byers, Tim, "Diet, Colorectal Adenomas, and Colorectal Cancer," *New England Journal of Medicine* 342, no. 16 (April 2000): 1206–7.

Craig, Winston J., "Phytochemicals: Guardians of Our Health," *Journal of the American Dietetic Association* 97, suppl. 2 (1997): S199–S204.

"Food," *New Bible Dictionary*, 2d ed. (Leicester, U.K.: Inter-Varsity; Wheaton, Ill.: Tyndale, 1982), 383–88.

Jacobson, Michael, *The Word on Health: A Biblical and Medical Overview of How to Care for Your Body and Mind* (Chicago: Moody Press, 2000).

Joshipura, Kaumudi J., Alberto Ascherio, JoAnn E. Manson, Meir J. Stampfer, Eric B. Rimm, Frank E. Speizer, Charles H. Hennekens, Donna Spiegelman, and Walter C. Willett, "Fruit and Vegetable Intake in Relation to Risk of Ischemic Stroke," *Journal of the American Medical Association* 282, no. 13 (October 1999): 1233–39.

Kant, Ashima K., Arthur Schatzkin, Barry I. Graubard, and Catherine Schairer, "A Prospective Study of Diet Quality and Mortality in Women," *Journal of the American Medical Association* 283, no. 16 (April 2000): 2109–15.

Lampe, Johanna W., "Health Effects of Vegetables and Fruit, Assessing Mechanisms of Action in Human Experimental Studies," *American Journal of Clinical Nutrition* 70, suppl. (1999): 475S–90S.

DIETS AND DIETING

What It Is

Dieting could be viewed as a national pastime (or obsession). Look at any magazine rack and you'll see the latest diet guaranteed to melt away the pounds as you sit and watch. "Lose weight while you sleep," calls the enticing ad.

In spite of all the "guaranteed" diets, the number of Americans who are overweight is growing. More than half of all adults in the United States and about a quarter of all children are overweight. About one in five adults is obese. And these numbers are getting worse.

In fact, the problem is worldwide. The World Health Organization, in an article in the October 1998 issue of the *Journal of the American Dietetic Association,* declared that obesity has become an "escalating epidemic" and "one of the greatest neglected public health problems of our time."

Obesity is spreading even as we learn more about the dangers of being overweight. Many chronic illnesses are caused or made worse by being overweight. Obesity puts people at higher risk for diabetes, high blood pressure, heart disease, gallbladder disease, stroke, and some cancers. Out of an average group of a hundred obese adults, eighty will have at least one of the following: diabetes, high cholesterol levels, high blood pressure, coronary artery disease, gallbladder disease, or osteoarthritis; twenty will have at least two of these problems. Over a quarter of a million Americans die every year because of obesity, making it the second leading cause of preventable death in the United States (only smoking causes more). Yet three-fourths of those who are seriously overweight are not concerned about how their weight could impact their health.

In response to this problem, a $35 billion dieting industry has sprung up in the United States. Of those who are trying to lose weight, a survey by Mary Serdula, M.D., found that only 20 percent were following the only well-established recommendations: eating fewer calories and engaging in two and a half hours of physical activity per week. Also of concern is a finding that almost one-third of United States women of *normal* weight are reportedly trying to lose weight.

Because of the difficulty of making lifestyle changes and the frustration of failed diets, dieting pills have become increasingly popular. The best-known pharmaceutical weight-loss medication was the combination called Fen-Phen (fenfluramine taken with phentermine). Prescriptions for these drugs soared from 60,000 in 1992 to 18 million prescriptions by 1996, even though the two drugs were never approved for use together. Tragically, reports of women developing valvular heart disease while taking the combination led to the "Fen" part (fenfluramine) of "Fen-Phen" being withdrawn by the manufacturer in 1997, along with a similar drug sold as Redux®. At the end of 2000, the FDA called for withdrawal of phenylpropanolamine (PPA), another drug present in over-the-counter diet pills as well as cold remedies, because of the increased risk of hemorrhagic stroke (bleeding in the brain).

Numerous herbal remedies and dietary supplements have stepped into the vacuum created by these withdrawals. (See reports on ephedra [or *ma huang*], chromium, pyruvate, and senna in chapter 13, "Herbal Remedies, Vitamins, and Dietary Supplements.") Many of these are formulated into complicated mixtures, such as Metabolife 356®. This mixture of eighteen herbs was literally cooked up in a man's kitchen for his ailing father. In spite of having no published controlled trials to support its effectiveness or safety, 1999 sales were approaching $1 billion.

In addition to diet pills, revolutionary, or fad, diets come and go every year. Many fall into the area of alternative therapies in that they often contain some grain of truth and hence work for some people. But then they are mass-marketed to help everyone lose weight. Some diets are said to be biblical; most are said to be scientifically based; all are guaranteed to work.

But do they? Will you shed those pounds in so many weeks? If you do, will you stay at your lower weight? Are there any precautions to be aware of before embarking on these diets?

The following chart gives a brief overview of some of the most popular fad diets.

Diet:	Description:	Claims:	Evidence:	Benefits:	Cautions:
Atkins Diet	This is the most famous low-carbohydrate, high-protein diet.The 1992 book *Dr. Atkins' New Diet Revolution* was an update of his 1972 classic.	Cutting down on carbohydrates is said to reduce blood sugar levels and decrease insulin production. Less insulin forces us to burn rather than store fat.	Insulin production is much more complicated. People who are overweight produce too much insulin, but not necessarily because of dietary carbohydrates. There is, in our opinion, virtually no reputable scientific evidence to support this diet.	Eliminating carbohydrates will reduce overall calorie intake. Fats are digested more slowly, meaning people feel full longer.	Large amounts of protein contain a lot of fat, which may contribute to high cholesterol levels and heart disease, and may be hard on the kidneys. There is little fiber in the diet, which may lead to intestinal problems. Many nutrients are lacking, leading the USDA to label this diet "nutritionally deficient." Bad breath can occur as excess fats are rapidly broken down into ketones.
Blood-Type Diet	People of different blood types should choose different diets.	Blood types reflect different evolutionary ancestry. For example, type O means your ancestors were Stone Age hunters, so you need lots of meat and intense exercise, but few grains and dairy products.	There is, to us, no convincing or reputable evidence that blood types are related to evolutionary ancestry or diet. People in the same family can have different blood types.	Some of the recommendations might be healthy. Type O people might start exercising more. Type A people are advised to cut down on meat, and that might be useful.	Some of the recommendations may be unhealthy. Type O elimination of grains and dairy products will reduce vitamin and nutrient intake. Type A people are told to reduce exercise, which will not help.

Diet:	Description:	Claims:	Evidence:	Benefits:	Cautions:
Cabbage Soup Diet	A soup made from cabbage, onions, peppers, tomatoes, and celery is eaten exclusively for one week. A short break is taken, then you restart with soup alone.	Drastically reduces your calorie intake and you lose weight.	It works to reduce weight rapidly, although much of this may be water loss. However, there is no evidence people keep this weight off.	Short-term, non-sustained weight loss.	Many essential nutrients and vitamins are lacking. Can cause serious problems if maintained for long periods.
Candida Diet	The goal is to eliminate all sources of yeast (like bread and beer) and sugar (sweets and fruit) from the diet.	Tiredness, allergies, and recurrent yeast infections are evidence of a yeast *(Candida albicans)* infection throughout the body. The claim is that yeast needs to be starved of all sugar and other yeasts need to be eliminated from the diet.	Candida is found in many healthy women. A small percent will have recurrent yeast infections that are difficult to treat. There is no convincing medical evidence that eliminating certain foods cures these infections.	Because so many foods are eliminated, people should lose weight.	Following this strictly will lead to deficiencies in many vitamins and nutrients.
Dean Ornish Diet	Stay away from fatty foods and eat natural, wholesome foods.	This is a balanced approach to eating healthy. The Ornish program also involves exercise, stress reduction, and group support, but can get into New Age ideas.	The Ornish program is probably the only diet with published research to support the program. Scientific evidence that the diet works is produced by primarily Ornish.	Other than being too low in fat, this program incorporates all of the aspects of recommended guidelines, but may be very difficult for many people to follow.	Because there is so little fat in this diet, it can taste very bland and requires much self-discipline. The USDA has labeled this diet as "nutritionally deficient."

Diet:	Description:	Claims:	Evidence:	Benefits:	Cautions:
Fasting	Completely abstain from any food, usually for a specific length of time. Water is usually consumed.	Fasting can be done to lose weight, to "detoxify" the body, or for religious reasons. The biblical rationale for fasting is to allow focused attention for prayer (Matthew 6:16–18; Acts 13:2; 14:23) and to empathize with the poor (Isaiah 58), not to earn God's favor.	Obviously, eliminating all calories will lead to weight loss. There is scientific evidence to support medically-directed fasting.	Weight can be lost, but for the first few days this is usually water loss. Proponents describe many spiritual benefits for Christians who fast.	Most Americans can easily afford to fast from time to time without any negative effects. However, extended use will lead to weakness (Psalm 109:24) and nutritional deficiencies, and may contribute to development of eating disorders.
Food-Combining Diet	This claims that we need to eat foods by category. Fruit should be eaten alone in the morning. Carbohydrates should be eaten with vegetables, but never with fat or protein, etc.	Health problems are caused by eating foods in the wrong combination. If mixed wrongly, our digestive enzymes are confused and the wrong ones produced. The food sits in the intestines, rots, and poisons us.	Few foods contain only one food group. Our digestive enzymes select the correct food and don't get "confused." There is no compelling evidence to support this diet.	The diet can lead to more fruit and vegetable intake, and a move toward smaller quantities.	This diet is highly structured and may lead some to an "all or nothing" approach. It may have some benefits, but do not neglect all mixed foods (especially dairy products).
Macrobiotics	Meals are composed of whole grains (50 to 60 percent), vegetables (25 to 30 percent), beans or soybean products (5 to 10 percent), with some nuts, seeds, miso soup, and herbal teas. Meat or seafood is allowed once a week.	Macrobiotics literally means "way of long life" and is a quasi-religious approach to diet. Foods are chosen based on *yin* and *yang*, pulse diagnosis, and life energy beliefs.	There is no evidence that a macrobiotic diet cures cancer and other diseases, as claimed. Weight loss occurs from calorie reduction.	Adherents will benefit from increasing plant products in the diet and reducing calories.	Nutrient deficiencies occur. Using macrobiotics to cure cancer may lead to neglect of effective treatments. People are at risk of great spiritual harm from Eastern religious teachings.

Diet:	Description:	Claims:	Evidence:	Benefits:	Cautions:
"Mayo Clinic" Diet	This diet has nothing to do with the famous Mayo Clinic. Eat half a grapefruit at every meal, other specific foods at every meal, and eight glasses of water and one of skim milk or tomato juice a day. Do this for twelve days; then eat freely for two days.	Grapefruit is said to act as a fat burner. The combination of foods is said to promote fat burning.	There is no evidence to support the diet, and no evidence that grapefruit has any specific dieting properties.	The plan is low on calories and high on vegetables and salads. The water is beneficial.	The diet contains quite a large amount of meat, which can contain significant amounts of fat and can be hard on the kidneys. It's low in calcium and quickly gets boring.
Sugar Busters!	Eliminate all sugar from the diet.	The goal is to eliminate white flour and all refined sugar. Lean meats, high in protein, are encouraged. Some carbohydrates are allowed, especially high-fiber vegetables.	Based on eliminating refined carbohydrates to prevent the insulin surge that occurs after eating sugars. There is very little compelling evidence to support this diet.	Eliminating these sugars will reduce calorie intake. Fat intake is controlled and usually reduced.	Eliminates some grains and fruits, so fiber level and vitamins need to be monitored.
Zone Diet	Lower the amounts of carbohydrates, and replace them with protein and fat.	Claims the perfect balance is 40-30-30, carbohydrate-protein-fat. Very detailed planning required.	No specific research, other than the importance of reducing fat and increasing vegetables and fruits.	Balanced approach should lead to calorie reduction.	Requires incredible attention to detail to follow exactly, and can be boring.

Study Findings

Why is it that every time you look at a magazine rack there's another new diet? Why does product after product claim to be the "breakthrough" dieters need?

If you've struggled with losing weight, you know the answer. Almost every fad diet brings initial success. The pounds start coming off. You feel better. But after a few weeks or months there's a night out. You splurge. There's cake at a birthday party. You smell your favorite food.

At first, it's just a little nibble. You deserve a reward. Then it's a "day off." Before you know it, the weight is coming back. You give up. The diet didn't work.

The most frustrating aspect of diets, weight-loss programs, and diet pills is that they all have a very high relapse rate. Studies show that the fad diets do not work over long periods of time for most users. One of the few studies with long-term follow-up found that 95 percent of those who lost more than thirty pounds regained that weight within five years. In another study of people who had lost eleven or more pounds, 52 percent had kept the weight off a year later, but only 11 percent still kept it off five years later. This type of "yo-yo" dieting has been shown to be particularly harmful. Whatever approach is going to work has to be one you can incorporate into your life long-term—even if that means the weight loss is slow but steady.

In spite of all the research on the effects of being overweight, and the benefits of losing weight, there has been little research into what works. At a summit meeting called by the Federal Trade Commission in 1998, commercial weight-loss programs admitted they are reluctant to gather the data that would help consumers figure out which programs work best. If companies are not willing to do this, it probably means they suspect their programs and products would not fare well in the analysis.

One interesting study surveyed people who had previously lost weight to figure out what worked best. The results are summarized in the following table. Kayman and colleagues wanted to see if there were significant differences between those who remained at a lower weight (called "Successful Maintainers") and those who regained lost weight (called "Unsuccessful Relapsers"). The results speak for themselves. More than 100 women were interviewed, during which they were asked to list all weight-loss methods they had used.

The Successful Maintainers used a small number of well-established and highly recommended approaches: exercise, a personal eating plan, and a support group. Those who regained weight used a large number of different approaches and, to a smaller extent, also followed the well-established recommended strategies. One of the more dramatic differences was that diet pills and shots were used by almost half of the Unsuccessful Relapsers, in contrast to only 3 percent of the Successful Maintainers.

Weight-Loss Method	Percent of Successful Maintainers Using It	Percent of Unsuccessful Relapsers Using It
At least 30 min. exercise, 3 times/week	90	34
Devised personal eating plan	73	39
Attended Weight Watchers®	76	36
Attended other program/groups	10	43
Followed doctor's orders	20	34
Took pills or shots	3	47
Fasted	3	11
Underwent hypnosis	0	9
Followed book or magazine diet	10	25
Total number of different methods used by those in each group	28	121

The only proven approach to losing weight and keeping it off involves three aspects.

- Reduce the number of calories and eat a balanced diet. The body needs fewer calories when it weighs less (estimated to be about ten calories less per day for every pound lost). The USDA says that most people can lose weight and keep it off if they consistently take in less than 1500 calories per day.
- Increase physical activity. Two and a half hours of moderate exercise per week is believed by some to be most effective. However, *any* increase in activity will help. Take the stairs instead of the elevator. Park farther away from where you're going. Walk and cycle. Mow your grass.
- Have social support. When someone is trying to lose weight, others can encourage and help with the necessary changes. In the study mentioned above, one-third of those who relapsed said they had no one helping or supporting them. This sort of support and encouragement is a practical way to love others during what can be a very difficult time. "And let us consider how we may spur one another on toward love and good deeds. Let us not give up meeting together, as some are in the habit of doing, but let us encourage one another—and all the more as you see the Day approaching" (Hebrews 10:24–25). This may be one of the reasons why group weight-loss programs, such as Weight Watchers®, seem to be more successful than "going it alone." Christian weight-loss programs (e.g., Weigh Down Workshop®, First Place™, and God's Weigh), which incorporate biblical resources and Christian insight, may prove to be successful; however, we are aware of no published scientific studies that have evaluated these programs.

These three strategies, taken together, have the best chance of helping someone make the lifestyle changes necessary to not only lose weight but keep it off. You must be able to live with these changes for the rest of your life.

Be realistic. How long do you think you could stay on any of the fad diets? Why not start with a plan that works? The three aspects of the only proven approach to losing weight and keeping it off consistently produce better long-term results than any of the drastic diets or the many dieting pills available on the market.

Cautions

Almost all the popular diets involve consuming fewer calories and can lead to initial weight loss. However, drastically reducing calorie intake can cause metabolic problems as your body uses up stored energy. Losing weight actually makes it harder for many people to lose more weight. With less food available, the body's metabolic rate is lowered, meaning your same activity level requires fewer calories. If your brain senses that your body is entering "starvation mode," it will often increase how much fat is stored (sort of long-range planning).

The diets that emphasize one food or food type can easily lead to a deficiency of essential nutrients and vitamins. For example, a vegetarian diet can lead to deficiencies in vitamin B_{12}, calcium, iron, and other nutrients, although all of these are readily available as supplements. Fats are important to give us a longer-lasting sense of having had enough to eat. Apart from being bland, low-fat diets lead to people being hungry sooner, putting them at higher risk of snacking too much or on the wrong foods. The best strategy is a balanced diet to ensure adequate amounts of all needed nutrients and vitamins. This is especially important with children and teenagers during these important growing periods.

Ineffective diets and dieting agents will lead to disappointment, but they can also make weight problems worse. People who go on diets and later give up often regain even more weight. Then the cycle repeats itself. More diets and products are developed. With this constant attention to dieting, children often get wrong impressions about their own weight. Eighty-one percent of ten-year-olds reported they were afraid of "being fat." Some may already have a problem with being overweight, but to some extent our society has generated a self-fulfilling prophecy. In a different study, teenage girls who reported using dieting agents and being concerned about dieting were those who were more likely to gain weight and become obese after their teenage years.

When considering a diet, ask the following questions. The more times you answer "yes" to these questions, the greater the chance that the diet is more of a fad than a reliable strategy for healthy eating. (Also see guidelines on pages 172–178.)

- Does the diet require eating a very small number of foods or focus exclusively on one food group?

- Does the diet focus on the *type* of food you eat rather than on amount of food and making lifestyle changes necessary for healthy eating?
- Are common foods rejected because people are said to be allergic to them or because they allegedly contain toxins?
- Is losing weight said to be easy or automatic or "guaranteed"?
- Is weight loss of more than a few pounds a week promised?
- Is weight loss promised without any increased activity (or even promised while you sleep)?
- Would you consider it unreasonable to ask the rest of your family to make the changes required by this diet?
- Are there other products and supplements being sold as part of the diet?
- Does the diet ignore the fact that a calorie is a calorie, no matter what food group it comes from?
- Does the diet exclude all tasty foods that appeal to you?

Recommendations

Almost any diet will work at first, giving you short-term improvement, if it reduces your calorie intake. Long-term improvements are much more important and harder to achieve. Successful weight loss can be difficult, but the benefits are well worth the investment. As an editorial in the November 1999 *Journal of the American Medical Association* noted: "Far too many people appear to have accepted the determinants of the problems of overweight and inactivity, and rely on 'treatments' in the forms of myriad ineffective diet remedies and nostrums. As with many health issues, it is essential to emphasize prevention as the only effective and cost-effective approach."

Christians should be especially motivated to keep their weight within healthy limits. Food is part of God's creation, to be received with gratitude and shared with others (1 Timothy 4:3–5). Food is one of God's general provisions through which we can experience his loving care for us. Jesus said, "So do not worry, saying, 'What shall we eat?' or 'What shall we drink?' or 'What shall we wear?' For the pagans run after all these things, and your heavenly Father knows that you need them" (Matthew 6:31–32).

Eating food can be a pleasant experience. Meals provide important times for building relationships among family and friends, socializing, and serving others.

But, like all good things, food can be abused. Overeating harms the body and can shorten the time we have been given on this earth to glorify God and serve others. People become overweight for many reasons, some of which are beyond their control. However, we cannot ignore the fact that overeating is more times than not an individual decision and sometimes plain old sin. The Bible views gluttony as immoral and links it with drunkenness. "Do not join those who drink too much wine or gorge themselves on meat, for drunkards and gluttons become poor, and drowsiness clothes them in rags" (Proverbs 23:20–21; see also Deuteronomy 21:20).

In condemning any sinful behavior, we must be quick to remember that "all have sinned and fall short of the glory of God" (Romans 3:23). Gluttony is just one of many ways we demonstrate our selfishness and rebellion. Instead of Jesus Christ being Lord of our lives, for some "their god is their stomach" (Philippians 3:19). This leads us into slavery to our appetites and neglect of others' needs.

We in the developed world have become so rich we are dying from eating too much. Millions of others are dying from having nothing to eat. To paraphrase 1 John 3:17, how does the love of God abide in those who have most of the world's food and close their hearts against those who are hungry?

Galatians 5 lists the sins of the flesh and the fruit of the Spirit. Among the sins is a Greek word translated "orgies" (v. 21), which actually describes wild parties involving drunkenness, fornication, and overeating. In contrast is "self-control" (v. 23), which involves keeping all our sensual appetites in check. The consequences of overindulging in alcohol, or not keeping our sexual appetites under control, are more serious and clearly visible. Yet we are called to allow the Holy Spirit to help us control our eating habits.

The fact that God is concerned about our weight should be a source of hope. God is with us in our attempts to get this area of our lives under control. We should approach this as we would any other area of character change, involving prayer, fellowship, and guidance from other Christians. We should also avoid legalistic approaches, or making ourselves feel guilty. Arbitrary rules and negative treatment of one's body "lack any value in restraining sensual indulgence" (Colossians 2:23).

Christ came to bring us freedom, not put us under bondage. But this does not give us license to do whatever we feel like doing. "Do not offer the parts of your body to sin, as instruments of wickedness, but rather offer yourselves to God, as those who have been brought from death to life; and offer the parts of your body to him as instruments of righteousness. For sin shall not be your master, because you are not under law, but under grace" (Romans 6:13–14). We need to show grace to ourselves and others who struggle with weight issues.

The best overall approach to losing weight is on low-tech, old-fashioned principles: eat fewer calories, become more active, enlist the support of others, and evaluate yourself for the sin of gluttony. Make the physical, mental, and spiritual changes that can help you eat a more healthy diet. Keep in mind the following:

- You are embarking on a challenging activity. Don't expect it to be easy, and don't be surprised that some days will be harder than others.
- Focus on changes that reduce "bad" fats, "bad" carbohydrates, and overall calories, especially by increasing consumption of "good" sources of protein and fat, and "good" or complex carbohydrates, such as stone-ground whole grains, as well as fruits and vegetables.

- Make changes that you can envision becoming part of your new lifestyle (like adding a fruit to your breakfast) as opposed to strategies you know cannot last long (like eating cabbage soup all day).
- Move your body more. Every activity uses up calories (walk over to talk to someone rather than using the phone). Find an exercise that you like and someone you like to do it with. Being accountable to another person helps.

As iron sharpens iron, so one man sharpens another.

Proverbs 27:17

If one falls down, his friend can help him up. But pity the man who falls and has no one to help him up!

Ecclesiastes 4:10

- Set reasonable goals and take small steps in that direction, rather than trying to take giant leaps (replace one of your daily cans of pop with sparkling water rather than quitting soda all at once).
- Enjoy the food you can eat, and give thanks for having it, as opposed to focusing on what you've chosen not to eat.
- If you slip up, don't give up. Admit what you did, show yourself some grace, and set a new goal.
- Find a way to keep yourself accountable, one which also allows you to see your progress (like a food journal, "coach," or support group).
- Enlist the help, support, and prayers of your spouse, family, and church members. The changes you are making should be healthy for everyone, and you will benefit from their support.
- Change your thinking from "I'm going on a diet" to "I'm going to improve my eating habits" or "I'm going to take better care of my body."
- Eat breakfast every day. Have a nutritious lunch. Keep dinner the smallest meal of the day and try to eat it as early in the evening as possible. Some call this the "royal" nutrition plan: eat breakfast like a king, lunch like a queen, and dinner like a pauper.
- Increase the amount of water you drink every day.

Further Reading

Cleland, Richard, Dean C. Graybill, Van Hubbard, Laura Kettel Khan, Judith S. Stern, Thomas A. Wadden, Roland Weinsier, and Susan Yanovski, *Commercial Weight Loss Products and Programs: What Consumers Stand to Gain and Lose* (Washington, D.C.: Federal Trade Commission, Bureau of Consumer Protection, 1998). Available at *www.ftc.gov/os/1998/9803/weightlo.rpt.html* (accessed March 23, 2001).

Kayman, Susan, William Bruvold, and Judith S. Stern, "Maintenance and Relapse after Weight Loss in Women: Behavioral Aspects," *American Journal of Clinical Nutrition* 52 (1990): 800–807.

Koplan, Jeffrey P., and William H. Dietz, "Caloric Imbalance and Public Health Policy," *Journal of the American Medical Association* 282, no. 16 (October 1999): 1579–81.

Mokdad, Ali H., Mary K. Serdula, William H. Dietz, Barbara A. Bowman, James S. Marks, and Jeffrey P. Koplan, "The Spread of the Obesity Epidemic in the United States, 1991–1999," *Journal of the American Medical Association* 282, no. 16 (October 1999): 1519–22.

Pierre, Colleen, "Is There Wisdom in Those Wacky Diets," *Prevention* 52, no. 6 (June 2000): 142–47, 208–11.

Rippe, James M., Suellyn Crossley, and Rhonda Ringer, "Obesity as a Chronic Disease: Modern Medical and Lifestyle Management," *Journal of the American Dietetic Association* 10, suppl. 2 (October 1998): S9–S15.

Serdula, Mary K., Ali H. Mokdad, David F. Williamson, Deborah A. Galuska, James M. Mendlein, and Gregory W. Heath, "Prevalence of Attempting Weight Loss and Strategies for Controlling Weight," *Journal of the American Medical Association* 282, no. 14 (October 1999): 1353–58.

Stein, Joel, "The Low-Carb Diet Craze," *Time* 154, no. 18 (November 1, 1999): 72–79.

ENERGY MEDICINE

What It Is

Energy medicine is a broad field covering a variety of therapies from many parts of the world. While each is based on the existence of a nonphysical energy pervading the universe, the nature of the energy, the form of the therapies, and how healing is believed to take place varies from culture to culture.

Energy medicine has traditionally been a part of Eastern medicine, little utilized or discussed in the United States until the 1970s. Then, with the opening of relations with China, the news media introduced the Western world to sights such as surgery where acupuncture seemed to be the only anesthetic. Acupuncture was heralded as a long-proven surgical anesthetic even though surgery itself was a skill very new to Chinese medicine, in contrast to its long history of use in the West. Reporters wrote glowing stories without carefully checking information that would have revealed that, in at least some cases, the acupuncture was used to *reduce* the amount of anesthetic required, not replace it. The reporters ignored the other supposed "miracle" of Chinese medicine:

doctors who claimed they performed surgical procedures on patients while the patients read aloud from the Little Red Book—*The Sayings of Chairman Mao*—to keep from feeling any pain.

The interest in everything Chinese was reinforced in 1977 with the release of the George Lucas movie *Star Wars.* With this came the idea of "The Force," an unseen, mystical, invisible energy or spirituality. The Force was both good and evil, the two being kept in balance, although at odds, and with either side able to triumph. Jedi knights embraced both sides, though in true Hollywood tradition, the knights were costumed like the actors in the early Western talking pictures. Westerns were frequently written as heroic morality tales, the bad guys dressing in black, the good guys dressing in white. The same was true for the costumes of the Jedi knights, the evil Darth Vader in black, his son and his son's teacher in white. The Force also did not allow for death. Instead, though your body was lost, you became one with the Force—stronger and able to communicate with the living when necessary.

The film quickly developed a cult following. Videotape was still in its infancy as a home entertainment medium, so cassettes were not yet available for purchase. It was common for teenagers to see the movie twenty-five, thirty times, and more. Status in some high schools was determined in part by how many times a student had seen the film in the first few weeks of its release.

Soon, the concept of the Force was being used in sermons and theological discussions by people apparently not well versed in theology. Some people started to refer to the Force as a reality, not the creation of a writer's imagination. Newspapers reported religious groups evolving around the idea, and though they were short-lived, the "truth" of the film as interpreted by the naïve and impressionable lingered. That generation has now grown to adulthood, and if you look at many who have sought one form of energy medicine or another, they are within that age group. It is presumed that though they are older, wiser, and probably now recognize the Force as a theatrical fantasy, they remain intrigued by the possibilities inherent in the philosophies of some of the different energy medicines.

Because energy medicine permeates so many different cultures, the names used for the energy vary from culture to culture. The energy is called *chi* (sometimes spelled *qi*) in traditional Chinese medicine, *prana* in Indian Ayurvedic medicine, *ki* in Japanese practices, and a variety of other names in Western history, like orgone and bioenergy. Biofield is a new term chosen for this energy by the National Center for Complementary and Alternative Medicine in the United States.

Although the details vary, this energy is believed to pervade the universe, but takes on a particular form in each person called the "human energy field" (HEF). According to these theories, the HEF, or human aura, contains a number of layers, each with energy of differing frequencies. The energy is transformed between layers, and eventually into the physical body, via structures called *"chakras."* These are shaped like a whirlpool, with seven major ones located around the spine and head. Illness is believed to begin with disturbances of the energy field that are eventually transferred to the physical or emotional realm. In energy medicine, the HEF must be treated first. According to practitioners, once the HEF is balanced and energy flows properly, true healing can occur.

Historical Development

Throughout the nineteenth and twentieth centuries, claims were made that the HEF had been detected and identified as a form of electromagnetic radiation (of which light, heat, and infrared radiation are familiar examples). Franz Anton Mesmer (1734–1815) claimed that health was dependent on "animal magnetism." He used magnets in his healing sessions, but later claimed he only needed his hands, engaging in the practice we today call hypnosis. His approach is the source of the contemporary term "mesmerized."

Wilhelm Reich (1897–1957), a psychiatrist and colleague of Freud's, also claimed to identify the HEF. He called his energy "orgone," saying it was a universal life energy that he could generate by devices he sold, called "orgone boxes." In a scandal around the time of his death, one of the orgone boxes, allegedly made to his specifications, was taken apart and examined. The box contained little more than a lightbulb activated when the box was plugged in. Whether Reich, a follower, or someone else was perpetrating such a scam is unknown. The orgone box fell into disfavor with even those individuals who followed Reich's theories, and manufacture was stopped. Reich had claimed he could use his orgone to heal and even produce living cells from inanimate matter. These claims were never independently verified.

In the early 1900s, Walter J. Kilner, a London physician, invented a special screen filled with a dye made from coal tar which he said allowed people to see one another's auras. Goggles based on these screens are still sold. When you look through these screens, people do have a colored aura. However, scientists have shown that this is caused by the dye used, which allows only blue and red light to pass through. Since these regions of the light spectrum do not exactly overlap, they give the impression of separate auras around a person. It is a little like the effect of looking at a 1950s 3-D comic book. Without the special glasses needed to look at the picture in three dimensions, the illustrations are merely a series of slightly separated lines of different colors.

"Proof" of the life energy field was again claimed by Semyon and Valentina Kirlian in the 1960s. These Russian researchers, working with concepts first developed in the 1890s, claimed to be able to photograph energy fields. What are now known as Kirlian photographs allegedly capture images of life energy, also called "bioplasma." These images show auras and streams of light coming out from people's hands or even from the leaves of plants. The intensity, shape, and color of these shapes are said to provide valuable information on the health of the person or organism.

Problems arise when these admittedly dramatic Kirlian photographs are investigated by independent scientists. The replication of the reported studies shows that the images have a completely physical explanation. For example, by varying factors such as the moisture level of the object photographed, the pressure exerted on the photographic film, the length of exposure, and the type of film used, the color, shape, size, and intensity of the resulting image changes. To be a diagnostic aid, recording the same life energy field using the same film should have a consistently reproducible result. This does not occur.

Additionally, Kirlian auras have been recorded for things like pennies, paper clips, and water droplets, none of which are said to have a life energy field. This shows that such auras are not solely related to features of living organisms.

In spite of all this evidence, proponents of energy medicine still claim that Kirlian photography provides objective evidence of the existence of the HEF. Some proponents of life energy therapies will admit there is no objective evidence for the existence of life energy or the HEF. Their belief becomes a faith issue that has no basis in demonstrable fact.

In contrast, electromagnetic radiation can be detected in, and does emanate from, the human body. Many conventional diagnostic techniques make use of these effects, such as EEGs and EKGs. However, these are not what energy medicine means by its HEF. Electromagnetic energies can be detected, generated, and studied objectively, while such studies have never been done with life energy.

The Human Energy Field

Since the HEF cannot be detected objectively, meditation becomes an important aspect of energy medicine. During meditation, practitioners are believed to reach a higher level of awareness that allows them to sense the HEF. Some practitioners claim that their use of meditation allows them to reach a state where they are more attuned to the universal energy field and better able to detect problems with someone's energy. Some claim that within this state they can then actually see the HEF and receive guidance for the healing. The guidance may be intuitive, along the lines of what Dr. Edward Bach believed when developing his Bach Flower Therapy, or it may be directly from spiritual guides who provide information to practitioners, such as with Reiki.

Many practitioners of energy medicine say that the HEF is divided into seven layers, or bodies. Each layer deals with different aspects of the person, some having more to do with physical, emotional, mental, or spiritual issues. The healing which a practitioner will suggest may have as much to do with emotional or spiritual issues as it does with the physical symptoms someone may be experiencing. (See other therapies based exclusively on energy medicine, such as Qigong, Reiki, Tai Chi, and Therapeutic Touch. These principles play varying roles in all other traditional Chinese and Indian medicine.)

Study Findings

While instruments may not be able to detect the HEF, it is still possible to design studies to test whether people can detect the HEF, whatever it might be. During the 1970s, a well-known English psychic healer, Matthew Manning, claimed to be able to see human auras even if he was separated from the subject by a closed door. A test was devised using such a closed-door technique, a test Manning felt was fair. Manning believed he would be able to see the aura of someone on the opposite side of the closed door, standing flush against it. He also believed he would be able to tell if the person moved away from the closed door because the aura would fade as the person walked away until it became undetectable.

If you or I took such a test and only had to state whether or not a person was close enough to see the aura, chance would ultimately allow us to make the right guess about half the time. Someone who really could see the aura should have a far higher success rate. When the Manning experiment was done (✘✘), he was found to have given the correct answer just half the time. His success rate was no better than that of someone guessing or flipping a coin (see Tart and Palmer's article, under Further Reading).

In a more recent test, ten people who claimed to be able to see human auras were given a chance to prove their abilities. Among the subjects were five individuals who earned some of their living as professional psychic healers.

Four identical screens were placed in a room with volunteers who took turns standing behind one or another of them. The people being tested believed they could detect each volunteer's aura and determine which screen he or she was behind. The results: 185 correct answers out of 720 attempts.

As a control, ten other people who made no claim to any special abilities and who had no experience with the HEF were tested in exactly the same way (✘✘✘). Again there were 720 attempts. This time, there were 196 correct attempts, eleven more than by individuals who were certain they could detect auras. The two best individual scores among all the people tested were 50 percent and 40 percent correct. These were achieved by two of the ten people in the control group, who claimed no ability to detect auras, not those who were convinced they could see auras.

The test of Therapeutic Touch practitioners by Emily Rosa, a fourth-grader, also counts as evidence against people's ability to detect the HEF. This study (✘✘) got much publicity after it was published in the April 1, 1998, *Journal of the American Medical Association*. Twenty-one Therapeutic Touch practitioners sat behind a screen with Emily on the other side. They put both their hands through the screen, palms open and facing up. They claimed they would be able to detect Emily's aura if she held one of her hands above one of theirs. They got the answer correct 44 percent of the time, which is again about what would be expected by chance.

Cautions

While scientific evidence does not support the existence of an HEF, or the effectiveness of many of energy medicine's therapies, there are still concerns. Energy medicine practitioners often do not separate spiritual from physical healing, and therefore spiritual practices are completely intertwined with the healing efforts of most of these practitioners. Therapies used in energy medicine often cannot be separated from the philosophical and religious beliefs underlying the practices. These practitioners will claim to rebalance one's aura by involving spiritual forces that they claim are poorly understood. While they may believe these are impersonal energies being used for our chosen purposes, there is no way to know if this is the case.

In our opinion, people who subject themselves to energy medicine are exposing themselves to real spiritual forces over which they have little control. This creates a serious problem for Christians who are told in 1 John 4:1 to "test the spirits to see whether they are from God, because many false prophets have gone out into the world." We should have no involvement with spiritual beings or forces other than those who clearly proclaim Jesus Christ as Lord and Savior.

While most concerns with the different energy medicine therapies are primarily spiritual, some specific therapies can have other adverse physiological and psychological effects. These are noted where appropriate in the discussions of the individual therapies.

Recommendations

The whole area of energy medicine is based on ideas and beliefs that are rooted in Eastern religions and esoteric Western philosophy. These beliefs are often in direct conflict with Christian teaching. The practices may expose people to spiritual forces that are not of God.

In general, Christians should completely avoid energy medicine. However, some therapies that have arisen within these belief systems include a physical component. Acupuncture is an example. We believe a therapy like acupuncture can be separated from the energy medicine philosophy. Medical doctors, including some Christian medical doctors, use this sort of therapy along with conventional medicine and reject the philosophy professed by its Eastern practitioners. In those cases where there is good evidence that these therapies work, they may be worth considering. However, you should remain alert to the possibility that you may hear some different religious ideas from some practitioners.

On the other hand, most therapies based on energy medicine do not involve physical contact, although sometimes it is used in addition to energy manipulation. Therapeutic Touch and Reiki are examples. These therapies are so completely intertwined with energy manipulating approaches that they should not be used by Christians under any circumstances. Practitioners who offer these therapies to patients should make the religious roots of the therapy very clear.

Treatment Categories

Scientifically Unproven
    For any indication   ☹☹☹

Scientifically Questionable

Energy Medicine

Quackery or Fraud
    In the hands of some practitioners

Further Reading

Albrecht, Mark, and Brooks Alexander, "The Sellout of Science," *Spritual Counterfeits Project Journal* 2, no. 1 (August 1978): 18–28.

Fish, Sharon, "Therapeutic Touch: Healing Science or Mystical Midwife?" *Christian Research Journal* 12 (1995): 28–38.

Tart, C. T., and J. Palmer, "Some Psi Experiments with Matthew Manning," *Journal of the Society for Psychical Research* 50 (January 1979): 224–28.

GERSON DIET THERAPY

What It Is

Dr. Max Gerson was a German physician during World War II when attention to routine medical research and pharmaceuticals was essentially put on hold. His focus was nutrition, an interest he had developed when plagued with migraine headaches. He discovered that he could manipulate his diet to ease or eliminate his headaches, a concept still in practice today now that we know the role of serotonin in migraine.

Next came a special diet for tuberculosis sufferers, and finally a diet for cancer patients. He fled the Nazis, came to the United States, and first published his research in English in 1945. However, the conventional medical community rejected his ideas so he moved to Mexico to found the Gerson Clinic. A cancer patient either had to travel to Mexico or attend a series of seminars he and his staff routinely gave in the United States. The latter were the result of his firm belief that he had found the answer to cancer in people's diet. He was convinced he could save lives that otherwise would be lost.

The Gerson Diet is actually the oldest of a group of alternative treatments called metabolic therapies, many of which are named for their creators: Kelley, Manner,

Contreras, and Gonzalez. Macrobiotics involves many similar approaches, but is based on the philosophy of traditional Chinese medicine.

Gerson's diet arose from his belief that cancer is primarily caused by changes in dietary patterns as countries become more developed and more affluent. People, he believed, simultaneously poison themselves with the chemicals found in foods grown using pesticides and artificial fertilizers, and starve themselves of vital nutrients and vitamins by using processed and poorly prepared food.

The Gerson Diet has the patient use freshly prepared vegetable juices made by pressing organically grown products. Until 1989, raw liver juice was also used, but this concept was abandoned after it was found that a number of patients suffered serious adverse reactions to contaminants in the juice.

About twenty pounds of fruits and vegetables are consumed each day by drinking a glass of freshly prepared juice every hour. Supplements are added to aid digestion or replenish vitamins. Castor oil is taken to cleanse the system, as are coffee enemas that are believed to relieve the pain from the cancer. The coffee enema routine starts with a rather intense cleansing ritual requiring their use every four hours. In addition, counseling, group therapy, and family support are strongly encouraged.

Claims

The most common claim for the Gerson Diet is that it cures cancer, but it is also said to cure many other diseases, and to lead to more vigor and vitality in those who are healthy.

Study Findings

Conventional medicine has remained skeptical of claims that the Gerson Diet actually cures cancer. There is no question that a change in diet can help many people feel better (✔✔✔), and diet has been shown to be an important factor in the *prevention* of cancer (✔✔). But *curing* cancer through dietary changes is a different matter.

The principal evidence for this diet was published in a book in which Max Gerson detailed fifty of his best case histories. This anecdotal information (✔) by the physician who developed the concept remains the most common form of evidence cited in favor of the diet. However, such personal stories are the least reliable form of evidence for a therapy because of all the other possible factors involved in causing improvement, especially with a disease like cancer.

In 1995, a more scientific study (✔✔) involving melanoma, a type of skin cancer, was published by Gar Hildenbrand and colleagues employed by the Gerson Research Center and a statistician. They found that melanoma patients had better survival rates using the Gerson Diet than those treated with conventional therapies. Criticism of the study was immediate because it was not a randomized, controlled trial that could be replicated by others. Rather, the researchers picked the charts of all Gerson Clinic patients with melanomas to investigate how they had fared after treatment. Approximately 25 percent of the patients had moved from their last known address and could not be interviewed, so they were left out of the analysis. It is possible that the patients who could not be found fared poorly on the diet, their change of address a result of deteriorating health or even death. These omissions could have considerably skewed the results in favor of the therapy.

Even with the information reported by the researchers, it is not possible to determine whether the diet was of benefit or not. The researchers admit that the patients used many other alternative and conventional therapies, including mind-body therapies, herbal remedies, homeopathy, and conventional surgery. They also admit that while at the Gerson Clinic, patients received psychological interventions and family support, and achieved a sense of control from mastering the diet. Any improvements that occurred may have had as much to do with these factors as with the diet. The researchers stated in their report: "These cases are not held out by us as evidence that here is a 'cure' for cancer, but rather that some patients can get well." Yet many claim the Gerson Diet is a cure for cancer, even though this is not supported by the evidence.

Cautions

Patients already weakened by cancer, and possibly by conventional therapies, should be very cautious about embarking on the drastic changes involved in the Gerson Diet. Patients often suffer diarrhea, vomiting, and skin sores. Frequent use of enemas can cause dehydration and damage to the colon, resulting in severe constipation. The diet, combined with enemas, can result in dehydration and electrolyte imbalances, which can cause serious problems. Adhering to the diet is burdensome and time consuming, and can be very expensive, especially if done as an inpatient at one of the specialized clinics.

Recommendations

Very little evidence supports the claims that the Gerson Diet or any of the other cancer diets listed earlier can cure cancer. The American Cancer Society urges people with cancer not to attempt these types of diets, especially if they are pursued in place of conventional therapies known to be effective.

Treatment Categories

Complementary Therapy
    For its psychological and relational component
        as well as the fact that it encourages dietary habits
        which may be more healthy than previous ones   ☺☺☺

Scientifically Unproven
    As a cure for cancer   ☹☹☹

Scientifically Questionable

Quackery or Fraud

In the hands of some practitioners

Further Reading

Cassileth, Barrie, "Metabolic Therapies," *The Alternative Medicine Handbook* (New York: W. W. Norton, 1998), 186–89.

Gerson, Max, *A Cancer Therapy: Results of Fifty Cases and the Cure of Advanced Cancer by Diet Therapy*, 5th ed. (Bonita, Calif.: Gerson Institute, 1990).

Hildenbrand, G. L. Gar, L. Christeene Hildenbrand, Karen Bradford, and Shirley W. Cavin, "Five-Year Survival Rates of Melanoma Patients Treated by Diet Therapy After the Manner of Gerson," *Alternative Therapies in Health and Medicine* 1, no. 4 (September 1995): 29–37.

HALLELUJAH DIET

What It Is

In 1976, the Rev. George H. Malkmus stopped eating meat, processed food, and cooked food. He had been diagnosed with colon cancer at the age of forty-two and was devastated. Having watched his mother die an agonizing death from colon cancer while undergoing conventional chemotherapy, he chose a different route. A Christian friend told him to eat only raw fruits and vegetables, especially lots of carrot juice. That's what he did, and a year later his cancer had gone from the size of a baseball to hardly detectable. What's more, he claimed the diet also got rid of his hemorrhoids, low blood sugar, allergies, sinus problems, high blood pressure, tiredness, pimples, colds, flu, body odor, and dandruff. He claims he has never been sick since, not visited a doctor, and not taken even an aspirin. The Rev. Malkmus reports a remarkable change in his health. He praises God for all these changes.

We provide a detailed evaluation of the Hallelujah Diet as an example of the problems that arise when Christians go beyond praising God for their recoveries and claim their improvements occurred because they discovered a new "Christian therapy." The Rev. Malkmus believes he is living the way God wants all people to live. He believes God's plan for all humans is found in Genesis 1:29: "Then God said, 'I give you every seed-bearing plant on the face of the whole earth and every tree that has fruit with seed in it. They will be yours for food.'" He interprets this verse as teaching that God designed humans to be vegetarians and that we poison our bodies when we eat other foods. We consider this teaching less than the full counsel of God's Word. Some have called this teaching a heresy.

Malkmus points out that of all the animals on earth, only humans cook their food. He believes cooking destroys 80 percent of the nutrients in the raw foods. Any preservatives, coloring agents, flavorings, and other additives, he believes, will poison us. We get sick and go to physicians who give us pharmaceuticals that he considers to be nothing more than additional toxins. Christians, he says, turn to God in prayer for healing, then wonder why he doesn't provide a cure. The problem, Malkmus says, is not with God, but with what we put into our bodies.

A diet of only raw fruits and vegetables. Malkmus promotes the Hallelujah Diet as his way to help all Christians restore their health. According to his diet plan, we need to eliminate everything from our diet except raw fruits and vegetables. Malkmus teaches (in newsletters available on his Website) that the nutrients are in the raw liquid part of fruits and vegetables. His March 17, 2000, newsletter stated: "Just as the life of the flesh is in the blood, the life of the plant is in the blood (or liquid part) of the plant." The fruits and vegetables must be put in a blender or juicer and consumed shortly after being prepared. Malkmus recently adjusted his recommendations to allow 15 percent of one's food to be cooked, the reasoning of which is not clear, given his theological assumptions.

Supplements. Malkmus recommends and sells two supplements: vitamin B_{12} and Barleygreen, a powder made from barley grass *(Hordeum distichon)*. The Barleygreen™ is made by making a juice from barley, adding maltodextrin (a carbohydrate), and drying the mixture through a process called "freeze-drying." He claims the maltodextrin prevents the juice's enzymes from decomposing the active ingredients. For some reason, this whole processing of the barley does not constitute the "food processing" Malkmus denounces.

The resulting green powder is believed by Malkmus to stimulate the immune system and rebuild all tissues of the body. He recommends people take three to four tablespoonfuls per day. He reports testimonies of many people claiming great medical benefits within just a few days of taking the supplement. The *PDR for Herbal Medicines* does not give any studies to support the medicinal use of barley, and reports only one unproven use: that some people claim barley is soothing on the digestive system.

Exercise. The final aspect to the Hallelujah Diet is exercise. Malkmus exercises for about an hour each day, varying his activity among walking, jogging, and exercise machines. He also recommends that people drink plenty of water, but only distilled water—as he believes regular water contains harmful contaminants.

All these dietary recommendations must be accompanied by a living relationship with Jesus Christ. Malkmus is very clear that the Hallelujah Diet does not connect someone with God or make someone more acceptable to God. In a Website article entitled "An Interview with Rev. George Malkmus," Malkmus stated: "Now I do acknowledge and believe that a raw vegetarian diet will heighten our awareness of God by cleaning out the body/temple and bringing us closer to His creation! But I do not believe that the vegetarian diet or lifestyle is the basis for our relationship or connection with God! This comes only by faith through Jesus Christ!"

Claims

In his February 25, 2000, newsletter, the Rev. Malkmus reported that he had already spoken twelve times that year. "In almost every meeting people told of cancers, diabetes, arthritis, fibromyalgia, high blood pressure, and other health problems simply going away after adopting the Hallelujah Diet. Many told of losing weight on our program, with at least a dozen who had lost over 70 pounds." He claims that just about every sickness and illness can be prevented or cured if people "change from the world's diet of dead food to God's Diet of living food."

It is one thing to claim that eating more fruits and vegetables will help make us healthier, or that people who eat more food from animals tend to have more of one disease or another. What Malkmus claims in a Web article entitled "God's Original Diet" goes well beyond this. "Almost every physical problem, other than accidents," Malkmus insists, "is caused by improper diet and lifestyle...and that if we will but change to a higher grade of fuel—raw food—the body will usually heal itself of whatever ails it!"

What Malkmus offers instead is equally dramatic. He states in another article, "God's Way to Ultimate Health," that he wants people, especially Christians, to believe that, "Truly, WE DON'T HAVE TO BE SICK! That disease and sickness are self-inflicted!" (emphasis in original).

Malkmus states in "The Hallelujah Diet FAQ" that the solution to all our health problems is simple: stop eating animal products and cooked food. "We see well over 90% of all physical problems just disappear in six months or less."

Study Findings

The Rev. Malkmus has in the past claimed to have research studies to back up his medical claims. However, in his January 25, 2001, newsletter, he gave the following reply to a letter writer who had requested research support for claims made regarding the Hallelujah Diet: "What you are seeking, for all intents and purposes, does not exist! It has been a great frustration to me through the years that practically no scientific research has been done to support or disprove RAW vegetarianism."

Malkmus offers only anecdotal evidence (✔). His literature focuses on stories from satisfied patients whose letters he quotes. These testimonials describe how, because of the Hallelujah Diet, people feel completely freed from old aches and pains, how most have more energy, and how people have been cured of heart disease, cancer, multiple sclerosis, and just about every disease imaginable.

Malkmus also takes anecdotal evidence from the Bible. He claims that all humans were vegetarians before the Flood and lived an average of 912 years without sickness.

Immediately after the Flood, God told Noah, "Everything that lives and moves will be food for you. Just as I gave you the green plants, I now give you everything. But you must not eat meat that has its lifeblood still in it" (Genesis 9:3–4).

Malkmus claims humans first ate meat at this point, and their health rapidly began to decline. Man's life span went from an average of 912 years to 100 years by the end of Genesis.

There is mounting evidence that a vegetarian diet can have health benefits. A 1999 review by Key of all the large epidemiological studies (✔✔) comparing vegetarians and nonvegetarians living in Western cultures found some interesting results. The death rate from ischemic heart disease (which includes atherosclerosis and angina) was 25 percent less for long-term vegetarians (those who had consumed no meat or milk for at least five years) than nonvegetarians. Ironically, those who had been vegetarians less than five years had a 20 percent higher death rate from heart attacks than nonvegetarians. One explanation could be that they became vegetarians because of heart problems. Overall, this is an important factor favoring vegetarianism.

However, this same review found no differences in the death rates of vegetarians and nonvegetarians from strokes, stomach cancer, colorectal cancer, lung cancer, breast cancer, prostate cancer, or all other causes combined. Overall, there was a 5 percent reduction in death rates among vegetarians, due completely to the lower death rate from ischemic heart disease. The Hallelujah Diet is more restrictive than the vegetarian diets used in these studies, so results may be somewhat different. However, these are very significant findings that directly contradict what Malkmus claims: that the Hallelujah Diet will eliminate all sickness.

Theological Evaluation

The question of whether God wants people to be vegetarians has come up again and again throughout the history of Christianity. The first thing to point out is that Genesis 1:29 declares that plants are given to humans as food. It does not command that humans eat only fruits and vegetables, nor does it forbid the eating of meat. Such an interpretation is as absurd as a teenager saying, after her father gives her the keys to her first car, "Oh, so this means I'm not allowed to drive any other car but this one?"

We are told nothing about how Adam and Eve fed themselves, but the first thing we are told about their children was, "Abel kept flocks, and Cain worked the soil" (Genesis 4:2). Cain sacrificed some of his crops to the Lord, while Abel sacrificed the firstlings of his flock. Theologians have assumed that each sacrificed to God what they used for food.

While we are not told that they ate meat, their actions are more understandable if meat was eaten. After Cain killed Abel, God's punishment included: "When you work the ground, it will no longer yield its crops for you. You will be a restless wanderer on the earth" (Genesis 4:12). Such wandering without crops suggests to many theologians that Cain would have to nourish himself, at least in part, from his livestock such as nomadic tribes still do to this day.

Six generations later, Jabal is described as "the father of those who live in tents and raise livestock" (Genesis 4:20). It is reasonable to infer that these herdsmen would have used some of the products from their animals as nourishment. And when Noah enters the ark, God tells him, "Take with you seven of every kind of clean animal, a male and its mate, and two of every kind of unclean animal, a male and its mate" (Genesis 7:2). The distinction between clean and unclean only seems to make sense if some were eaten and others were not.

We admit that the evidence is not conclusive that humans ate meat before the Flood, and some theologians believe that humans were vegetarians before the flood of Noah. However, all the comments we just reviewed show that we cannot rule out the possibility that some humans did eat some meat.

After the Flood, God makes a declaration just as clear as his one about plants in Genesis 1: "The fear and dread of you will fall upon all the beasts of the earth and all the birds of the air, upon every creature that moves along the ground, and upon all the fish of the sea; they are given into your hands. Everything that lives and moves will be food for you. Just as I gave you the green plants, I now give you everything. But you must not eat meat that has its lifeblood still in it" (Genesis 9:2–4).

Again, this does not command people to eat meat, fish, and fowl, but states that they may be eaten, so long as their blood is not consumed. Soon afterward Abraham, the father of the Israelites, welcomes three guests whom many theologians believe were the Lord and two angels. As was the custom of the day, Abraham and Sarah (his wife) prepared a meal to honor the guests.

> So Abraham hurried into the tent to Sarah. "Quick," he said, "get three seahs of fine flour and knead it and bake some bread." Then he ran to the herd and selected a choice, tender calf and gave it to a servant, who hurried to prepare it. He then brought some curds and milk and the calf that had been prepared, and set these before them. While they ate, he stood near them under a tree.
>
> Genesis 18:6–8

This group of heavenly visitors ate meat and other cooked food, washing it all down with milk—an animal product.

When Abraham's son Isaac was an old man, he called for his son Esau: "Now then, get your weapons . . . to hunt some wild game for me. Prepare me the kind of tasty food I like and bring it to me to eat, so that I may give you my blessing before I die" (Genesis 27:3–4). Without moral qualms, Isaac soon ate meat (Genesis 27:25).

During the exodus from Egypt, the Israelites complained about their food, so God said, "I have heard the grumbling of the Israelites. Tell them, 'At twilight you will eat meat, and in the morning you will be filled with bread. Then you will know that I am the

LORD your God'" (Exodus 16:12). That night, God sent them quail, an edible bird. Later, Moses received much direction from God about which animals could be eaten and which should not be eaten (e.g., Leviticus 11). Under God's law (the Mosaic covenant), the animal and grain sacrifices were to be the food for the priests. Meat was eaten at many of the special feasts and holidays, such as during Passover. God even instructed the Israelites how to cook the lamb: "Do not eat the meat raw or cooked in water, but roast it over the fire—head, legs and inner parts" (Exodus 12:9; see also Leviticus 6:24–26). If it was God's intention that humans never eat meat, it seems strange that he would provide such painstaking details in a number of places telling the Israelites which meats they should eat, which they shouldn't, and how to cook the meat.

We see numerous examples in the Gospels of people eating food that is not from plants. Concerning John the Baptist, "His food was locusts and wild honey" (Matthew 3:4). Jesus not only ate animal products, he gave them to others to eat (Matthew 15:32–38; John 21:12–13). The prophet Isaiah predicted of the Messiah, "He will eat curds and honey when he knows enough to reject the wrong and choose the right" (Isaiah 7:15). Curds are made from milk, and are similar to yogurt or butter.

The eating of clean and unclean animals was controversial during the early years of Christianity. Jewish Christians wanted to remain faithful to their traditional laws, but weren't sure if Gentile Christians should also be required to abstain from unclean foods. Peter received a vision of a large sheet. "It contained all kinds of four-footed animals, as well as reptiles of the earth and birds of the air. Then a voice told him, 'Get up, Peter. Kill and eat'" (Acts 10:12–13). Many of the animals were unclean, and when Peter pointed this out, he was told, three times, "Do not call anything impure that God has made clean" (Acts 10:15).

Peter explained that the dream showed that the Gentiles were not unclean in God's eyes: "But God has shown me that I should not call any man impure or unclean" (Acts 10:28; see also Acts 10:34; 11:1–15). Peter immediately began interacting with the Gentiles and even eating with them (Galatians 2:12).

This Scripture also shows that God removed the distinction between clean and unclean animals. Some of the Jewish Pharisees who became Christians taught that Gentile converts should keep the law of Moses. Peter used his dream to argue, "Now then, why do you try to test God by putting on the necks of the disciples a yoke that neither we nor our fathers have been able to bear?" (Acts 15:10).

As a result of these discussions, the apostles sent a letter to the Gentile converts in Asia Minor noting that they knew that messages instructing them to keep the dietary laws were disturbing the believers. The apostles' letter declared: "It seemed good to the Holy Spirit and to us not to burden you with anything beyond the following requirements: You are to abstain from food sacrificed to idols, from blood, from the meat of strangled animals and from sexual immorality. You will do well to avoid these things" (Acts 15:28–29). This would have been the perfect opportunity to tell the Gentiles not to eat meat, if that was to be the Christian teaching, but instead we find no prohibition of meat.

In Romans 14, Paul attacked the issue of eating meat directly by explaining that questions about diet (and which day to worship on) were "disputable matters"—in other words, there is no clear teaching from the Lord, and Christians can operate in these areas as led by the Holy Spirit. Both of these issues (the Sabbath and kosher dietary laws) were extremely important to practicing Jews. Paul, it seems to us, is teaching that no food, in and of itself, is unclean for Christians. He also seems to teach that restricting diet as a matter of faith may be evidence of a weak faith—not of a deep faith. To put your faith in a diet and not in God would be antithetical to Paul's teaching. Finally, Paul teaches that one's choice of food has to be kept in perspective. "For the kingdom of God is not a matter of eating and drinking, but of righteousness, peace and joy in the Holy Spirit, because anyone who serves Christ in this way is pleasing to God and approved by men" (Romans 14:17–18).

Elsewhere, Paul gives similar principles in responding to asceticism, where people deny themselves pleasures in the belief this makes them more acceptable to God. Paul tells Timothy to reject teachers who, among other things, call on people "to abstain from certain foods, which God created to be received with thanksgiving by those who believe and who know the truth. For everything God created is good, and nothing is to be rejected if it is received with thanksgiving, because it is consecrated by the word of God and prayer" (1 Timothy 4:3–5). Could Paul have been predicting teachers such as the Rev. Malkmus?

Elsewhere, Paul calls on Christians not to submit to those who declare, "Do not handle! Do not taste! Do not touch!" (Colossians 2:21). He goes on to point out that "such regulations indeed have an appearance of wisdom, with their self-imposed worship, their false humility and their harsh treatment of the body, but they lack any value in restraining sensual indulgence" (Colossians 2:23).

We see this borne out in the lives of those in the Bible who, according to the Rev. Malkmus, adhered to the Hallelujah Diet most closely. If we accept that those who lived prior to the Flood were strict vegetarians, we see that this brought them no advantage in terms of their overall spiritual health. In spite of eating only plants, and living hundreds of years, they became completely wicked. Their every intention was evil, so that "the LORD was grieved that he had made man on the earth, and his heart was filled with pain" (Genesis 6:6). As a result, he decided to judge and execute every human except Noah and his family.

Jesus explained to his followers that true righteousness has essentially nothing to do with what one puts in one's mouth. He taught that food does not defile us, but our heart does. He said, "What goes into a man's mouth does not make him 'unclean,' but what comes out of his mouth, that is what makes him 'unclean.' Don't you see that whatever enters the mouth goes into the stomach and then out of the body? But the things that come out of the mouth come from the heart, and these make a man 'unclean.' For out of the heart come evil thoughts, murder, adultery, sexual immorality, theft, false testimony, slander. These are what make a man 'unclean'; but eating with unwashed hands does not make him 'unclean'" (Matthew 15:11–20; see also Mark 7:1–23).

Should people today, for health reasons, not eat those animals listed in Scripture as unclean? The two of us do not agree on that issue. One of us (Walt Larimore) believes it is still a good health practice to reduce the consumption of or avoid these unclean animals; the other (Dónal O'Mathúna) does not. However, our preferences in this "disputable matter" are exactly that: our preferences. We should never teach either position as doctrine. Further, we should never let this preference be a stumbling block for others or, worse, a cause for division with others in the church. Jesus commanded his disciples to "eat what is set before you" (Luke 10:8). In teaching about eating meat and drinking wine, Paul says: "So whatever you believe about these things keep between yourself and God" (Romans 14:22).

The problem with Christian vegetarianism is not so much what Christians eat and don't eat. The problem is that it easily leads people to an external focus on factors that are not what the Bible teaches are the most important factors in this life. Jesus commanded us, "Do not worry about your life, what you will eat or drink; or about your body, what you will wear. Is not life more important than food, and the body more important than clothes?" (Matthew 6:25).

It is too easy to become overly consumed with eating the perfect foods and drinking the perfect beverages. Instead, we should "seek first his kingdom and his righteousness, and all these things will be given to you as well" (Matthew 6:33).

If God were so concerned about Christians being vegetarians, he would have made that clear to us in his Word. Yet throughout the Bible we see references to the eating of meat and animal products without any condemnation (1 Kings 4:22–23; Nehemiah 13:16; Proverbs 27:27; Luke 15:29). While we cannot be absolutely certain it was the Lord eating meat when visiting Abraham, we can be sure that Jesus cooked and ate fish and gave fish to others for them to eat. In so doing, Jesus was violating the Hallelujah Diet.

Even if we were to agree that humans were designed by God to be vegetarians, and are healthiest if we live that way, it seems to us that the Rev. Malkmus is not consistent in applying his interpretive principle. If we look back at the Genesis account, we learn some other things about Adam and Eve. We learn that Adam and Eve were naked until they sinned. Were humans designed not to wear clothes? Should Christians be nudists? Adam and Eve lived in a garden, and Adam spent his time naming the other creatures. Is this how all humans should spend their days? Should all Christians be farmers? Clearly, the interpretive principle upon which Malkmus bases his argument is flawed.

What the Rev. Malkmus ignores is the clear biblical evidence that God does not expect humans to adhere to something like the Hallelujah Diet. Paul declares: "Eat anything sold in the meat market without raising questions of conscience" (1 Corinthians 10:25). Scripture states that Christians can even eat meat that has been sacrificed to idols! Instead of declaring that Christians should not eat meat, Paul encourages the Corinthians to "eat whatever is put before you" (1 Corinthians 10:27).

Cautions

People consuming only plants for food must be careful not to develop deficiencies in certain nutrients. The Hokin and Butler study of Seventh-day Adventist ministers who had been vegetarians for many years found that almost three-quarters were deficient in vitamin B_{12} (called "cobalamin"). The only medical study published on the Hallelujah Diet (by Donaldson, a researcher employed by Malkmus) found that about half of a group of forty-nine people on this diet for two to four years were vitamin B_{12} deficient. Although the daily requirement for vitamin B_{12} is very small (about 1 to 2 micrograms per day), plants contain none. This raises the question of why God would want people to be vegetarians if he also created them requiring a vitamin available only from animal foods.

Vitamin B_{12} deficiency can lead to anemia and neurological problems, with symptoms progressing from numbness and tingling in the hands and feet, unsteadiness, moodiness, mental slowness, poor memory, confusion, agitation, and depression, all the way to delusions, hallucinations, and even psychosis. Women who are pregnant or nursing, and small children, are especially prone to develop vitamin B_{12} deficiencies when eating a purely vegetarian diet like the Hallelujah Diet.

To their credit, the authors of the Hallelujah Diet's Website acknowledge the risk of vitamin B_{12} deficiency, and recommend the use of supplements, especially sublingual tablets, which are conveniently sold on the site. (To our knowledge, there is no medical reason to take vitamin B_{12} in this expensive form.) Although these supplements are made in the same way as pharmaceutical drugs, the Rev. Malkmus recommends and sells them despite his teachings against drugs and processed foods.

Vegetarians must also be diligent to ensure they obtain an adequate dietary intake of calcium, vitamin D, and iron. This can easily be accomplished today because many foods are fortified with vitamins and minerals, but those following the strictly vegetarian Hallelujah Diet may not get enough of these nutrients. The Rev. Malkmus addressed issues related to calcium and vitamin D in his September 21, 28, and October 5, 2000, newsletters. He claims that since we need these nutrients, God must have put enough of them in plant foods. He claims that the belief that milk is essential for calcium and vitamin D is the result of a marketing conspiracy by the dairy food industry. He claims that animal and processed foods contain minerals in a "toxic" form. While we agree that many minerals are available from plants, and a vegetarian diet can be healthy, the Rev. Malkmus's approach may scare people away from some nutritious foods.

Another danger with the approach of the Rev. Malkmus is the way he discredits and discourages appropriate use of pharmaceuticals and physicians, as in a Web article entitled "Drugs: A Killer of Mankind." We readily admit that too many pharmaceuticals are used in the United States, and that some physicians fail to practice good medicine. But the Rev. Malkmus claims that the biblical teaching on physicians is summed up in Mark 5:25–26: "And a woman was there who had been subject to bleeding for twelve years.

She had suffered a great deal under the care of many doctors and had spent all she had, yet instead of getting better she grew worse." The Rev. Malkmus maintains that conventional medicine is dominated by false ideas and motivated by financial incentives.

He goes even further in discrediting pharmaceuticals, claiming that the biblical teaching on drugs is summed up in Revelation 18:23. This passage talks about the overthrow of Babylon, the epitome of evil, of how God will judge Babylon because of how negatively it influenced the world: "By your magic spell all the nations were led astray." The Greek word here for "magic spell" ("sorcery" in other translations) is *pharmakeia*. This is the word from which we get pharmacy in English.

This word did originally mean a drug (usually a poison). But long before the New Testament was written, the word *pharmakeia* came to mean "magical material" (sometimes including drugs) which was used for purposes of hate (see the article by biblical scholar Dr. Edwin Yamauchi). The word *pharmakeia* and those closely related to it are used only five times in the Bible (Galatians 5:20; Revelation 9:21; 18:23; 21:8; 22:15). The best translation of these words in all these instances is as "sorcery" or "sorcerer," as all major Bible translations render it. Virtually all the theologians who have published on this topic indicate that there is no good interpretive reason to believe that this verse denounces the use of medicinal agents. Another reason against that interpretation is that numerous other passages talk about the use of available medicinal agents in a positive light.

> From the sole of your foot to the top of your head
>   there is no soundness—
> only wounds and welts
>   and open sores,
> not cleansed or bandaged
>   or soothed with oil.
>
> Isaiah 1:6

> Babylon will suddenly fall and be broken.
>   Wail over her!
> Get balm for her pain;
>   perhaps she can be healed.
>
> Jeremiah 51:8; see also 8:22; 46:11

> [The Good Samaritan] went to him and bandaged his wounds, pouring on oil and wine.
> Luke 10:34

> Is any one of you sick? He should call the elders of the church to pray over him and anoint him with oil in the name of the Lord.
>
> James 5:14

We are concerned that the complete dismissal of conventional medicine and modern pharmaceuticals can and will lead to much harm. Most of the scriptural references to physicians say nothing negative (Jeremiah 8:22; Matthew 9:12; Luke 4:23) and Luke, who wrote both a Gospel and the book of Acts, was a physician (Colossians 4:14). Although certainly some modern therapies can cause harm, and all can be overused, many modern therapies do much good. What is needed is appropriate use of effective and safe therapies for those conditions for which they are indicated.

Recommendations

There are numerous ways in which people can and should change common dietary practices (see Diet and Nutrition, page 171). Many people could benefit from eating a more healthy, balanced, and a more natural diet, with fewer processed foods. But to do so does not necessitate becoming a vegetarian. Nor does it require abandoning the cooking of all foods. Christianity should bring new freedom to God's people. The life of Jesus fulfilled the Old Testament rituals and ceremonial laws so that now Christians are free. "It is for freedom that Christ has set us free. Stand firm, then, and do not let yourselves be burdened again by a yoke of slavery" (Galatians 5:1). The slavery mentioned here is to arbitrary laws and dogma regarding foods and other practices.

We must be careful how we exercise our freedom. In the context of dealing with the eating of meat, Paul states: "'Everything is permissible'—but not everything is beneficial. 'Everything is permissible'—but not everything is constructive" (1 Corinthians 10:23). We believe that the Bible clearly teaches that Christians have the freedom to eat meat, but not to overindulge in it. We should eat a healthy, balanced diet so that we can enjoy good health in this life, and thereby glorify God and serve others.

Our primary concern is not with vegetarianism. Christians are free to be vegetarians if they so choose. Our concern is with the way the Hallelujah Diet is presented as being "God's diet," giving scant biblical evidence and using questionable methods of interpretation. Paul told the Corinthians that when someone spoke out in God's name (as a prophet), "the others should weigh carefully what is said" (1 Corinthians 14:29). The Hallelujah Diet, and all others of that type, claim to give dietary guidance with the imprimatur of God. We feel obligated to disagree theologically and scientifically.

As in all areas of health, what is needed is balance. The Hallelujah Diet may bring some benefits, and probably will to those who previously ate inappropriately. In "God's Way to Ultimate Health," Malkmus claims, "All we have to do to be well is eat and live according to the way God intended!" By this he means adhere to the Hallelujah Diet. We respectfully disagree.

The focus for good health in the Hallelujah Diet is placed completely on the choices we make. Yet the reasons why we get sick are many and complicated, and often have nothing to do with our diet. We cannot realistically avoid all sickness and disease.

We concur with Dr. Michael Jacobson's ten "Warning Signs of Deception" when it comes to diets like the Hallelujah Diet, specifically, and to Christian alternative therapies in general:

1. Are people taught that God's ideal for man today is found only in Genesis 1:29, that is, that man is to be vegetarian? Or, that the therapy is "God's will for His church," even though it is not explicitly taught in Scripture?
2. Do people think or feel that they are not biblically free to eat flesh, animal products, or even "unclean" meat?
3. Do people believe that certain foods defile the body?
4. Do dietary practices interfere with fellowship or relationships? Do they become a divisive factor between the members of families or the congregation?
5. Is the therapy (or the diet) a common focus of conversation—even eclipsing a focus on Jesus?
6. Is the diet or the therapy promoted as *the* answer to anyone's health problem(s)?
7. Is the diet or therapy given the credit when healing takes place?
8. Is there a critical spirit toward others who do not use the diet or therapy?
9. Is there a critical spirit toward any in the medical profession who do not use or prescribe the diet or therapy?
10. Is there other evidence of involvement in deceptive practices?

The Hallelujah Diet offers some nutritional benefits, but there also are dangers—physically and spiritually. Before starting such a diet, understand the limitations of a vegetarian diet and the essential nutrients it does not provide, the risks you take. Make sure your decision to try the diet is based on health concerns, not the belief that God wants Christians to be vegetarians exclusively. We do not see that taught in the Bible.

If you decide to try the Hallelujah Diet, do so with joy, wisdom, and understanding. Do not do so dogmatically. And do not follow the teaching against conventional medicine and pharmaceuticals.

Treatment Categories

Complementary Therapy
    Physical   ☺
    Spiritual   ☹☹☹☹

Scientifically Unproven

Scientifically Questionable

Quackery or Fraud
    In the wrong hands

Further Reading

Donaldson, Michael S., "Metabolic Vitamin B_{12} Status on a Mostly Raw Vegan Diet with Follow-Up Using Tablets, Nutritional Yeast, or Probiotic Supplements," *Annals of Nutrition and Metabolism* 44, no. 5–6 (December 2000): 229–34.

Hokin, Bevan D., and Terry Butler, "Cyanocobalamin (Vitamin B-12) Status in Seventh-Day Adventist Ministers in Australia," *American Journal of Clinical Nutrition* 70, suppl. 3 (September 1999): 576S–578S.

Jacobson, Michael, *The Word on Health: A Biblical and Medical Overview of How to Care for Your Body* (Chicago: Moody Press, 2000).

Key, Timothy J., Gary E. Fraser, Margaret Thorogood, Paul N. Appleby, Valerie Beral, Gilliam Reeves, Michael L. Burr, Jenny Chang-Claude, Rainer Frenzel-Beyne, Jan W. Kuzma, Jim Mann, and Klim McPherson, "Mortality in Vegetarians and Nonvegetarians: Detailed Findings from a Collaborative Analysis of 5 Prospective Studies," *American Journal of Clinical Nutrition* 70, suppl. 3 (September 1999): 516S–524S.

Malkmus, George H., *Why Christians Get Sick* (Shippensburg, Penn.: Treasure House, 1995); Website at *www.hacres.com* (accessed March 23, 2001).

Willett, Walter C., "Convergence of Philosophy and Science: The Third International Congress on Vegetarian Nutrition," *American Journal of Clinical Nutrition* 70, suppl. 3 (September 1999): 434S–438S.

Yamauchi, Edwin M., "Magic in the Biblical World," *Tyndale Bulletin* 34 (1983): 169–200.

HERBAL MEDICINE

What It Is

Many people who practice herbal medicine think of it as a "no-brainer." For thousands of years people went into the woods and selected plants they had learned had healing or soothing qualities. They would make infusions, poultices, or eat the plant alone or in a soup or stew. The plants used varied with the part of the world in which people lived, but when the plants were later analyzed scientifically, they were sometimes found to contain a component that did, indeed, have medical utility. Thus, when a Native American made a tea from willow bark, for example, he or she was actually getting a form of the chemical that today we call aspirin. Thus, rather than risk the changes and adulterations that exist with the chemical equivalent of an herb or other plant (along with binders, coloring, and other additions), why not go back to the herbs themselves?

The theory seems good to many, but the reality is not. At least not yet. An estimated 1,400 different plants are used to make about 20,000 different herbal remedies in the United States. Few of these have been scientifically tested in humans using controlled studies. Most ancient groups of indigenous people whose medical practices are well understood used a lot fewer remedies. In addition, there is no consistency in how the herbs are selected and used. One practitioner of herbal medicine might use one part of a plant, while a different practitioner uses a different part of the same plant. Sometimes the plant material is dried and powdered, others insist the fresh plant must be used. Some use the powder to make capsules, others say it's best to make the powder into a tea.

The active ingredients are sometimes removed from the plant material by extraction, a process similar to brewing coffee from coffee grounds. The liquid is usually water, although alcohol or steam can also be used. An alcohol extract is called a "tincture." Herbal remedies are sometimes given as injections in Europe, but this is rare in the United States. How the remedy is made, and the plant part used, influence what the final preparation contains and what its potential uses may be, even though the same basic herb has been used to make the preparation.

Claims

Herbal medicine is growing in popularity. *Prevention* magazine's 1999 survey of herbal and other dietary supplement usage by adults in the United States was conducted by Princeton Survey Research Associates, with the FDA providing technical assistance in developing the survey. The survey found that 49 percent of adults reported using an herbal remedy in the previous twelve months, and 24 percent reported using herbal remedies on a regular basis. The most common regularly used herbs were garlic (13 percent), ginseng (8 percent), ginkgo (7 percent), St. John's wort (4 percent), and echinacea (2 percent).

The most common reasons that people use these products are: to ensure good health (75 percent), to improve energy (61 percent), to prevent or treat colds and flu (58 percent), to improve memory (43 percent), to ease depression (35 percent), and to prevent or treat serious illness (29 percent). The survey also reported the reasons why people prefer herbs over prescriptions: prefer natural products (43 percent), fewer side effects (21 percent), more effective (14 percent), allowed self-treatment (11 percent), less expensive (8 percent), and more gentle or mild (6 percent).

As can be seen from the results of this survey, many believe that because herbal remedies are natural, they are less harmful than pharmaceutical drugs. There is some truth to this because, in general, herbal remedies are milder, less concentrated. However, herbs are not harmless. Under the individual entries for herbs, we will point out that virtually all herbal remedies can have adverse effects. People have overdosed on popular herbs like ephedra, leading to serious problems and even deaths. Some herbs like pennyroyal and chaparral cause more harm than good, leading us to conclude they should never be used. Many herbal products also cause interactions with drugs, other supplements, or even foods. Natural is not necessarily safe.

Study Findings

Studies of herbal remedies vary widely in quality, as will be seen in the entries on specific herbs later in this book. Herbal medicine relies primarily on traditional usage, sometimes ignoring the fact that different indigenous people have sometimes used the same herb in radically different ways for quite different healing practices. Basically, many assume that if an herb has been used for a long time, it must be somewhat effective. That assumption is not necessarily valid.

The recent interest in herbal medicine is leading to more clinical trials, but the focus is on a small number of herbs that show promise, leaving the majority of preparations not tested. Research in Europe is usually done on standardized products that differ from products available in the U.S. In addition, some promoters of herbal medicine argue that when a traditional herbal remedy is found to be ineffective in testing, the problem is with the test. They argue that if an herb was tested in the strength they use, the results would be quite different. Since such tests have often not been conducted, it is impossible to argue with their logic.

Some claim that conventional medicine is incompatible with herbal medicine. However, it should be remembered that more than one-quarter of the pharmaceutical drugs on the market today were originally isolated from plant material; over half came from natural sources, when you include microorganisms and animals. Throughout the rise of conventional medicine, departments of pharmacognosy were found in major schools of pharmacy. Here, herbs and other natural products were examined for their potential therapeutic benefits. Their approach was to isolate the active ingredients because of a number of difficulties with herbal medicine.

For example, when willow bark was shown to relieve pain, or foxglove to help with congestive heart failure, standardized preparations were sought. However, plants vary widely in how much active ingredient they produce. The particular variety of plant, where it is grown, the weather during growth, when it is collected, how the collected plant is treated and stored, and many other factors influence the contents of the plant. Foxglove (Digitalis purpurea) was found to contain drugs that have a powerful effect on the heart, but many of them were also toxic. Plants closely related to foxglove were examined for similar drugs, leading to the discovery of digoxin. Specific doses of digoxin must still be used for it to be effective without causing toxicity. To ensure that each dose contained the same amount of digoxin, the active chemical was isolated and prepared in pure form, thus removing the need to use the crude herb.

This variation in the active ingredients in plants became apparent in the 1960s during the Vietnam War. At the time, marijuana had become a popular recreational drug. It was (and is) illegal, but was frequently grown both in backyards and in wilderness areas, including isolated sections of national parks. The drug was smoked, as it still is, for its "buzz," or mellow high.

When American soldiers were sent to fight in Vietnam, some of them sought the local marijuana for recreational drug use. They assumed all marijuana was the same. The leaves of a plant in Vietnam were identical in appearance to those back in the United States. What the soldiers did not realize was that the climate, soil, growing, and harvesting conditions in Vietnam created a very different drug. The marijuana they encountered was hallucinogenic, much like LSD. It was also fat soluble, so stayed in the body.

A fairly heavy user would experience flashbacks well after he or she had last smoked the marijuana.

Herbal remedies can be prepared in what are called "standardized formulations." In these a specific amount of one active ingredient is contained in a dose. For example, the "Australian Standard" of tea tree oil contains at least 30 percent terpinene-4-ol (an active ingredient) and no more than 15 percent 1,8-cineole (a skin irritant). Australian regulators hold manufacturers to this standard, so that high-quality products are ensured. However, standardized products are more expensive, and regulation is required to enforce them. In the United States, no such regulation exists. Therefore, huge variations will be found in the amount of active ingredient in products on the U.S. market.

There is growing evidence to support this concern. ConsumerLab.com is an independent company that tests herbs, vitamins, and supplements sold in the United States against generally accepted testing standards. Initial tests have shown that many products contain levels of key ingredients that are lower—and in some cases *much* lower—than the package claims. In testing preparations from different companies, the laboratory found, for example, that 63 percent of saw palmetto preparations did not contain the amount of active ingredient listed on the label. The lab reported similar findings with 46 percent of glucosamine-chondroitin products, 100 percent of chondroitin, 23 percent of ginkgo, and 15 percent of vitamin C products. You can find out which products did pass muster by subscribing to the lab's Website (*www.consumerlab.com*). The company continues to release new tests every year.

In 1995, *Consumer Reports* studied a number of ginseng products. The different product labels listed different amounts of ginseng: anywhere from 100 mg to 700 mg of ginseng per capsule. Chemical tests of the capsules found very different amounts of ginsenosides, the chemicals believed to be the active ingredients in ginseng. (Note: With some herbs, we know what causes change in humans. Willow bark contains salicylic acid, the key ingredient in aspirin and the reason a willow bark tea will reduce or stop some pain. We do not know the specific aspect of ginseng that causes change for humans, though we suspect it is the ginsenosides.) An even bigger problem found by *Consumer Reports* was that the capsules with larger amounts of ginsenoside were not labeled as having more ginseng. In fact, there was no correlation between the labels and what was actually found in the capsules.

This type of variation in products from different manufacturers is one reason why some products are less effective than others. They don't contain enough of the active ingredient. *Consumer Reports*, in May 2000, published a massive survey of 46,806 of their readers that in part measured how people subjectively perceived the effectiveness of various therapies. A very high percentage of survey respondents reported some, little, or no help from a number of herbal products that medical studies have demonstrated to be effective. For example, the percent of adults reporting they had some, little, or no help with various disorders included: 82 percent using garlic for high cholesterol, 75 percent using echinacea for the treatment of colds or flu, 82 percent using melatonin for sleep, 76 percent using glucosamine for arthritis, 76 percent using St. John's wort for depression, and 76 percent using saw palmetto for prostate problems.

These high levels of dissatisfaction were disturbing, but not unexpected for those aware of the great variability in these products. It is reasonable to conclude that the products, if taken correctly, simply did not work. Why? The most likely explanation would be poor product quality. These products are virtually unregulated in the United States.

Another problem with unregulated herbal remedies has been contamination. More than 100 cases of severe kidney damage have occurred in Belgium because *Stephania tetrandra* was mistakenly replaced by *Aristolochia fangchi* in a Chinese herbal remedy. Of those women whose kidneys were removed because they no longer worked, more than half had developed cancer in the surrounding tissues. *Aristolochia* species are known to contain compounds that are poisonous to the kidneys and cause cancer. This terrible tragedy probably happened due to a simple mistake: the Chinese names of the two unrelated species are very similar.

Other problems are more suggestive of deliberate actions. Synthetic drugs are regularly found in herbal remedies. Some ephedra products have been found to contain mixtures of compounds not found naturally in any *Ephedra* species.

Regulation of herbal remedies and supplements is needed. Consumers have come to expect the highest quality in health products. But until changes are made, consumers cannot be assured that the herbal remedies they buy contain what is listed on the label.

Cautions

Uncertainty often exists about whether any particular herbal remedy works, how much active ingredient it contains, and whether there are any toxic effects. For example, ephedra, used to lose weight or improve athletic performance, has caused at least forty-four deaths and is proving to be very difficult to remove from the market. Cases of deliberate adulteration of herbal remedies have been reported. Relatively inexpensive pharmaceutical drugs such as aspirin, antihistamines, or steroids have been found in herbal remedies in what would appear to be attempts to make the herbal remedies seem effective.

Another area of concern is how herbal remedies interact with other herbs and drugs. Many herbs and drugs are eliminated from the body by the liver. If the liver is tied up metabolizing components of herbal remedies, less of the drug will be eliminated and may even reach toxic levels. Other herbs (like St. John's wort) stimulate the liver to more actively eliminate other drugs, leading to those drugs being less effective. That's why it is important to let all your health care providers, conventional and alternative, physicians and pharmacists, know about *all* the medicines and remedies you are taking, including drugs, over-the-counter products, herbs, vitamins, and dietary supplements.

Very little is known about the long-term effects of taking herbal remedies. Most traditional uses of herbs involve short-term use for a specific condition, although practitioners in one country sometimes follow guidelines not used in others. For example, many practitioners of herbal medicine in Europe say that their experience requires that ginseng not be used for more than two weeks at a time. Yet in the United States, practitioners seem to feel comfortable recommending its use for months or years as an energy booster. Current use of herbal remedies and dietary supplements is often for conditions, such as for mild depression, general anxiety, antiaging, and as energy boosters, for which the remedies would be taken for years. There is no information on how the body will tolerate this extended use.

Given the general lack of information on the toxic effects of many herbs, some general guidelines can be proposed. Women who are pregnant, or who are sexually active and thus might become pregnant, should be extremely cautious about using any herbal remedy. The same is true for nursing mothers. Very little is known about how herbal remedies affect the unborn and children, but their potential for causing them harm is even higher than with adults. We do not know the exact amount that can be considered a safe dose for an adult. We know even less for the unborn and the newborn. Because of this lack of knowledge, babies and children should not be given herbal remedies (see chapter 7, "Alternative Medicine and Children").

Adults taking herbal remedies should limit their use to only short periods of time unless long-term studies have been done (which is beginning to be the case for a few herbs). Never assume that just because something is natural, it is safe. The opposite might be true. Take only reasonable amounts of any herbal remedy. If things don't improve relatively quickly, see your physician and report what you've been taking. Don't fall into the trap of assuming that if a small dose helps a little, a large amount will help a lot. This is not the case with pharmaceutical drugs, and it's not the case with herbal remedies.

Only use standardized preparations bought at reliable stores. *The United States Pharmacopoeia* (USP) is a volunteer organization of pharmaceutical experts that evaluates the standards by which any drug or herbal remedy has been manufactured. Look for its stamp of approval as a way of determining which products at least say that they are made according to high standards. They will theoretically be the safest, though that does not mean that the manufacturer's claim for its effectiveness, or the actual amount in the bottle, will be accurate. Consider subscribing to *www.consumerlab.com* to see if the brand you're considering has been tested by this independent company. And when you find a reliable brand, don't shop around. You may be better off sticking with a brand that is giving you the results you want rather than trying to save a few dollars.

All of what we have discussed here applies to "herbal medicine," where herbal remedies are used in ways similar to how prescription drugs are used. Another term sometimes found in these discussions is "herbalism." This term is usually found within a pantheistic world view that sees herbal remedies as an essential part of humanity's one-ness with nature, not as chemicals that have certain physical effects on the body. Rather, herbal remedies are believed by these practitioners to be one of the ways that Mother Earth, or the Universal Consciousness, cares for humanity. For example, David Hoffman, a well-known herbalist, writes, "The Earth is not a physico-chemical mechanism but a living entity with the equivalent of senses, intelligence, memory and the capacity to act." In other words, the Earth is a living, personal being. For many of these practitioners, she is also the object of their worship.

Herbalism varies with the culture, but the common view is that herbs are believed to balance or strengthen a person's vital force or life energy. Thus, herbs are chosen by how they are believed to rebalance a person's vital force or trigger natural healing mech-anisms. In this way, the same herbs may be used in completely different ways in differ-ent cultures, or even between different patients within the same community.

Herbalism is a religious or magical approach to herbs. One form of magic uses the similarity of objects to allegedly cause desired effects. Thus, herbs that grow with shapes similar to parts of the human body gain magical reputations for healing those body parts. For example, mandrakes have fleshy, forked roots that resemble the lower parts of the human body and have been used, since biblical times, to promote fertility. Jacob's wife Leah collected mandrakes to use this way (Genesis 30:14–17). This passage demonstrates the futility of herbalism's approach, although the main teaching is that fertility is a gift from God. Leah gives her mandrakes to Rachel, Jacob's other wife. Leah then becomes pregnant, while Rachel uses the mandrakes and remains barren for the time being.

Since the approach is clearly at odds with Christian worship of the One True God, Christians should not use herbal remedies within this context. If you seek out an expert in herbal remedies, make sure you are not exposing yourself to those who practice in this way.

Recommendations

Herbal medicine has been the source of people's drugs for most of human history. Given the diversity of God's creation, it is unlikely we have discovered all the potential blessings contained in the plant kingdom. In fact, one of the tragedies of the rapid destruction of the rain forests is that we may be losing indigenous plants capable of cur-ing some of our most devastating diseases, including certain forms of cancer. However, while we certainly have not yet discovered all that God has given us, it seems safe to assume that it is unlikely that every plant will cure something.

Traditionally the herbal market has been portrayed as an unorganized group of Mom-and-Pop operations trying to fight against the big, bad pharmaceutical giants. No longer is this the case. Herbal remedies are a multibillion-dollar market, with all the dangers that accompany this type of giant enterprise. Common sense and careful investigation are needed before wandering into a field as dangerous as any shark-infested waters.

Additionally, some herbal remedies, such as the Bach flower remedies (see Bach Flower Remedies, page 303), are believed to work because they have been "spiritually vitalized." Others make use of herbal remedies within the context of a sort of religious practice called "herbalism." A number of hallucinogenic herbs and other preparations are used in witchcraft and shamanism to access the spirit world. In all these contexts, herbal remedies are tools to promote occult activities and should be avoided. What seems to be more important in these situations is to have discernment about those manufacturing and promoting the preparations.

Treatment Categories

Conventional Therapies
   A growing number of specific herbs for specific indications—discussed under the heading of each herb

Complementary Therapies
   A small, but growing, number of herbal products and indications

Scientifically Unproven
   Many herbs, and some preparations of those used as conventional therapies

Scientifically Questionable
   Many herbal products

Quackery or Fraud
   In the hands of some practitioners

Further Reading

Blumenthal, M., J. Gruenwald, T. Hall, C. Riggins, and R. Rister, *German Commission E Monographs: Medicinal Plants for Human Use* (Austin, Tex.: American Botanical Council, 1998).

DerMarderosian, Ara, ed., *The Review of Natural Products* (St. Louis, Mo.: Facts and Comparisons, various years).

Fetrow, Charles W., and Juan R. Avila, *Professional's Handbook of Complementary and Alternative Medicine* (Springhouse, Penn.: Springhouse, 1999).

Foster, Steven, and Varro E. Tyler, *Tyler's Honest Herbal: A Sensible Guide to the Use of Herbs and Related Remedies*, 4th ed. (London: Haworth Press, 1999).

"Herbal Roulette," *Consumer Reports* 60, no. 11 (November 1995): 698–705.

Hoffman, David, *The Elements of Herbalism* (New York: Barnes & Noble, 1997).

Jellin, Jeff M., Forrest Batz, and Kathy Hichens, *Pharmacist's Letter/Prescriber's Letter: Natural Medicines Comprehensive Database* (Stockton, Calif.: Therapeutic Research Facility, 1999). Also available by subscription at *www.naturaldatabase.com.*

Johnston, Barbara A., "*Prevention* Magazine Assesses Use of Dietary Supplements," *HerbalGram* 48 (2000): 65.

"Mainstreaming of Alternative Medicine, The," *Consumer Reports* 65, no. 5 (May 2000): 17–25.

PDR for Herbal Medicines, 2d ed. (Montvale, N.J.: Medical Economics, 2000).

HOMEOPATHY

What It Is

German physician Samuel Hahnemann (1755–1843) was typical of many compassionate medical practitioners working during a time when medicine was harsh and unpleasant. Treatments could be quite severe, such as bloodletting, blistering, and purging. Worse, the efforts were usually ineffective, and patients suffered needlessly.

Dr. Hahnemann wanted to find a milder, safer system. He and his assistants began experimenting on themselves with a series of tests called "provings." Each was an experiment based on a theory he developed from observation.

For example, malaria had been a scourge in Europe for many years. Eventually it was found that the use of cinchona bark could effectively treat malaria, and by the time Dr. Hahnemann was practicing, quinine had been isolated as the active ingredient in cinchona. Dr. Hahnemann noticed that if you gave a healthy person quinine, he or she developed malaria-like symptoms. It was an observation that led him to develop his Law of Similars. According to this concept, if a substance produces a specific set of symptoms in a healthy person, it will cure people of the illness that has those same symptoms—provided it is diluted repeatedly. For example, since quinine given to healthy people produces symptoms similar to those experienced by malaria sufferers, extremely diluted solutions of quinine (called "homeopathic quinine") are felt to cure malaria. Likewise, belladonna given to healthy people produces fevers, flushing, and other flu-like symptoms, so homeopathic belladonna is used to treat colds and flu.

Over the course of his career, Hahnemann tested hundreds of substances and meticulously observed the symptoms elicited. He wrote the *Homeopathic Pharmacopoeia*, a text still highly respected by homeopaths and consulted regularly.

One of the reasons some patients like homeopaths is because the practitioner makes many of the remedies in the office, adding a sense of personal medicine. The remedies are made by dissolving plant, mineral, animal, or chemical products in water and alcohol. Unlike drugs and herbal remedies, though, extremely dilute solutions must be used. This is because Hahnemann's observations led him to propose another, highly controversial law, the Law of Potentization.

The Law of Potentization claims that the more diluted a substance, the higher its potency. Homeopathic remedies are diluted again and again in the belief that this increases their potency and effectiveness. This law contradicts the generally accepted finding in pharmacy and medicine that the more dilute a solution, the weaker its effect on the body.

Homeopathic remedies are labeled as so many "x" or "c." For example, a 15x potency means the substance was diluted 15 times at a ratio of 1 in 10 (1 drop of the original solution is mixed with 9 drops of alcohol or water). A 12c potency means the substance was diluted 12 times at a ratio of 1 in 100. Some of these remedies are so diluted that homeopaths acknowledge there is practically no chance of even one molecule of the original substance remaining.

A variety of hypotheses are proposed to explain how such diluted solutions could have any effect on the body. A popular one, based on a 1988 article by French scientist Jacques Benveniste and published in the prestigious journal *Nature*, claims that the substances leave some sort of electromagnetic imprint on the water molecules. Very few scientists accept this idea of "water memory," and no one has been able to repeat Benveniste's experiments. Such repetition is an important test of any theory.

The more traditional explanation for homeopathic effectiveness is based on life energy theories and vitalism. Hahnemann used the term "vital energy" for the same life energy that is called *chi* in traditional Chinese medicine and *prana* in Ayurvedic medicine. Hahnemann explained this energy's role in his 1810 book, still regarded as the bible of homeopathy, *Organ of the Art of Healing* (also called *Organon*). "In the state of health the spirit-like vital force (dynamis) animating the material human organism reins in supreme sovereignty."

According to this view, the symptoms of an illness are signs that the body's life energy is fighting against an illness. Thus a substance that produces those same symptoms works with the body's vital energy to promote self-healing. Eliminating those symptoms (a common factor in conventional medicine) is thus counterproductive, according to homeopathic theory. Thus homeopathy does not seem to be compatible with conventional medicine because they are fundamentally at odds with one another in their approaches to healing.

Hahnemann's explanation for the effectiveness of such diluted solutions focused more on the way the dilutions were done. At each dilution, the mixture must be shaken vigorously. Hahnemann believed this shaking released "the spiritual vital force" of the healing substance. Thus, more shaking releases more energy and gives stronger effects. According to Dana Ullman, president of the Foundation of Homeopathic Education and Research, this energy is similar to *prana* (see Ayurveda), "the inherent, underlying, interconnective, self-healing process of the organism." Thus although some claim homeopathy works through some unknown natural mechanism, its core principles are based on life energy beliefs. The scientifically questionable premises in homeopathy are understandable only by introducing life energy concepts.

Claims

Homeopaths vary considerably in what they claim to be able to treat. Some limit their claims to chronic illnesses or those for which conventional medicine offers only limited symptom management. The most common ones in this area are allergies, flu, cold, arthritis, and asthma. However, other homeopaths claim to be able to cure almost every known disease, including diabetes, cancer, heart disease, and other serious illnesses. Thousands of different homeopathic remedies are made from many different substances in accordance with the particular mixture of symptoms a patient reports.

Claims of effectiveness are often backed up by the consistent popularity of homeopathy in Europe (in particular, the long-standing endorsement by the British royal family), and the growth in sales in the United States. According to *Time* magazine, homeopathic sales rose 25 percent annually from the late 1980s through 1995 when sales exceeded $165 million a year. However, even while the National Health Service in Britain is paying for more alternative therapies, a number of local health authorities have stopped paying for homeopathic remedies because of a lack of evidence to support their effectiveness.

Study Findings

Clinical studies (✗✗) have not consistently found that homeopathic remedies are any better than placebos. A *Consumer Reports* study reported the percent of adults who reported some, little, or no help with homeopathy for allergies was 64 percent, with only 34 percent saying it helped "much"—about what would be expected of a placebo response. A number of studies (✔✔) have reported significant improvements with a variety of illnesses. A very small number of these studies were of good quality. Some had results favoring homeopathy, others did not.

However, others have pointed out significant problems in many of these studies that make their results very tenuous. One 1991 review of more than a hundred homeopathic studies concluded that the research methods were so poor, clear conclusions could not be drawn. A 1997 review concluded that while all of the results in homeopathic studies could not be explained by the placebo effect, there was insufficient evidence to conclude that homeopathy is effective for any particular clinical condition. The problem is that every study is designed differently and examines different conditions. A 1999 review of six studies (✗✗✗) that compared homeopathy to conventional therapies concluded that all were seriously flawed and could therefore give no reliable evidence about homeopathy's effectiveness. When researchers compared the quality of the studies to their results, they found an interesting pattern. Studies (✗✗✗) of higher quality tended to find homeopathy ineffective, while low-quality studies tended to find it somewhat effective. Results like this make it difficult to accept that homeopathy works by anything other than a complex placebo effect.

In spite of these results in clinical research, many people continue to believe that the remedies work. Some claim this comes from a powerful placebo effect stemming from the positive interactions patients have with homeopaths. The initial visit will involve an extensive interview to determine which preparation most closely matches the patient's combination of symptoms. Some homeopaths also believe it is important to classify a patient according to a set of constitutional types. The same problem might be treated with different remedies in people of different constitutional types, or the same remedy might be used to treat different problems in different people. The individualized attention needed to determine which remedy is used may be very therapeutic in itself.

Cautions

Since homeopathic remedies are extremely diluted (to the point of having no active ingredients at all), and only very small amounts are given, harmful side effects are not likely. However, there have been some reports of contamination of products. Homeopathic preparations are not regulated or standardized in the United States because of an exemption granted by law in 1938. In spite of the theoretical close connection between patient and homeopathic practitioner, most sales are directly to consumers by mail or from health food stores. A lot of people are self-diagnosing their problems and self-prescribing homeopathic (and herbal) remedies. The danger is in neglecting diagnosis and treatment of conditions which conventional medicine can cure or alleviate.

Recommendations

The scientific evidence that homeopathy works any better than a placebo is small and, in our opinion, very weak. For homeopathic remedies to work as proposed, many core tenets of conventional medicine would have to be completely overhauled—or even thrown overboard. For this reason, most within conventional medicine remain highly skeptical of homeopathy. Those who use homeopathy tend to believe very strongly that it works. Given that it is relatively safe and harmless, homeopathy might help those who believe in it because of the placebo effect. However, Christians who decide to use homeopathy must be discerning about the homeopaths they choose. Belief in homeopathy as a method of manipulating life energy is incompatible with Christian beliefs.

Treatment Categories

Complementary Therapy
Possibly due to placebo effects from patient-homeopath interactions ☹☹☹

Scientifically Unproven
For most indications

Scientifically Questionable

Energy Medicine
Depending on the practitioner

Quackery or Fraud
In the hands of some practitioners

Further Reading

Bopp, H. J., *L'Homeopathie*, translated from French and available at *http://logosresourcepages.org/homeopat.html* (accessed March 23, 2001).

Ernst, E., "Classical Homoeopathy versus Conventional Treatments: A Systematic Review," *Perfusion* 12, no. 1 (1999): 13–15.

Linde, Klaus, Michael Scholz, Gilbert Ramirez, Nicolas Clausius, Dieter Melchart, and Wayne B. Jonas, "Impact of Study Quality on Outcome in Placebo-Controlled Trials of Homeopathy," *Journal of Clinical Epidemiology* 52, no. 7 (1999): 631–36.

Linde, Klaus, Nicolas Clausius, Gilbert Ramirez, Dieter Melchart, Florian Eitel, Larry V. Hedges, and Wayne B. Jonas, "Are the Clinical Effects of Homoeopathy Placebo Effects? A Meta-Analysis of Placebo-Controlled Trials," *Lancet* 350 (September 1997): 834–43.

"Mainstreaming of Alternative Medicine, The," *Consumer Reports* 65, no. 5 (May 2000): 17–25.

O'Mathúna, Dónal P., and Dennis McCallum, "Postmodern Medicine: Miracle or Menace?" *Today's Christian Doctor* 27 (Fall 1996): 28–32.

Toufexis, Anastasia, "Is Homeopathy Good Medicine?" *Time* (September 25, 1995), 47–48.

Ullman, Dana, *Discovering Homeopathy: Medicine for the 21st Century*, rev. ed. (Berkeley, Calif.: North Atlantic, 1991).

HYPNOSIS

What It Is

Hypnosis (formerly called "hypnotism") has been seen by some as the illegitimate child of both medicine and psychology. Teenagers growing up in the 1950s would discover advertisements on the back of comic books where anything from 10 cents to 25 cents could buy a booklet that would teach them how to "control the minds of others" using "hypnotism." Earlier, in the 1930s, Dr. George Estabrooks, head of the Psychology Department at Colgate University, was adamant in his belief that hypnosis could be used to create a double agent or a secret assassin, or be used for interrogation. Despite this seemingly sinister potential, many experts in the field believe that only one in five individuals makes a good subject for hypnosis no matter how it is used.

It is hard to get a firm grasp on exactly what hypnosis involves. Different methods are used to "induce" hypnosis, and there is some disagreement among experts about how to verify that someone is in a hypnotic trance as opposed to other similar states of altered consciousness.

Many of the effects of hypnosis can be obtained without hypnosis, leading some to question whether a unique state of hypnosis even exists. Disagreement also exists over whether hypnosis is ever appropriate for Christians. There are Christian hypnotherapists, and there are Christians who vehemently oppose the practice. What almost everyone agrees on, though, is that hypnosis is a method of inducing what is commonly called an "altered state of consciousness" (ASC)—when the mind is not under the usual control of rational, logical faculties or consciousness. Daydreaming, tuning out, even sleeping can be referred to as types of altered states of consciousness. You're reading and find yourself drifting in and out of full awareness. You even turn a page and realize you've no idea what you've just read. Yet you were awake—reading—in an altered state of consciousness.

People under anesthesia, under the influence of drugs or alcohol, or engaged in various mystical experiences are in other forms of an ASC. Perhaps the most common experience of this type that most of us share is when we are deep in thought about some problem while driving or taking a long walk. Suddenly we find ourselves at our exit ramp off the highway, several miles from our office, with no memory of getting there. Or we realize we have walked all the way around a park and cannot recall anything about what we've just done. In both instances, we were functioning effectively. We drove and walked safely, not endangering others or ourselves, yet our awareness was on our thoughts, the problem we were trying to solve. This, too, is a form of ASC.

These ASC experiences can be objectively verified by measuring changes in breathing patterns, body temperature, and responses to stimuli, and through electroencephalography (EEG, which measures the electrical activity of the brain). Behavior can change, and the person responds differently to external stimuli. The student in class who has "drifted into another world" no longer hears the teacher's voice, though the voice is as loud and clear as before.

Hypnosis is another form of ASC, though difficult to define. Some experts say people in hypnotic trances are alert and "in control," while other experts believe that people "in trance" are not fully alert, yet they are not asleep either. Rather than give a one-sentence definition of hypnosis, John Court, a Christian counselor and educator who uses hypnosis, describes the characteristic features of ASCs in general, and hypnosis in particular.

Court explains that having a person focus attention and filter out external distractions can induce hypnosis—or a hypnotic state or trance. Repetition helps here, for example, with rhythmic drum beating used in religious ceremonies, or therapists ask clients to count backwards. As the focus narrows, left-brain thinking (that which is logical and rational) becomes less dominant, and right-brain thinking is facilitated. This may leave a person open to imagery and visualization, which are commonly used during hypnosis. Therapists will often ask people to picture themselves in a relaxing scene, such as lying on a warm, pleasant beach.

While in the hypnotic trance, people are more passive than active. They wait and listen for things to happen, rather than actively seeking to do something. They are very open to suggestion, to the ideas (and, possibly, the persuasion) of others.

And therein lies the basis for both the uses and concerns of hypnosis. A therapist might tell someone during hypnosis that her arm is numb and insensitive, so she feels no pain while a physician is doing minor surgery on the arm. A psychologist may use hypnosis to help clients discuss some painful memories that they would not allow themselves to even think about while fully conscious. Or a stage hypnotist could tell someone to act like a dog, and the person starts running around the stage barking.

Even those who practice hypnosis agree that it should be practiced only within a trusting relationship. Court acknowledges, "To be in a state of heightened suggestibility is to be at risk from any unscrupulous person who might seek to exploit the situation." During hypnosis, the person is under great pressure to respond to the expectations of the therapist. When hypnosis is being used to examine past memories, Court writes, "The hypnotist can find what is being looked for, whether grounded in reality or not."

Allegations of childhood abuse based on memories recovered during hypnosis have been very controversial. Even more controversy arises, in both Christian and non-Christian circles, when the memories are said to come from past lives, and thus used as evidence for reincarnation. Because of how open to others' suggestions people become, hypnosis should never be entered into lightly.

A useful definition of hypnosis can be found in a Christian publication, the *Baker Encyclopedia of Psychology*: "Hypnosis is clearly not a power or force that one possesses to control another. Rather, hypnosis appears to involve a shift in concentration, executed in a passive manner (such as occurs in daydreaming or sleeping), resulting in a state of consciousness distinguishably different from alertness or ordinary sleep. It is characterized by narrowing of attention, reduced rational criticalness, and increased responsiveness to suggestion. It appears to provide a clearer access to the functioning of the mind, allowing understanding of that which is subconscious or dissociated." So, while hypnosis is induced in somewhat similar ways to how we fall asleep, the resulting state is distinguishable from sleep. During hypnosis people have greater "access" to their subconscious minds, but are less under the control of their conscious minds.

History of Hypnosis

Hypnosis has been practiced for centuries in the Far East, but in the West, the first prominent promoter of hypnosis was Franz Anton Mesmer (1734–1815), an Austrian physician. He originally used magnets in his healings, believing that these assisted in the flow of "animal magnetism," a fluid he believed was present in all people. He later dropped the use of magnets, and his subjects were believed to be healed by being "mesmerized."

As mesmerism fell into disrepute, hypnosis gained some followers. Jean-Martin Charcot (1835–1893) used it to explore and alleviate hysteria in patients. He taught hypnosis to his students, including Sigmund Freud, who used it to explore hidden memories, but later stopped using it in favor of what would become known as psychoanalysis.

British physician James Braid (1795–1860) coined the term "hypnotism" (which has since been replaced by "hypnosis") and noted that people usually don't remember what happened during hypnosis. A British surgeon, James Esdaile, used hypnosis as an anesthetic during surgery. Hypnosis seemed poised to find a number of applications, but faded rapidly after Freud's psychoanalytic methods replaced it as a psychological tool, and drugs became available to induce anesthesia.

At the same time, Mesmer's form of hypnosis grew in popularity among a number of new spiritual groups, especially in the United States. Mesmerism was seen as a way to bring people into "harmony" with unseen spiritual forces. It was also seen as a useful technique to help people develop clairvoyant skills. Phineas Quimby (1802–1866) used mesmerism, and his results led him to believe that all sickness is illusory. His system developed into the New Thought movement and was taken up by Mary Baker Eddy, who had been treated by Mesmer at one time and became a part of Christian Science (although Court notes that Eddy later rejected hypnosis).

All of these associations with unorthodox religious or spiritualist movements have left many Christians wary of hypnosis. More recently, the New Age movement adopted hypnosis as an important technique for spiritual enlightenment. Coupled with the entertaining, though also somewhat frightening, scenes of stage hypnotists getting people to do all sorts of strange and uncharacteristic things, some Christians see nothing but danger in hypnosis. Some even claim that the list of occult practices forbidden in Deuteronomy 18:10–11 includes hypnosis when it refers to one who "casts spells."

In light of these concerns, those considering hypnosis must look at both scientific and theological issues. Some might conclude that hypnosis can be embraced. Others might believe it should be rejected. Our answer is more complicated. After a careful examination of all sides of the argument, our conclusion is that "It depends!"

Claims

The claims about hypnosis can be divided into four groups according to the primary goal of its use: entertainment, medical conditions, counseling, or for spiritual growth and experiences.

Entertainment. Stage hypnosis involves entertainers getting people to do things they normally wouldn't, all for the benefit of giving the audience some laughs. True hypnosis, even done for pure entertainment, demonstrates its real power.

Stage hypnotists are highly skilled at recognizing who in the audience is most likely to enter a hypnotic trance. It is widely recognized that among any group of a hundred people, ten will be easily hypnotized, ten will be very difficult to hypnotize, and the rest fall somewhere in between. Yet some stage hypnosis may be fraudulent or illusionary. John Court quotes from a training manual for stage hypnosis that admits this: "Experience has shown down through the years that the hypnotic show must be faked, at least partially so, to hold audience interest and be successful as entertainment. . . . The successful hypnotic entertainer of today is actually not interested whether or not the subjects are really hypnotized—his basic function is to entertain. He is interested in his ability to con his subjects into a pseudo-performance that appears as hypnotism."

These shows and party "games" demonstrate how open to a hypnotist's suggestions people can be during a hypnotic trance. They show how a hypnotist can dramatically influence behavior. They show the power and the danger of naïvely becoming involved with hypnosis.

Medical conditions. Hypnotherapy in medicine is used primarily for the relief or prevention of pain, and for anesthesia, diverting attention from the pain. This use has become so commonplace that some medical schools require all students to learn the practice and use it during minor surgery and during labor and delivery.

Counseling. The psychological use of hypnotherapy is to help people deal with phobias and unwanted habits, to uncover repressed memories, to treat dissociative conditions, and to enhance sports or arts performances. Hypnosis also has been used abusively, according to John Court, as a "brainwashing" procedure.

Spiritual. The final area of interest in hypnosis is as a spiritual or religious practice. Those in favor of hypnosis, including Christian hypnotherapists, point to the similarities between the hypnotic trance and many religious practices and experiences. Worship services often include repetition, rhythmic singing or music, focused attention on an altar or pulpit, visual and verbal imagery, and distinctive odors. People report an openness to words in a sermon or song, and often sense a spiritual presence. The Bible, for example, records people of faith having visions (Daniel, Peter, and many of the prophets) sometimes recorded as trances, as was the case with Peter: "I was in the city of Joppa praying, and in a trance I saw a vision. I saw something like a large sheet being let down from heaven by its four corners, and it came down to where I was" (Acts 11:5; see also Acts 10:11; 22:17).

The hypnotic trance is viewed by these Christian hypnotherapists as a legitimate and natural way for anyone to achieve a greater sense of the transcendent, and to become more open to spiritual encounters. The *Baker Encyclopedia of Psychology* puts it this way: "The value of hypnosis is that it provides a means of achieving a special state in which the person can go beyond the bounds of usual rational thinking to affect both mental and physical processes. . . . Such experience taps into the spiritual and unconscious resources of the individual and also into that part of the psyche that is open to the influence of God and the cosmos."

Study Findings

Studies of hypnosis for pain management have been conducted for more than thirty years. A review of these in the *Textbook of Pain* found that pain perception diminished and pain tolerance improved during hypnosis. Much of the early research in this area was not controlled effectively. We found eleven controlled studies (✔✔✔) on headache pain, all of which showed short-term improvements in pain intensity and headache frequency.

The more recent studies (✔✔✔) found that analgesia similar to hypnosis occurred using various relaxation techniques or teaching patients to focus on something other than their pain. We also examined six studies (✔✔✔✔) involving pain during labor. All reported less pain in those women undergoing hypnosis, although no study compared hypnosis with a nonhypnotic relaxation technique as was done in the headache studies.

Hypnosis has also been studied for acute pain relief with dental work, surgery, and care of burns. Six controlled studies examined the effect of hypnosis on pain after surgery. Three (✔✔✔✔) found hypnosis better than no treatment, one (✘✘✘) found no differences, one (✘✘✘) found local anesthesia better than hypnosis, and one (✘✘✘) found no differences between hypnosis and a nonhypnotic relaxation technique. Three studies (✔✔✔✔) with burn patients found hypnosis produced better pain relief than no treatment, but none of these included a nonhypnotic relaxation group.

The largest study of this type (✔✔✔) was reported in April 2000 in the British journal *Lancet*. More than 200 patients were divided into three groups, one receiving normal treatment, another receiving hypnosis, and the third group received extra attention from someone who ensured nothing negative was said during their surgery. All patients could give themselves as much pain medication as they needed. About half the patients in both the extra attention and hypnosis groups needed no pain medication at all, and those who did used half the amount used by those in the no-treatment group. Those receiving hypnosis also reported that their pain did not get worse, they had no blood pressure problems, and their surgeries finished seventeen minutes earlier. The time savings were thought to have occurred because there were fewer complications. However, this study did not compare hypnosis with a nonhypnotic relaxation group to determine if the benefits were specifically due to hypnosis or just to a general relaxation response.

Hypnosis has also been used for chronic pain relief, especially with cancer sufferers. Again, most of the research has been uncontrolled (✔✔). In the few controlled studies (✔✔✔✔), hypnosis did produce significantly more pain relief than no-treatment controls. However, in those limited cases (one with cancer pain, one with jaw and facial pain) where a nonhypnotic relaxation technique also was used, this was as effective as hypnosis. In one case testing hypnosis on nonspecific chronic pain (✘✘✘), the relaxation technique was significantly better than hypnosis.

The review in the *Textbook of Pain* concluded: "In short, the available clinical data provide no support whatsoever for the oft-heard but unsupported contention that hypnotic procedures are intrinsically more effective than other psychological procedures at reducing clinical pain." In other words, according to these experts, hypnosis is no more effective than other "psychological procedures" such as meditation, guided imagery, stress-reduction techniques, or relaxation techniques. This conclusion is echoed by an April 2000 review published in the *International Journal of Clinical and Experimental Hypnosis* which stated: "In many of the studies reviewed, there is empirical evidence to support the effectiveness of psychological treatments that include hypnotic interventions. . . . To date, it is unclear whether hypnosis adds anything to treatment effectiveness above and beyond information, relaxation training, or suggestions provided without a hypnotic induction."

This conclusion, however, contrasts with what appears to be a more positive view of the studies found in the *Baker Encyclopedia of Psychology* under "hypnotherapy." This entry claims that all of the above applications are positively affected by hypnosis. However, only one study was actually cited, that by Barber. This study (✔✔) found a dramatic 99 percent success rate in performing routine dental procedures without anesthesia in patients who used hypnosis. However, as the *Textbook of Pain* review points out, Barber's was an uncontrolled study, and another 1984 study (✘✘) was not able to reproduce its results (obtaining a 51.7 percent success rate). Even the 1984 study had neither a no-treatment group nor a nonhypnotic group, making it difficult to know if relaxation alone may have been the source of the benefits.

Controlled studies on the use of hypnosis in psychological or behavior counseling are difficult to conduct. Most reports are case studies (✔✔), usually finding some benefit from hypnosis. Court's book describes a number of cases involving patients with depression, phobias, and earlier traumatic incidences. Court reports significant healing using hypnosis in conjunction with counseling, medication, and prayer. As with any form of counseling or behavior modification program, it is difficult to tease out the precise role of any one aspect of the treatment plan.

One review of hypnosis for smoking cessation demonstrates the difficulty of evaluating particular strategies in this area. *The Cochrane Library,* a British review of all published randomized clinical trials, found that among case reports and uncontrolled studies of hypnosis, the success rate for smoking cessation varied from 4 to 88 percent. This is an extremely wide margin. Nine randomized controlled studies were found, although there were many differences in the way hypnosis was induced and in how many treatments were given. Overall, the review found that six months after undergoing hypnosis, the percent of patients who were still not smoking was the same as in the group receiving any other treatment or those in a no-treatment group. A couple of studies did find hypnotherapy more beneficial, but these were the smaller and more poorly designed studies. The authors concluded, "There is insufficient evidence to recommend hypnotherapy as a specific treatment for smoking cessation."

Another area which has received more research than most is hypnosis for the treatment of obesity. Three meta-analyses of this research were published in the *Journal of Consulting & Clinical Psychology*. The first (✔✔✔) found that when hypnosis was added to cognitive-behavior therapy, obese patients lost significantly more weight than with therapy alone. The second (✘✘✘) reexamined the data from the first, added other studies that the first had not included, and concluded that there was no benefit from adding hypnosis. The third (✔✔✔) added new data obtained directly from the researchers (which had not been in the published research) and concluded that hypnosis was of benefit. These inconsistencies show how unclear the research data are at the moment. It is extremely difficult to evaluate psychological therapies, and this is reflected in the various conclusions of researchers.

Cautions

The use of hypnosis during medical procedures seems to be very safe, with few adverse effects reported. Probably the biggest concern about hypnosis arises from its other uses. Some believe that hypnosis gives control of one's mind over to someone else. If this occurs, people may be deceived into doing things they don't want to do, they may be taken advantage of (sexually or spiritually, in particular), or they may even be exposed to evil spiritual beings. Court, the Christian hypnotherapist, warns: "The inherent dangers of a powerful technique that affects thinking, feeling, and behaviour cannot be discounted since anything powerful is open to abuse. The possibility of being open to demonic influence in this setting cannot be dismissed as fanciful if we believe in the presence of evil."

Kurt Koch, a widely respected Christian authority on the occult, has had much experience with hypnosis as practiced in East Asia. In his books, he recounts numerous cases of hypnosis bringing people into contact with occult spirits. While these sometimes occurred as part of religious practices, some occurred after people innocently engaged in hypnosis at parties and shows. During this type of hypnosis, people are unduly under the influence of others whom they may not know. They may not have the degree of control over their minds which is expected of Christians who are called to be alert at all times. "So then, let us not be like others, who are asleep, but let us be alert and self-controlled" (1 Thessalonians 5:6). "Be self-controlled and alert. Your enemy the devil prowls around like a roaring lion looking for someone to devour" (1 Peter 5:8). For this reason, we believe that Christians should not engage in any form of hypnosis for purely entertainment purposes.

Christian hypnotherapists claim that fear of being controlled by another human is based on stage hypnosis and older authoritarian forms of hypnotherapy that are no longer commonly practiced. They claim that the primary purpose of hypnosis as a therapy is to give patients increased control over themselves and their behavior, not less control. Court states: "Most Christians will acknowledge that they have less control than they wish over some areas of their lives—habits, addiction, fears, sins—and are seeking to enhance control." Hypnosis, for Court, is a way to help Christians develop self-control. He points out that we are called to do this in Galatians 5:23.

Court describes this approach to hypnotherapy as one that empowers patients to have more control over their lives: "This non-directive approach, involving conversation rather than formal induction, indirect allusion and metaphor rather than commands, together with agreed goals and purposes, provides quite a different environment from that which traditionally has been feared. It is based on the skillful use of communication at various levels, by words, gestures and metaphors. . . . The person with specific fears over control issues can be helped to see that, far from losing control, an increase in control can occur as areas of life which were previously chaotic become manageable."

Recommendations

Christians are divided over the appropriateness of using hypnosis. It has been successfully used for pain control, allowing the avoidance or reduction of medication. It has been used to aid in relaxation without resorting to sleep medication for individuals recovering from psychological and physical trauma. Its use is limited and always will be, even under the best of circumstances, because only one in five individuals appears to be a good candidate for any type of hypnosis.

Case reports for the medical uses of hypnosis for anesthesia and analgesia are prolific, though there are questions about what is happening. Is it hypnosis that occurs or a deep state of relaxation? Does the difference even matter if the doctor using hypnosis is a Christian with no ulterior motives?

The fact that a form of self-hypnosis can occur naturally in an experience of religious ecstasy does not mean hypnosis should be artificially induced. It is never wise for a Christian to participate in stage hypnosis. Likewise, unless you know the practitioner and his or her methods and religious beliefs, it is unwise to experience any form of hypnosis. But if the practitioner is a Christian with no thought of anything other than using hypnosis to aid healing, there is evidence that the technique may bring positive changes in some, but not all, people.

Other areas associated with hypnosis are less certain. Age regression through hypnosis is a tool sometimes used to allow a patient to discuss early childhood traumas that might otherwise be forgotten. But how the hypnosis is induced, and how the individual is questioned, will determine whether the memory is real or created by suggestive questioning. This is an area that must be looked at with great caution and with the wisdom of mature Christian counsel.

Treatment Categories

Complementary Therapy
    Analgesia ☺☺☺
    Anesthesia ☺☺☺
    Pain management ☺☺☺
    Headache management ☺☺☺
    Labor pain management ☺☺☺
    Chronic pain management ☺☺

Scientifically Unproven
    Psychological indications

Scientifically Questionable
    Smoking cessation ☹☹☹
    Weight control ☹☹
    Other indications

Energy Medicine
>Used by some practitioners to generate spiritual experiences

Further Reading

Abbot, N. C., L. F. Stead, A. R. White, J. Barnes, and E. Ernst, "Hypnotherapy for Smoking Cessation (Cochrane Review)," in *The Cochrane Library*, no. 2 (Oxford: Update Software, 2000).

Barber, Joseph, "Rapid Induction Analgesia: A Clinical Report," *American Journal of Clinical Hypnosis* 19, no. 3 (January 1977): 138–47.

Benner, David G., ed., *Baker Encyclopedia of Psychology* (Grand Rapids: Baker, 1985).

Court, John, *Hypnosis: Healing and the Christian* (Carlisle, U.K.: Paternoster, 1997).

Koch, Kurt E., *Occult ABC* (Grand Rapids: Kregel, 1986), 95–100.

Lang, Elvira V., Eric G. Benotsch, Lauri J. Fick, Susan Lutgendorf, Michael L. Berbaum, Henrietta Logan, and David Spiegel, "Adjunctive Non-Pharmacological Analgesia for Invasive Medical Procedures: A Randomised Trial," *Lancet* 355 (April 2000): 1486–90.

Marks, John, *The Search for the "Manchurian Candidate"* (New York: Dell, 1977 and 1988).

Pinnell, Cornelia M., and Nicholas A. Covino, "Empirical Findings on the Use of Hypnosis in Medicine: A Critical Review," *International Journal of Clinical and Experimental Hypnosis* 48, no. 2 (April 2000): 170–94.

Schwarz, Ted, and Duane Empey, *Satanism: Is Your Family Safe?* (Grand Rapids: Zondervan, 1988).

Spanos, Nicholas P., Sharon J. Carmanico, and Jacqueline A. Ellis, "Hypnotic Analgesia," in *Textbook of Pain*, ed. Patrick D. Wall and Ronald Melzack (Edinburgh and New York: Churchill Livingston, 1994), 1349–66.

IRIDOLOGY

What It Is

Iridology is a way of examining the iris of the eye to obtain health information. This method is at least 100 years old and is based on the assumption that diseases manifest themselves in patterns visible in different parts of the iris. Practitioners feel that the iris is divided into sections, each one connected in some manner to a particular body part. Very specific areas are assigned to each organ and tissue. For example, if the eye is looked at like the face of a clock, changes in the kidneys would manifest themselves in the right iris where the hour hand would be at about five-thirty; thyroid changes would be seen where the hour hand would be at about two-thirty.

Iridology seems to have a basis in scientific knowledge in that certain diseases, such as rheumatoid arthritis, do lead to changes visible in the iris. However, these are general changes throughout the iris, not the isolated changes described in iridology.

Claims

Iridologists claim to be able to diagnose the existence of a wide variety of diseases in the organs of the body. They claim they also can determine if an organ has a tendency to develop an illness at some point in the future, since these weaknesses will manifest as changes in the iris before symptoms occur. These diagnoses can be made either by examining the iris directly or by using photographs. Other alternative practitioners use these same assumptions to make diagnoses based on the examination of only a small area of the body. For example, some practitioners will try to diagnose a patient's illness based on the shape and pattern of the tongue, the sole of the feet, the palm of the hand, the pulse, or the ears.

Traveling iridologists go to health food stores and conventions, taking close-up instant photographs of customers' irises. Then they examine the photos and provide the customer with a list of concerns diagnosed by studying the eyes. They often also suggest herbal remedies they sell. The customer usually buys whatever is deemed appropriate to prevent a problem from starting or to reduce an existing problem. Such traveling iridologists are often held in disdain by those who practice iridology in offices under what they feel are more scientific and accurate conditions.

Study Findings

No scientific evidence supports any of the connections proposed between the patterns of the iris and the parts of the body. A small number of studies (✗✗) found that the diagnoses made by iridologists are neither accurate nor consistent from one iridologist to another. In a 1979 study (✗✗), three iridologists examined iris photographs of patients who were known to have either severe to moderate kidney disease, or no kidney disease. One of the iridologists was a world-renowned expert who had written the authoritative book on iridology at the time. None of the iridologists correctly determined which patients had kidney disease with statistical reliability. In other words, their results were no better than chance.

The iridologist with the best results was correct only 2.5 percent of the time when he concluded that someone had kidney disease (as verified by other conventional tests). Three ophthalmologists with no experience in iridology examined the same photographs, and had results similar to the iridologists. The best ophthalmologist correctly diagnosed kidney disease 3 percent of the time. In contrast, the standard conventional medical test at the time for kidney disease (plasma creatinine) had an accuracy level of 98 percent.

A small number of other studies (✗✗) have examined iridology objectively, and found similar results. One (✗✗) particular study tested three iridologists, and none of them noticed that one of the photographs was of a glass eye.

Cautions

Iridology itself is harmless, as the practitioner examines only the eyes. However, harm can occur if iridology is used in place of effective diagnostic tools. Someone with an actual illness or disease will be given information based on nothing more than intuition. People with serious illnesses may be told they don't have an illness and may delay effective treatment. Others will be told they have illnesses when they don't, and will go through the worry and disturbance of dealing with a misdiagnosis. Misinformation has practical consequences—negative health effects and the inappropriate use of time and money. In addition, when iridology is used to sell herbal remedies, these herbal remedies may have an adverse effect on the health of someone who did not need them.

Recommendations

Iridology is based on principles that go against well-established scientific knowledge and approaches. Objective tests have found no evidence that it reliably helps in making diagnoses. There is no reason to spend time and resources using iridology.

Treatment Categories

Scientifically Questionable
    For any indication   ☹☹☹☹
Probably Quackery

Further Reading

Knipschild, Paul, "Looking for Gall Bladder Disease in the Patient's Iris," *British Medical Journal* 297 (1988): 1578–81.

Simon, Allie, David M. Worthen, and John A. Mitas II, "An Evaluation of Iridology," *Journal of the American Medical Association* 242, no. 13 (September 1979): 1385–89.

LIGHT THERAPY

What It Is

Many factors affect the way we feel, but one of the more common involves the presence or absence of full spectrum light. The awareness of this impact began when studying people who live in northern climates where the winter hours of daylight are severely limited. Psychologists and psychiatrists found a direct relationship between increased depression and periods of limited daylight. Further studies have indicated that people who are isolated from this type of light due to working at night or staying indoors during daylight hours also suffer from depression more than those whose jobs and lifestyles regularly take them outdoors during daylight.

Light therapy evolved as an artificial way to help people who have inadequate exposure to actual daylight to achieve the same effect indoors. Through the use of full spectrum lightbulbs, often placed in special multibulb holders, they bring the equivalent of noonday light indoors. The bulbs are the same type of bulb sold by garden supply centers for growing warm-weather outdoor plants inside in the winter.

Light is measured in degrees Kelvin, K (without the little degree symbol). Household lightbulbs, regardless of their brightness, are in the range of 3200 K and 3500 K. A full-spectrum lightbulb (both fluorescent and standard incandescent) is rated at approximately 6500 K, the same as noonday sun. These full-spectrum lightbulbs are quite safe because, where a tanning booth uses ultraviolet (UV) rays to make up much of the radiation, full-spectrum lights emit very few UV rays.

Light boxes are used as deemed appropriate in treating light deprivation symptoms. Someone who is severely depressed from being in an area where the winter days are extremely short may be suffering from seasonal affective disorder and be told to use a multibulb light box for eight or more hours a day. Other people find that their mood improves when the office or factory light is replaced with full-spectrum bulbs. These may be used in a desk lamp or overhead light.

Other forms of therapy use light of different colors to treat specific illnesses believed to be associated with particular colors (also called "color therapy"). Sometimes UV radiation and even lasers are used in light therapy.

Claims

One of the most common uses of light therapy is to relieve depression that occurs during periods of little sunshine (called "seasonal affective disorder"). This approach has become standard therapy recommended by many psychiatrists, especially those practicing in areas with limited winter daylight hours. Light therapy is also considered standard therapy for a number of skin disorders, such as psoriasis (although in conventional therapy for psoriasis, the light includes UV rays).

There are many other claims concerning the therapeutic value of light. For example, in color therapy, each cell and tissue is said to respond differently to different colors. Diseases are said to relate to energy imbalances in the tissues that can be rebalanced by light of different colors.

A radical form of cancer treatment involves injecting dyes into skin cancer tumors based on the belief that the dyes absorb certain colors of light and kill the cancer cells.

Study Findings

Numerous studies (✔✔) have shown that people living in more northerly latitudes, where the winters are longer and darker, suffer more from depression. Elsewhere, people report (✔✔) more depression when their exposure to daylight is limited, both because of hours of available sunlight and because of when and how they work. Studies (✔✔✔) have shown that introducing full-spectrum light boxes into people's homes can relieve depression related to these issues. Replacing workplace lighting with full spectrum bulbs can have a similarly therapeutic result.

Light (✔✔) affects body temperature, hormone production, and sleep patterns. Light (✔✔✔✔) is needed to produce vitamin D in skin, and is used to treat jaundice in newborns. Additionally, adequate light (✔✔✔✔) is important to avoid eyestrain and fatigue, especially when reading and working.

However, when light therapists claim to treat and cure other diseases, they have little or no evidence to support them. Color therapy is usually based on the principles of life energy and *chakras* (see Energy Medicine, page 193). Each *chakra* is associated with certain tissues and emotions, but also with a particular color. Practitioners claim (✔) to be able to determine if certain colors are missing. Light of specific colors is then believed to be useful in the treatment of those conditions. Crystals are sometimes used to direct light of different colors and energies to the person. In addition, some practitioners claim to be able to "send" healing colors to the person just by visualizing them. There is no scientific evidence to support the use of light to treat or cure illnesses in this way.

Cautions

Light therapy that increases someone's exposure to full-spectrum light has not produced adverse reactions. Standard light boxes filter out UV radiation, but if this is not done, overexposure can lead to sunburn, premature wrinkling, and skin cancer. While additional light can relieve some forms of depression, talking to others about the issues and seeking professional help remain important.

Color therapy should not be used instead of conventional treatment, especially for any serious illness. Christians should be particularly aware of color therapy practitioners who base their ideas on Eastern philosophy and life energy.

Recommendations

People thrive on an adequate balance of many natural substances. We realize the importance of rest, exercise, diet, and water for our health, but we also need adequate daylight. With our hectic lifestyles and increased time spent indoors, people need to work at spending enough time outside in sunlight. If this is not possible, making use of full-spectrum light boxes may bring some general relief to seasonal depression caused by the lack of sunlight. However, the use of light or color therapy to treat or cure most diseases is not supported by the evidence.

Treatment Categories

Conventional Therapy
Depression ☺☺☺☺
Avoiding eye strain ☺☺☺☺
Jaundice in newborns ☺☺☺☺
Some skin disorders ☺☺☺☺

Scientifically Unproven
Color therapy

Scientifically Questionable
Color therapy

Energy Medicine
As practiced by some therapists

Quackery or Fraud
In the hands of some practitioners

Further Reading

Cassileth, Barrie R., *The Alternative Medicine Handbook* (New York: W. W. Norton, 1998), 276–79.

Woodham, Anne, and David Peters, *Encyclopedia of Healing Therapies* (London and New York: Dorling Kindersley, 1997), 186–88.

MAGNET THERAPY

What It Is

Magnet therapy is based on the belief that magnets have healing properties. The concept dates back to the 1500s, but its most famous proponent was Franz Mesmer, an eighteenth-century Austrian doctor. Mesmer later promoted hypnosis as a therapy and gave his name to the term "mesmerized" (see Hypnosis, page 226). Mesmer claimed that all illness was caused by problems in the flow of "animal magnetism." He moved magnets around a patient's body to allegedly correct the flow of this magnetic energy.

Elisha Perkins was a prominent New England physician at the end of the 1700s who became a proponent of magnetic healing. He moved metallic rods, called "tractors," over an area where a patient was afflicted with a problem, such as rheumatism. He was convinced the rods worked because patients spoke so highly of the relief they experienced. Perkins did not realize that the relief was due to what is now called "the placebo effect." A person believes he or she feels better because of faith in the treatment, not because of anything the treatment itself does. Those who respond positively to an object that looks like medicine but has no possible biochemical effect on the body are said to be responding to the placebo.

John Haygarth, a physician practicing at the same time as Perkins, demonstrated the placebo effect of Perkins' tractors. Haygarth made copies of the tractors out of wood, and painted them to look like the metal rods that were supposedly influencing the magnetic fields. He treated patients using the tractors, but used the metal tractors on one day, the wooden ones the next. With either procedure, his patients reported feeling better. They had convinced themselves that the tractors he was using were helping them, even though, if Mesmer's ideas of magnetic fields were correct, the days they were "treated" with the wooden tractors should have given them no relief.

Today there are two forms of magnet therapy. Recent interest has primarily been on permanent magnet therapy, where magnets are strapped on the body, put in mattresses, or placed in shoes. A second form is pulsating electromagnetic field therapy based on the electromagnetic effect discovered by English physicist Michael Faraday. He noted that passing electricity through a wire coil produces a magnetic field. He also observed that by changing a magnetic field around an object, electric voltage could be generated. The pulsing of the magnetic field is essential for this effect, and is thus completely different from the effects of permanent magnets.

Electrical signals are found throughout the body. For example, an EKG is a tracing of the electrical signals of the heart, and an EEG is a tracing of the electrical signals of the brain. Hence, pulsating electromagnetic field therapy has been studied as a way to promote healing by generating electrical currents in the body. The most widely studied application of electromagnetic field therapy has been in the healing of broken bones. Results are promising, and the U.S. Food and Drug Administration approved this therapy.

The therapy just described is quite different from the popular use of permanent magnets that don't involve any pulsing electric current. There is no known way for a permanent magnet to induce electrical current, yet promotional materials for permanent magnets often cite the promising results of the very different pulsating electromagnetic therapy.

Claims

The claims for permanent magnet therapy are very broad. They are most commonly promoted for the relief of aches, pains, headaches, and arthritis. For this purpose, magnets are placed within a variety of straps and wraps. Magnetic insoles are worn inside shoes to promote better overall health.

Proponents of permanent magnet therapy say that the magnets promote a better flow of charged electrolytes in the blood. Some manufacturers claim their magnets cure cancer, relieve enlarged prostates, and heal almost every ailment known to humanity.

In August 2000, the Consumer Justice Center, a nonprofit corporation, brought a lawsuit against one magnet manufacturer alleging its promotional material violated California's state consumer protection statutes (Superior Court of the State of California Case 00CC09419). The manufacturers claimed their Magneforce™ Shoe "generates a deep-penetrating magnetic field which increases blood circulation; reduces leg and back fatigue; and provides natural pain relief and improved energy level." These, and many similar claims, are alleged to be false, deceptive, and misleading, and through them "the General Public is scammed out of substantial money." Almost immediately, the company removed these claims from its Website. At the time of writing, the case was pending.

Study Findings

Claims that permanent magnets increase blood flow are based on two studies, one done in saline (salt water) contained in glass tubes and the other on horses. However, these studies had a number of major flaws. Furthermore, many other studies have found no increase in blood flow. In addition, MRI scanners are widely used today and these expose people to magnetic fields two to four times stronger than magnet pads. Yet no changes in blood circulation have been reported with the widespread use of this technology.

Magnets are most commonly promoted (✔) for the relief of aches and pain. One study (✔✔✔) has reported better relief from magnets than from a placebo treatment of arthritis-like pain in patients who had polio. However, another study (✘✘✘) found no relief from shoulder and neck pain from wearing a magnetic necklace. Yet another study (✘✘✘) found no difference in relief of heel pain between patients wearing a magnetic insole or a nonmagnetic insole. In the latter study, 60 percent of patients in both groups reported improvement, which demonstrates the importance of the placebo effect. (Note: Treatments for pain are known to be highly susceptible to placebo effects, indicating that the mind is a major factor in controlling some forms of pain.) The most recent study (✘✘✘) as of this writing, only the second to be double-blinded, found permanent magnets were no better than placebo in twenty patients with chronic back pain.

There is another general problem with static magnet therapy. Calculations have demonstrated that the level of magnetism to which the body is exposed by these magnets is extremely tiny, much less than would be needed to influence the flow of ions in the blood. Additionally, some static magnet therapy uses pads that are made by placing strips of magnets together and alternating the north and south poles. This is also how refrigerator magnets are made and gives much more flexibility in the overall shape of the magnet. The problem is that this design results in the strength of the magnetic field dropping off rapidly as you move away from the magnet. This is why refrigerator magnets will support only a few pieces of paper.

In some cases, the padding or belt around the therapeutic magnet is thick enough to prevent a paper clip from "sticking" to it. This makes it extremely unlikely that enough magnetic field will enter the body to influence anything.

Cautions

Magnets have not been found to cause any side effects. Those with heart pacemakers must avoid strong magnetic fields such as exist in MRI facilities, but the magnets we are evaluating are too weak to interfere with pacemakers. However, using them instead of effective therapies may delay finding actual relief. With serious illnesses, this can have disastrous consequences.

Recommendations

Many people are convinced that magnets help relieve a variety of conditions, which resulted in annual sales of over $5 billion. However, simply wearing a belt, pad, or insert may be enough to produce a beneficial effect. In addition, the placebo effect is very powerful with the types of conditions for which magnets are commonly recommended. Magnet therapy has repeatedly come and gone in popularity over the last few centuries, suggesting that it becomes popular briefly because of the placebo effect, then loses support when patients do not get better. No demonstrable physiological mechanism adequately explains how this therapy might work.

Much of the popular use of magnets is allegedly based on scientific principles, though not ones that hold up under close scrutiny. However, some proponents drift into life energy ideas from magnet therapy. Mesmer stopped using magnets when he found he could influence people in similar ways by hypnotizing them. This led him to describe animal magnetism in terms very similar to life energy. Promoters of theosophy later used magnetism in this same way. (Theosophy is a philosophical-religious approach that blends ideas from the occult and Eastern religions, and laid much of the foundation for the New Age movement.) Whenever people discuss magnets in terms of their influence on generalized energies of the body, Christians should be alert to the concerns we raise about energy medicine.

Treatment Categories

Scientifically Unproven
Any indication

Scientifically Questionable

Energy Medicine
    In the hands of some practitioners

Quackery or Fraud
    In the hands of some practitioners

Further Reading

Collacott, Edward A., John T. Zimmerman, Donald W. White, and Joseph P. Rindone, "Bipolar Permanent Magnets for the Treatment of Chronic Low Back Pain: A Pilot Study," *Journal of the American Medical Association* 283, no. 10 (March 2000): 1322–25.

Livingston, James D., "Magnetic Therapy: Plausible Attraction?" *Skeptical Inquirer* 22, no. 4 (July/August 1998): 25–30, 58.

Ramey, David W., "Magnetic and Electromagnetic Therapy," *Scientific Review of Alternative Medicine* 2, no. 1 (Spring/Summer 1998): 13–19.

MASSAGE THERAPY

What It Is

Mention massage to a group of people and you are likely to notice one of two reactions. Some think in terms of a soothing back rub either by a loved one or in a setting such as a health club. Others think in terms of something sexual, knowing that advertisements for massage in some counterculture publications are really euphemisms for offers of prostitution. When talking about massage therapies, neither is accurate, though the soothing back rub comes far closer to reality.

Massage properly refers to a broad group of medically valid therapies that involve rubbing or moving the skin. Ancient writings and drawings document that massage has long been valued. The famous Greek physician Hippocrates wrote, "The physician must be experienced in many things, but assuredly in rubbing."

Massage was part of the foundation of the physical therapy profession, but its use in health care faded during most of the twentieth century. Some of this relates to the availability of other therapies, but the association of massage with sexual touching was also significant. Physical touch was seen as less appropriate in medical settings, while massage parlors gained reputations that had little to do with health care. However, by the end of the twentieth century, massage was receiving renewed interest and respectability because it was again understood in its historic, medical context.

Today different types of massage are available, and massage is incorporated into a number of other therapies. The best known form is probably Swedish massage in which the hands move over the skin in long, gliding strokes (also called "effleurage"). The muscles may be kneaded, or light friction is applied to the skin.

Some other forms of massage include Shiatsu massage, a much deeper and more aggressive form of massage (see Shiatsu Massage, page 271), and Rolfing, which uses significant amounts of pressure to rebalance joints and restore elasticity to the fascia (the connective tissue surrounding all muscles). In addition, craniosacral therapy, reflexology, and acupressure involve putting pressure on specific parts of the body.

Bodywork is another name for various forms of massage that also tend to include life energy healing. Some of these are only slight modifications of Reiki, Healing Touch, and Therapeutic Touch (none of which necessarily involve physical contact).

Claims

Your skin is the body's largest sensory organ, and, as such, touch in general is important to how you feel. The primary claim made for massage is that it relaxes people, directly leading to reduced muscle tension, lower heart rate, and lower blood pressure. Massage is also said to be helpful during infant development, to remove edema caused by swelling, and to relieve pain.

Study Findings

Even though massage is one of the oldest therapies on record, research on its effectiveness is sparse. However, some studies are starting to verify what most people know through experience.

Studies (✔✔✔) with premature infants who were gently massaged showed that they gained weight quicker and left the hospital earlier than those who were not deliberately touched in this manner. Other studies (✔✔✔) have documented the relaxing effects of massage, including the lowering of anxiety levels and, to some degree, the reduction of some pain. Forms of chest massage have also been shown (✔✔✔) to help patients with respiratory problems. While all of these benefits are significant, no studies support any claims that massage can cure or treat more serious illnesses.

Cautions

Massage itself is very safe and effective for relaxation. The main danger arises if people think it actually cures an underlying disease. Some of the more aggressive forms of massage can cause bruising and pain afterward, and should be used carefully on children and those who are frail. Given that some forms of massage can be intermixed with life energy therapies, Christians should inquire about all that will happen during a massage.

Recommendations

As a form of helping oneself to relax, massage is an old and valued therapy. Giving a massage or shoulder rub to a friend or family member can be a loving way to help him or her release some stress. Having a professional massage may bring extra relief so long as the underlying cause of the stress is also dealt with appropriately.

Treatment Categories

Conventional Therapy
    Premature infants   ☺☺☺☺
    Relaxation   ☺☺☺☺
    Lowering anxiety levels   ☺☺☺☺
    Reduction of some types of pain   ☺☺☺
    Respiratory problems   ☺☺

Complementary Therapy
    For other indications involving stress reduction

Scientifically Unproven
    For other indications, in particular to cure any illness

Energy Medicine
    Certain types or by some practitioners

Further Reading

Woodham, Anne, and David Peters, *Encyclopedia of Healing Therapies* (London and New York: Dorling Kindersley, 1997), 56–61.

MEDITATION

What It Is

Meditation is a word that has been so broadly applied to an array of both healthy and harmful activities that it is difficult to get consistent agreement about its impact on health. For example, one person's idea of meditating may be to sit quietly while forcing his body to relax. He will inhale deeply, exhale slowly, and create a moment of restful quiet in the midst of an otherwise hectic day. Another person's idea is to tune out all else while daydreaming or concentrating on something that is not the primary concern of the moment. One advertising agency account supervisor talks of going on a long walk while she meditates on her client's problem, the focused attention helping her to establish creative solutions. And for others, meditation can be a means of contacting spirit beings or demons. Meditation offers a whole range of practices generally designed to take our minds off everyday business and stressful activities, helping us become more relaxed and reflective.

The type of meditation recommended as an alternative therapy sometimes can have its origin in Eastern religions and mysticism. Transcendental Meditation (TM) is a recent adaptation of these older concepts. In general, the meditator wants to relax in a peaceful environment. Most sit comfortably, focusing their thoughts on something that minimizes troubling or distracting thoughts. Some focus on their own breathing, concentrating on the movement of air in and out of their lungs. Others repeat a mantra—a sacred word or formula given by a spiritual master—or just an ordinary phrase. With practice, people can consciously relax their muscles and learn to control other bodily functions not usually under their control.

Claims

The initial goal with meditation is to induce a state of relaxation. Herbert Benson has documented the many health benefits of what he calls the "relaxation response." This can bring about relief from much of the stress and anxiety experienced by people today. Since this stress can underlie numerous health problems, meditation has the potential to bring about many health benefits.

Eastern meditation and mystical meditation were not developed for their health benefits. They are primarily means toward spiritual enlightenment. The goal is to quiet or empty the rational mind so that people become more aware of their inner selves. This occurs as they enter a state of altered consciousness and come in contact with what those who believe in these practices call the Universal Oneness. Here they claim to receive information about their health problems and the healing needed. Alternative therapies place great emphasis on intuition and the insight gained during meditation, encouraging people to trust their own intuitions rather than the rational ideas of others.

Study Findings

Clinical studies (✔✔✔) have confirmed that meditation can provide short-term results in reducing stress, relieving chronic pain, and reducing blood pressure. Studies (✔✔✔) also have shown that meditation can give some people a better sense of happiness and control of their bodies. However, what has not been shown is whether these changes have long-term health benefits. A number of studies are being conducted in this area, but no conclusions can be given at this writing.

Cautions

Meditation has been documented to cause problems. Transcendental Meditation, initially promoted by the Maharishi Mahesh Yogi, was very popular in the 1960s and did much to familiarize Americans with meditation and Hinduism. But studies (✗✗) have found that its results were not always positive. Almost half of those active as TM trainers reported episodes of anxiety, depression, confusion, frustration, mental and physical tension, and inexplicable outbursts of antisocial behavior. Other studies (✗✗) have documented adverse effects as serious as psychiatric hospitalization and attempted suicide. The problems come from viewing meditation as a simple exercise, when in fact it has considerable power to deeply impact a person psychologically and spiritually.

The spiritual enlightenment some maintain occurs in meditation can involve contact with spirit guides. Even the attempt to rely more on one's own intuition counters the biblical declaration that our own intuition leads to falsehood and deception. In many ways, humanity's problems stem from our reliance on ourselves to know what is best. God told Moses to have the Israelites sew tassels onto the corners of their garments to remind them of this important teaching. "You will have these tassels to look at and so you will remember all the commands of the LORD, that you may obey them and not prostitute yourselves by going after the lusts of your own hearts and eyes" (Numbers 15:39; see also Deuteronomy 12:8; Judges 17:6).

Insight received during meditation is especially problematic. Divination and visions are altered states of consciousness used to gain spiritual insight. Yet unless this insight comes from God, it only reveals the futility and deception of people's own minds. "Then the LORD said to me, 'The prophets are prophesying lies in my name. I have not sent them or appointed them or spoken to them. They are prophesying to you false visions, divinations, idolatries and the delusions of their own minds'" (Jeremiah 14:14; see also 23:16–17, 25–32). "The word of the LORD came to me: 'Son of man, prophesy against the prophets of Israel who are now prophesying. Say to those who prophesy out of their own imagination: "Hear the word of the LORD! This is what the Sovereign LORD says: Woe to the foolish prophets who follow their own spirit and have seen nothing!"'" (Ezekiel 13:1–3).

Recommendations

Christians should relax and reduce unnecessary stress in their lives. "Be still, and know that I am God; I will be exalted among the nations, I will be exalted in the earth" (Psalm 46:10). The Bible tells us to meditate. "Do not let this Book of the Law depart from your mouth; meditate on it day and night, so that you may be careful to do everything written in it. Then you will be prosperous and successful" (Joshua 1:8; see also Psalms 1:2–3; 19:14; 49:3; 104:34; 119:97, 99). But Christian meditation is not emptying one's mind or focusing on one's inner self. Rather, it is filling one's mind with biblical truth while focusing on the Creator, God of the Universe. We will gain insight when we meditate on biblical truth. But this insight is based on the revealed Word of God, and should lead to a life more in conformity with his ways.

Christians should make every effort to retain control over their thought life. "We demolish arguments and every pretension that sets itself up against the knowledge of God, and we take captive every thought to make it obedient to Christ" (2 Corinthians 10:5). Altered states of consciousness open people to spiritual suggestion, making them vulnerable to demonic or other unwholesome influences.

Treatment Categories

Complementary Therapy

Short-term therapy for reducing stress or anxiety ☺☺☺☺

Chronic pain ☺☺☺

Reducing blood pressure ☺☺☺☺

Giving some people a better sense
of happiness and control of their bodies ☺☺

Scientifically Unproven

For other indications

Energy Medicine

In the hands of many non-Christian practitioners

Further Reading

Haddon, David, and Vail Hamilton, *TM Wants You! A Christian Response to Transcendental Meditation* (Grand Rapids: Baker, 1976).

Heide, Frederick J., "Relaxation: The Storm Before the Calm," *Psychology Today* (April 1985), 18–19.

NATUROPATHY

What It Is

Naturopathy is the system of health care usually practiced by naturopathic doctors (N.D.s). Their focus is on "natural" means of preventing and curing illness as opposed to using "unnatural" pharmaceutical drugs and surgeries. The naturopathic approach tries to be holistic, taking into consideration body, mind, and spirit. According to the National College of Naturopathic Medicine, illness demonstrates that the body is trying to heal itself via its "inherent vitality." This concept pervades the naturopathic approach to medicine, but is defined in different ways. For some, it simply means a natural tendency toward health, but for others it reflects the same sort of life energy we have seen in Ayurvedic and traditional Chinese medicine. Regardless, naturopaths see their primary role as assisting nature to bring about healing, or removing obstacles to healing.

In some ways, naturopathy seems like a sensible approach to health and healing. The roles of diet, exercise, relationships, and other lifestyle issues in health are recognized. The emphasis on using only natural approaches to healing has a strong impact on many of the therapies recommended—herbal remedies, supplements, homeopathy, and

Bach flower remedies. Instead of surgery, exercise and chiropractic therapy are used or recommended. Naturopaths often oppose immunization because it is not natural. In this way, while naturopathy can address some important dimensions of health and healing, it often neglects other valid issues and approaches.

Naturopathic training is varied. Some N.D.s have attended a four-year degree program, with much of the first two years similar in content to that received by students in medical schools. The last two years focus on the "natural" treatments that N.D.s use most often—including homeopathy, herbal remedies, acupuncture, biofeedback, counseling, diet, and physical manipulations. Some states in the United States license N.D.s, and the number is growing. A licensed N.D. is permitted to practice all therapies associated with naturopathy after passing certification examinations given after four years of training. Of great concern is that an N.D. degree can be obtained in much less rigorous ways. It is very important to determine how an N.D. obtained his or her degree.

Claims

Naturopaths claim they can treat most general and chronic illnesses, and say that they refer patients requiring complicated surgeries or high-technology treatments to conventional medical doctors. The emphasis in naturopathy is on preventive medicine and teaching people healthy lifestyles. However, some naturopaths have an antagonistic relationship with physicians and are very reluctant to refer patients to a physician. Likewise, many physicians are antagonistic toward N.D.s. These physicians are concerned that since naturopaths receive much less training in medical diagnosis, they may not recognize a serious health problem. In spite of this, some health insurance plans cover N.D. services, treating them as primary care providers in the same manner as a physician's assistant or nurse practitioner.

Study Findings

Studies related to naturopathy itself have not, to our knowledge, been published. However, studies related to specific therapies used by N.D.s are relevant and show much diversity. Homeopathy has little scientific support, while some herbal remedies and supplements have a growing body of research support. However, the vast majority of the herbal remedies used by N.D.s are supported by only anecdotal evidence. Recent research has affirmed the importance N.D.s place on diet, exercise, and relaxation.

Naturopathic literature places a much greater emphasis on anecdotal evidence than controlled clinical trials. A long tradition of use within naturopathy counts as significant evidence of effectiveness for many N.D.s. For example, the Summer 2000 *Naturopathic Newsletter,* published by the University of Bridgeport College of Naturopathic Medicine, lauded a number of alternative therapies on which little or no controlled research has been done. It stated that Bach flower remedies can treat "any emotional or mental condition," that Chinese herbs are effective for a huge variety of conditions ranging from infertility to allergies and asthma, that acupuncture should be considered along with herbs, and that chiropractic can assist with pregnancy problems, heart conditions, and many other illnesses. The newsletter also promoted Ayurvedic medicine, hypnosis, and regression therapy. This type of uncritical promotion of everything "natural" concerns us and leaves us questioning the reliability of the recommendations made by many N.D.s. Not all N.D.s buy into every therapy, but that places a great burden on patients to be very discerning in choosing an N.D.

Cautions

Naturopathy as an approach has few demonstrated harmful effects—if its limitations are accepted and adhered to. With serious illnesses like cancer, or emergencies like heart attacks, good N.D.s recognize the need to refer patients to others for specialized care. They will instead focus on issues related to general healthy lifestyles and prevention of illness. However, if an N.D. fails to diagnose a serious illness or delays referral to a physician, harm could arise.

Some naturopaths claim illnesses arise from the accumulation of toxins in the body. These N.D.s recommend cleansing, sometimes through diet or exercise, but also with purgative methods or chelation therapies, some of which are very severe and can be both physically and psychologically harmful. In addition, since naturopathy is tied into vitalistic beliefs, some naturopaths promote New Age approaches to health and spirituality. Discernment is needed when any practitioner moves into philosophical and religious discussions.

Recommendations

Naturopathy emphasizes a holistic approach to health care that can be compatible with a biblical approach. However, naturopathy can sometimes include New Age spirituality and vitalism. In general, naturopathy recommends some practices and lifestyle changes that can be beneficial. In our opinion, there is a risk with any N.D. who is antagonistic toward physicians because that antagonism could lead to delays in patients getting effective treatments for serious conditions. Since some naturopathic treatments have not demonstrated clinical effectiveness, they should not replace therapies with established positive results. We would encourage naturopaths to apply the scientific method to their therapies. Furthermore, we believe that the publication of studies demonstrating both the safety and effectiveness of any particular N.D. therapy will increase its acceptance both by the lay public and conventional physicians.

Treatment Categories

Complementary Therapy
For some indications

Scientifically Unproven
> For many indications

Scientifically Questionable
> For some indications

Energy Medicine
> In the hands of some naturopaths

Further Reading

Cassileth, Barrie R., *The Alternative Medicine Handbook* (New York: W. W. Norton, 1998), 47–52.

Woodham, Anne, and David Peters, *Encyclopedia of Healing Therapies* (London and New York: Dorling Kindersley 1997), 118–21.

PRAYER FOR HEALING

What It Is

Christian prayer is talking to God and listening to his answers. The Bible records numerous instances where God, in answer to prayer, directly intervened to bring healing. King Hezekiah was near death when he prayed and received this reply from God, "I have heard your prayer and seen your tears; I will heal you" (2 Kings 20:5).

Prayer contributes to health benefits generally (see page 260). Prayer for personal comfort and endurance during illness and as death approaches is integral to Christian spirituality.

The Bible promises comfort during sickness and pain. "Praise be to the God and Father of our Lord Jesus Christ, the Father of compassion and the God of all comfort, who comforts us in all our troubles, so that we can comfort those in any trouble with the comfort we ourselves have received from God" (2 Corinthians 1:3–4).

People differ in what they mean by prayer. The Bible is very specific: prayer is communicating with God. Requests made to God in prayer should, according to the Bible, always be saturated with humility, prayed in accordance with God's will and in the name of Jesus. "This is the confidence we have in approaching God: that if we ask anything *according to his will*, he hears us" [emphasis added] (1 John 5:14). Ultimately, what we want will come about only if it is God's will.

Larry Dossey, the author of *Healing Words*, describes his view of prayer as "far different" from the "old biblically based views of prayer." He claims that biblical prayer arises from a world view that "is now antiquated and incomplete" and constitutes a "uniquely 'pathological mythology.'" For Dossey, praying is a general attitude of leaving things in the hands of fate, or some Universal Consciousness.

A researcher in the field of spirituality and healing, Elisabeth Targ, called prayer a form of "distant healing" which is "any purely mental effort undertaken by one person with the intention of improving physical or emotional well-being in another." Intercessory prayer is offered for a specific result to occur in someone else. But biblical prayer is more than "mental effort." We humbly ask God to intervene and cure Joe of cancer or speed Susan's recovery from surgery.

James 5:13–16 directly addresses prayer for healing.

Is any one of you in trouble? He should pray. . . . Is any one of you sick? He should call the elders of the church to pray over him and anoint him with oil in the name of the Lord. And the prayer offered in faith will make the sick person well; the Lord will raise him up. If he has sinned, he will be forgiven. Therefore confess your sins to each other and pray for each other so that you may be healed. The prayer of a righteous man is powerful and effective.

The oil mentioned here may have had two roles. John Wilkinson, a physician and theologian, points out that oil was used for its medicinal properties—the elders may have been applying a medication. But oil also had important symbolic value. The disciples who were sent out by Jesus "drove out many demons and anointed many sick people with oil and healed them" (Mark 6:13). As in the Old Testament, oil was closely associated with the work of God, and may have been a reminder that God could bring about healing.

The emphasis in biblical prayer is not what we must *do* to convince God to answer, but on God's *will*. An answer to prayer is dependent on God's power and God's will, not ours. There has been much interest recently in evaluating whether intercessory prayer really works. Medical researchers are conducting clinical studies in the hope of proving scientifically whether prayer brings healing.

Study Findings

Interest in research involving intercessory prayer (which we will refer to as "prayer research") is not new. In 1872, John Tyndall proposed that all Christians pray for the patients of one London hospital for at least three years. Skeptical of Christianity, Tyndall believed his study would provide scientific evidence that prayer is ineffective.

The experiment was never conducted, but it generated a storm of controversy, with articles flying off the presses raising scientific, theological, and ethical concerns. Francis Galton, a cousin of Charles Darwin, noted that people frequently pray for clergy and royalty, in particular that they be granted long lives. He found they actually lived shorter lives than "less noble" professionals. To Galton, this was clear evidence that prayer doesn't work.

In 1988, Randolph Byrd, M.D., published a study on the effects of intercessory prayer on almost 400 cardiac patients in an intensive care unit in San Francisco General Hospital. Half of the patients were prayed for by "born-again" Christians, and the other half made up a control group. The intercessors prayed for a rapid recovery, prevention of complications, and prevention of death. The patients prayed for did significantly better in six ways than those in a control group who received no prayer through the research. However, twenty-three other measurements made during this study showed no statistically significant differences. In fact, when all the results were grouped together, the prayer group did only a little better overall.

Measuring twenty-nine different outcomes, instead of only six, would seem to be a more thorough way of doing research, but it generates problems. The more outcomes measured, the greater the risk of finding a positive result just by chance. Also, if all twenty-nine outcomes are only slightly different (and not significant individually), adding them together could produce an overall result that is statistically significant. Byrd admitted that his individual results "could not be considered statistically significant because of the large number of variables examined." Only when the results were combined were they statistically significant.

Another team of researchers, led by William Harris, Ph.D., set out to repeat Byrd's study. This time 990 patients admitted to a coronary care unit in Kansas City, Missouri, were randomized into two groups. Half were prayed for by teams of five Christians (Protestant and Catholic) for twenty-eight days. Thirty-five different medical outcomes were measured.

Their study failed to reproduce Byrd's findings. Byrd had developed a research tool for ranking and evaluating his different measurements and producing an overall result. When Harris's team used Byrd's tool, the differences between the two groups were not significant. They also found no statistically significant differences for any individual measurement. But then they developed a new tool that found that the prayer group scored 10 percent better than the control group. This difference is statistically significant, but Harris concluded that "there is no known way to ascribe a clinical significance to it." In other words, they don't know how much difference this makes in people's actual lives.

Intrigued by these results, we searched for any controlled study of the health effects of intercessory prayer or related practices. We found nineteen in all. All of these, except the two studies already described, were very different, using different types of prayer in patients with many different health conditions. We've grouped these studies as follows:

- Small studies examining physical conditions
- Higher quality studies of physical conditions
- Studies of psychological conditions

Small studies of physical conditions

In this group of six small studies, all with less than ideal designs, two had positive results and four showed no benefits from prayer. These studies (with between sixteen and fifty-three subjects) examined the effects of intercessory prayer on conditions such as diabetes, blood pressure, rheumatoid arthritis, pain and wound healing after hernia surgery, and leukemia. Three used Christian prayer; the other three used a variety of energy-directing forms of prayer. Of the two studies where those who were prayed for did significantly better than the control group, one involved Christian prayer, the other a combination of Reiki and LeShan prayer.

Reiki is a method of calling on spirit guides to assist in a life energy type of healing (see Reiki, page 266).

LeShan proponents believe the universe is interconnected and that when people achieve a certain state of consciousness, they can stimulate and enhance another person's natural capacity for self-healing. Although they claim their approach is not based on life energies, the concept is similar. LeShan is said to be completely natural, meaning it does not involve anything supernatural.

Higher quality studies of physical conditions

This group of eight studies, which included the two cardiac studies by Byrd and Harris, were all designed according to current standards of high-quality clinical research. Most had large numbers of subjects. Two studies involved a form of laying on of hands in addition to prayer. One of these, involving "paranormal" healers, showed no significant healing. The second involved patients with rheumatoid arthritis and had two parts. Some patients reported much improvement after Christian prayer, laying on of hands, and Christian teaching. However, this part had no control group. The second part was randomized and double-blinded, but the group prayed for showed no benefits compared to the control group.

Two other studies examined "spiritual healing," a form of energy therapy, though even the researchers were unsure what the therapy involved. No significant benefits were found in either study.

The last two studies in this group involved patients receiving a combination of Christian, Jewish, New Age, and Buddhist prayer. One was a pilot study that had "encouraging" results but, because of the small number of participants, was not statistically reliable. Based on the findings of that pilot study, researchers have started a larger project with 1500 cardiac patients. The second study, involving AIDS patients, had mixed results (some positive, some negative) using a variety of prayer types. Of the eleven outcomes measured, AIDS patients in the prayer group did significantly better in six.

Studies of psychological conditions

In the studies of psychological conditions, three randomized, double-blind studies published during the 1990s showed no benefits. One used LeShan prayer, the second a general form of prayer to God, and the third involved prayer by Jewish and Christian volunteers. Two earlier studies showed some benefits, but both were poorly designed and were not controlled studies. The improvements found in those who were prayed for could have been the result of a number of other factors.

Overall, from a purely scientific perspective, no clear conclusions can be drawn from these studies in spite of the improvements found in some. Two systematic reviews of prayer research came to this same conclusion (see Astin and Roberts, page 260).

Cautions

Prayer research is controversial. Some see it as a form of testing God that should not be done. We disagree. We do not believe this research is inappropriate, though we have reservations about its helpfulness. The story of Gideon's fleece in Judges 6:36–40 is an example of God answering a specific request for evidence of his reality and power.

When the disciples of John the Baptist asked Jesus if he was the Messiah, Jesus told them to believe him because of what they could verify by observation. "At that very time Jesus cured many who had diseases, sicknesses and evil spirits, and gave sight to many who were blind. So he replied to the messengers [from John the Baptist], 'Go back and report to John what you have seen and heard: The blind receive sight, the lame walk, those who have leprosy are cured, the deaf hear, the dead are raised, and the good news is preached to the poor'" (Luke 7:20–22).

But the results of prayer research are far from conclusive. We disagree with those, either Christian or otherwise, who make these inconclusive results the primary pillars of their theological or philosophical claims. We also are concerned about those researchers who use their studies merely as an opportunity to find support for their particular beliefs about the nature of prayer—either to support or refute the power of prayer. Scientific research, to be valid, must be conducted in such a manner that results are not skewed by some preconceived idea.

Prayer research is not without risks. The inconclusive results might lead some people to turn away from prayer—and even from God himself—especially if they approach him strictly on the basis of scientific evidence. The great variability in what people mean by prayer is problematic not only scientifically but also spiritually. Non-biblical types of "prayer" are often used. In some research, prayer means sending impersonal healing energy to another person. Elaine Harkness and colleagues claim healing from prayer comes "from the 'channeling' by the healer of an as yet undefined 'energy' from a 'source' to the patient." Those who view prayer this way often call it "distant healing" or "spiritual healing."

Various occult activities have also been defined as "prayer" to allow their inclusion in prayer research. Marilyn Schlitz and William Braud equate prayer with sorcery, shamanism, psychic healing, and telepathy. Harkness includes meditation, magic, and using mediums or "spirit doctors" as forms of distant healing. A popular author, Rosemary Guiley, views prayer as a vibrating inner connection with the divine that leads her to view prayer as control over esoteric powers.

People are being exposed to occult activities labeled as "prayer," possibly without their knowledge. Researchers tend to ignore or avoid these spiritual concerns, but they are crucial to how Christians evaluate this research and make decisions about whether to get involved in various types of prayer offered in health care settings.

Theological Assessment

The fundamental theological flaw with all prayer research is the assumption that only humans impact the results. In this view, if prayer works, what people pray for will come about.

Dossey and others believe prayer follows some natural law, and science will help us understand that law, just like it did the law of gravity. Under this view, negative results or inconclusive results count as evidence against prayer being effective.

Such an assumption holds true only if prayer is *impersonal*, based on some energy or thought-power or unknown force. But that's not biblical prayer. Prayer, according to the Bible, is not an energy that, once emitted, takes on a life of its own with predictable outcomes. Scientific research could easily measure whether such an energy "works," but this is not what Christianity means by prayer. Biblical prayer is an inherently *personal* encounter with a personal and loving Father. In fact, inconsistent research results are precisely what we should expect with prayer, given the biblical teaching on prayer for healing.

After James instructs Christians to pray for healing, he presents Elijah as an example of a righteous man whose prayer was "powerful and effective" (James 5:16–18). We can learn how to pray from Elijah's example and, in particular, from an incident involving him and the prophets of Baal (1 Kings 18:16–40).

This incident contrasts Elijah's effective prayer with the ineffective prayer of the prophets of Baal, a god worshiped by the nations around ancient Israel. At that time, the people of Israel were undecided about whether to follow God or Baal. Elijah proposed a test to show whose god was the true God. He told the prophets of Baal to sacrifice a bull, place it on a stack of wood, and then pray to Baal to send fire from heaven to burn up their offering. Elijah said he would do likewise, but pray to the God of Israel.

The prophets of Baal built their wooden altar, placed their sacrificed bull on it, and prayed to Baal. From morning until noon, they repeated, like a mantra, the words "O Baal, answer us! O Baal, answer us!" They danced and leaped around the sacrificial altar, working themselves into a greater and greater frenzy. They eventually slashed themselves with swords and spears until blood gushed from their wounds. This continued until evening.

The narrator sums up the pathetic picture of their attempts to get an answer from the heavens: "But there was no response, no one answered, no one paid attention" (1 Kings 18:29).

Elijah took over. He repaired the altar of the Lord, which was in ruins. He arranged wood on the altar, sacrificed another bull, and placed it on the wood. He had the people soak everything with water, even filling a trench he had dug around the altar. Then Elijah prayed: "O LORD, God of Abraham, Isaac and Israel, let it be known today that you are God in Israel and that I am your servant and have done all these things at your command. Answer me, O LORD, answer me, so these people will know that you, O LORD, are God, and that you are turning their hearts back again" (1 Kings 18:36–37).

All of a sudden, everything on the altar burst into flames. Even the stones Elijah used to build the altar were consumed by fire. "When all the people saw this, they fell prostrate and cried, 'The LORD—he is God! The LORD—he is God!'" (1 Kings 18:39).

The theology in this story is particularly relevant to prayer research. It reminds us that the Bible forbids certain spiritual practices—and demonstrates their ineffectiveness in comparison to the power of God. Christians should refuse to participate in prayer research that involves non-Christian prayer.

The prophets of Baal believed that the more they prayed, and the louder they prayed, and the more they worked themselves into a frenzy, the more likely it was that their prayers would be answered. They focused on what they had to *do* to get an answer from Baal, their god.

A serious problem with prayer research is that it may foster such a mechanical approach to prayer. It uses and studies prayer as if it were just another impersonal "therapy" to try when needed. Prayer, spirituality, and even God himself can become viewed as things to be used to get what we want. Faith in God and his provision is thus trivialized and demeaned.

Prayer already becomes mechanical too easily. While we may not slash ourselves with swords to impress God, how often do we think God will be more inclined to answer our prayers if we do something extra or deny ourselves something? Do we think God will be more likely to hear us if we get up earlier, or stay up later, or pray longer? Do we hope some study will show us the best way to pray or the right words to say?

Elijah didn't relate to God through impersonal rituals, or rote prayers. He prayed to God directly and personally. He asked God to let the people know that same day that he was the God of Israel. Elijah was not so much concerned that his prayer produce certain results (like flames from heaven), but that God would be glorified. And God answered his prayer.

God is not interested in meaningless repetition. The Bible affirms persistence in prayer (Luke 18:1–5), but Jesus gave us the Lord's Prayer while rejecting rote prayer. "And when you pray, do not keep on babbling like pagans, for they think they will be heard because of their many words" (Matthew 6:7; see also Isaiah 29:13). Sadly, even the beautiful Lord's Prayer can be recited in meaningless ways. We should humbly make our requests to our Father in heaven, and lay the burdens of our hearts at his feet.

For Christians, the inconclusive results of prayer research can be discouraging. Does this mean that God doesn't answer prayer? Or, worse still, does he just arbitrarily pick and choose whose prayer to answer? Why would God not heal us physically in answer to our prayers for healing?

Prayer research will never answer these questions. Clinical research on the effectiveness of prayer is designed to control the impact of human factors on the results. It cannot take into account God's decision—whether or not to answer a particular prayer—or even to delay an answer.

God may choose not to heal people of great faith despite their prayers for healing. (Part Two of our book elaborates on this topic.) God may use an illness to assist us in our spiritual growth and to remind us of our need to depend on him. Paul's prayer to remove his "thorn in the flesh" was not answered the way he first wanted. This "thorn" is widely believed to have been a physical ailment.

> *Three times I pleaded with the Lord to take it [the thorn] away from me. But he said to me, "My grace is sufficient for you, for my power is made perfect in weakness." Therefore I will boast all the more gladly about my weaknesses, so that Christ's power may rest on me. That is why, for Christ's sake, I delight in weaknesses, in insults, in hardships, in persecutions, in difficulties. For when I am weak, then I am strong.*
>
> 2 Corinthians 12:8–10

The inconclusive results from prayer research may also be due to another factor: researchers cannot ensure that those in a control group receive no prayer. We would have ethical problems with any such attempt to block prayer. A whole host of other people could be praying for the research subjects in both groups. Because of such lack of controls, some scientists think this type of research will never reveal clear-cut answers.

Recommendations

The inconclusive results of these experiments should not be viewed as evidence against the power of prayer. God never promised to answer every prayer immediately or in the affirmative. Like any loving parent, God can answer "No!" and still be just, loving, and righteous. God can answer "Just wait. Be patient." "Wait" and "No" are both answers to prayer that cannot be measured by the scientific method.

The inconclusive results of prayer research are consistent with the fact that God's will differs from one person to another. He may have a reason to heal someone in one situation, but not heal someone else. As more studies are published, the results will continue to vary because God cannot be forced to act within the controls of scientific research.

We believe in the power of prayer because Scripture teaches us to pray. We recommend prayer for healing on the basis of our theological beliefs, not scientific research. This research makes it clear that Christians must be discerning about what is meant by "prayer" before welcoming it into modern health care or participating in its practice.

As we learn to cope with our illnesses, disabilities, and the knowledge of our eventual death, prayer to God can make a huge difference in our lives. But as we pray for healing, we must remember that God does not promise to heal us of every disease, though he does make a number of remarkable promises:

- Salvation to anyone who is willing to turn to him for forgiveness.
- A personal relationship with those who initiate one with him.
- His unceasing presence in this life to comfort his people in their trials.
- Eternal life in his presence for those who put their faith in him.

We can, and should, pray for all of these promises when we are sick and suffering. We can know that he will answer these prayers. He will give us the strength to endure what we must bear. We also can, and should, pray for healing. In spite of not having a guarantee of physical healing, we have something even greater: the knowledge that the Lord of the universe will be with us in our suffering. Knowing these promises, and trusting in God, we will be able to say along with Paul:

> *For I have learned to be content whatever the circumstances. I know what it is to be in need, and I know what it is to have plenty. I have learned the secret of being content in any and every situation, whether well fed or hungry, whether living in plenty or in want. I can do everything through him who gives me strength.*
>
> Philippians 4:11–13

Treatment Categories

Complementary Therapy
In all situations, because of biblical teaching   ☺☺☺☺

Further Reading

Astin, John A., Elaine Harkness, and Edzard Ernst, "The Efficacy of 'Distant Healing': A Systematic Review of Randomized Trials," *Annals of Internal Medicine* 132, no. 11 (June 2000): 903–10.

Byrd, Randolph C., "Positive Therapeutic Effects of Intercessory Prayer in a Coronary Care Unit Population," *Southern Medical Journal* 81, no. 7 (July 1988): 826–29.

Dossey, Larry, *Healing Words: The Power of Prayer and the Practice of Medicine* (New York: HarperSanFrancisco, 1993).

Galton, Francis, "Does Prayer Preserve?" *Archives of Internal Medicine* 125 (April 1970): 580-81, 587; excerpt from "Statistical Inquiries into the Efficacy of Prayer," *Fortnightly Review* 12 (1872): 125–35.

Guiley, Rosemary E., *Prayer Works: True Stories of Answered Prayer* (Unity Village, Mo.: Unity Books, 1998).

Harkness, Elaine F., Neil C. Abbot, and Edzard Ernst, "A Randomized Trial of Distant Healing for Skin Warts," *American Journal of Medicine* 108, no. 6 (April 2000): 448–52.

Harris, William S., Manohar Gowda, Jerry W. Kolb, Christopher P. Strychacz, James L. Vacek, Philip G. Jones, Alan Forker, James H. O'Keefe, and Ben D. McCallister, "A Randomized, Controlled Trial of the Effects of Remote, Intercessory Prayer on Outcomes in Patients Admitted to the Coronary Care Unit," *Archives of Internal Medicine* 159 (October 1999): 2273–78.

Letters to the Editor on Intercessory Prayer Study, *Archives of Internal Medicine* 160 (June 2000): 1870–78.

Roberts, L., I. Ahmed, S. Hall, and C. Sargent, "Intercessory Prayer for the Alleviation of Ill Health (Cochrane Review)," in *The Cochrane Library,* no. 4 (Oxford: Update Software, 2000).

Schlitz, Marilyn, and William Braud, "Distant Intentionality and Healing: Assessing the Evidence," *Alternative Therapies in Health & Medicine* 3, no. 6 (November 1997): 62–73.

Targ, Elisabeth, "Evaluating Distant Healing: A Research Review," *Alternative Therapies in Health & Medicine* 3, no. 6 (November 1997): 74–78.

Wilkinson, John, *The Bible and Healing: A Medical and Theological Commentary* (Edinburgh, Scotland: Handsel; Grand Rapids: Eerdmans, 1998), 248–55.

QIGONG

What It Is

Qigong (pronounced CHEE-guhng) literally means "energy work." Within traditional Chinese medicine (TCM), *qi,* or *chi* (both pronounced CHEE), is believed to be vital to keep a person healthy. There are Chinese hospitals where only Qigong is available, though most Chinese hospitals also have other health services, including an increasing amount of Western conventional medicine.

TCM focuses on preventive measures: physical moderation, exercise, diet, and breathing techniques. When President Richard Nixon visited China, news crews filmed millions of Chinese arising each morning in order to practice breathing and movement techniques, such as the popular martial art Tai Chi. These practices seemed to fit into Western concepts even though they are all based on spiritual life energy concepts and run counter to Christian teachings.

The Chinese term for human life energy is *chi. Chi* is believed to be a mix of inherited energy, passed from parents to children at the time of conception, and energy derived from the food and air that sustain us throughout life. The transportation system for *chi* is believed by the Chinese to be a series of meridians that extend throughout our bodies and link our skin with our internal organs in order to assure our well-being. (For more information on Chinese health beliefs, see Traditional Chinese Medicine, page 279, and Acupressure, page 144.) It is *chi* that is believed to provide protection from illness and promotes health.

Qigong consists of meditation, breathing exercises, and gentle repetitive movements. Tai Chi and other Chinese martial arts are based on these same principles except that the physical movements get progressively more active and assertive.

Qigong exercises involve slow, rhythmic movements of parts of the body while sitting or standing. The movements can also be done from wheelchairs or a bed, making this a type of exercise that can literally be used throughout a person's life. Legend has it that the movements were inspired by watching the instinctive movements of wild animals.

Practitioners of Qigong focus on their breathing while doing the exercise movements, and visualize *chi* flowing smoothly through their bodies, or accumulating in areas that may be depleted.

Qigong is practiced in two very different ways. Internal Qigong involves balancing and manipulating the flow of *chi* within oneself. External Qigong is a skill only master therapists can develop. Qigong masters are said to be able to direct *chi* externally to either heal other people or move objects without touching them. These Qigong masters perform great feats by what they claim involves manipulating and directing this non-physical energy. Skeptics claim these are conjuring tricks, involving either sleight of hand or true magical powers.

Claims

Practicing internal Qigong is said to induce relaxation, promote general well-being, and reduce stress—effective as a complement to conventional therapies for patients with heart problems and cancer. The exercises can be a helpful and gentle regimen for those who are physically unfit or weakened by illness.

The claims made for external Qigong are much broader and more dramatic. Qigong masters are said to have cured every form of serious illness and even to have brought people back from the dead. This aspect of Qigong practice and belief raises significant concerns for Christians.

Study Findings

Many reports (✔) on Qigong have come from China, though Chinese studies on Qigong have not been systematically reviewed in the West. The studies that have been seen (✔✔) are often criticized for being nothing more than reports of one or two patients—anecdotes, case histories, or case reports too limited to be used as proof of value. They also lack the controls needed to assure that any observed changes were due to Qigong and not a host of other factors influencing people and their health.

There is no evidence that Qigong increases resistance to illness, or that it can cure any illness. Evidence from other studies (✔✔✔) of gentle, regular exercise support the beneficial effects of that component of the practice. However, randomized, controlled studies of Qigong compared to other exercise regimens are needed to show if Qigong has any benefits in the treatment of any illness or if those benefits extend beyond those of exercise alone.

Cautions

In some ways, Qigong introduces people to the importance of taking time to relax and develop some sort of regular, gentle exercise routine. However, as with yoga, meditation, and other Eastern practices, we should never forget that the ultimate goal of many of these practices is religious. These practices are designed to help people become more unified with the universal energy field and to develop one's awareness of that energy. While the breathing and movement exercises may be innocuous at first, Qigong is an introduction to a world view and religious system completely different from Christianity (see Energy Medicine, page 193).

Qigong is not without problems. Numerous reports exist (✖✖) of people suffering side effects—from relatively mild symptoms of headache, dry mouth, and muscle twitching all the way to hallucinations and psychotic breakdowns. Most of these symptoms cease within a couple months of stopping Qigong, although others have taken a couple years to resolve. With the growing popularity of Qigong in China, specialized clinics have opened there to treat the increasing numbers of patients with what are now called "Qigong-induced mental disorders."

A Chinese book, *Qigong: Chinese Medicine or Pseudoscience?*, was recently translated into English. The authors interviewed many of those involved in the studies that allegedly demonstrated amazing feats using external Qigong. They concluded that most of these claims were based on hoaxes or conjuring tricks. If Qigong masters were able to do what they claim, in our opinion they would have to be tapping into some form of psychic or spiritual power. Since this clearly is not of God, it is most likely of the Evil One and antithetical to what Christians should be involved with. We should assume that the more benign manifestations of Qigong are simply less powerful examples of the same occult energy.

Recommendations

Christians should take a holistic approach to their health. This recognizes the importance of exercise, stress reduction, and taking time out of a busy schedule to allow our bodies and minds to recuperate. But since we can easily do all of these things without getting involved in practices and techniques that are infused with non-Christian beliefs and concepts, there should be no reason to practice Qigong. Given the alleged paranormal abilities of Qigong masters, Christians should be very reluctant to participate in their therapies at any level.

Treatment Categories

Complementary Therapy
   Exercise and breathing technique   ☺☺

Scientifically Unproven
   For other indications   ☹☹☹☹

Scientifically Questionable

Energy Medicine
   In the hands of most practitioners

Further Reading

Cassileth, Barrie R., *The Alternative Medicine Handbook* (New York: W. W. Norton, 1998), 145–48.

Ng, Beng-Yeong, "Qigong-Induced Mental Disorders: A Review," *Australian and New Zealand Journal of Psychiatry* 33, no. 2 (April 1999): 197–206.

Sancier, Kenneth M., "Medical Applications of Qigong," *Alternative Therapies in Health and Medicine* 2, no. 1 (January 1996): 40–46.

Zixin, Lin, Yu Li, Guo Zhengyi, Shen Zhenyu, Zhang Honglin, and Zhang Tongling, *Qigong: Chinese Medicine or Pseudoscience?* (Amherst, N.Y.: Prometheus, 2000).

REFLEXOLOGY

What It Is

Dr. William H. Fitzgerald, an ear, nose, and throat physician, created the American forerunner of reflexology back in 1915. He had an idea that he described as "zone therapy," though a variety of relaxation techniques and healing therapies similar to reflexology date back to Africa, Egypt, India, and parts of Asia. Originally, these were related to life energy concepts such as the Chinese *chi* or the Indian *prana*.

Reflexology, as it evolved from Dr. Fitzgerald's work, looks like a foot massage, but is said to be much more. In its twentieth-century form, the body was divided into ten vertical zones running from the feet to the head, and down each arm. The belief was that "energy" flows through each zone and must be balanced in order for the organs of that zone to be healthy. The zones on the left side of the body have reflex points on the left hand and foot; zones on the right correspond to reflex points on the right hand and foot. Imbalances in energy lead to the accumulation of waste material (uric acid and calcium crystals) at the reflex points.

Today the practice of reflexology involves the application of pressure at the reflex points to break up the granular accumulations. Practitioners claim this allows free and balanced flow of energy, which allegedly restores health.

In the 1930s, Eunice Ingham, a nurse and physical therapist, mapped out all the reflex points on the feet. She showed which part of each foot corresponded to which organ. For example, the brain can be assisted by putting pressure on the tips of the three largest toes on both feet. The left pelvis corresponds to the heel of the left foot, and so on. Today some reflexologists have come to believe that emotional problems can also be resolved by applying pressure to certain reflex points.

Claims

Practitioners claim reflexology aids almost every part of the body and relieves more than a hundred ailments. These include acne, asthma, cirrhosis of the liver, colds, fatigue, impotence, infections, and stress. It is said to work by improving the flow of blood to the corresponding parts of the body and eliminating toxic accumulations. Although this system sounds just like the energy therapies of traditional Chinese medicine (one of its historic roots), some proponents say it is based on a completely different type of energy. Others make no distinction, utilizing the same concept of life energy as used in Therapeutic Touch, acupuncture, and other energy therapies.

Study Findings

Reflexology may benefit people in the same way massage helps people relax and reduce their stress levels. However, little scientific evidence supports claims that the benefits exceed basic massage techniques. Most of the reports in the literature are case studies or anecdotal reports (✔). A small number of pilot studies (✔✔) have found reflexology to be of some help, but large-scale, well-controlled research does not exist.

Cautions

A number of practitioners claim reflexology can elicit a "healing crisis." This is a common claim in any therapy that involves "detoxification." Flu-like symptoms—lightheadedness, disturbed sleep, and diarrhea—are said to result from the elimination of the toxic buildup that caused whatever problems led a patient to the practitioner. There appear to be no other serious side effects, though standard precautions should apply. Reflexology should not be pursued instead of proven effective treatment, but may be a welcome, relaxing adjunct to therapy, in much the manner of massage easing the stress of someone with heart problems, cancer, and the like.

Some reflexologists interpret their work in terms of life energy manipulation. Christians should be discerning about the beliefs being promoted by the person offering this type of foot massage.

Recommendations

Reflexology seems to be a form of therapy that may help with relaxation. But given its unproven efficacy and the potential for life energy involvement, there seems to be no reason why a Christian would pursue such therapy. Have an ordinary foot massage instead.

Treatment Categories

Complementary Therapy
Relaxation, for people with anxiety or tension ☺☺☺
Relaxation, for people with headaches or pain ☺

Scientifically Unproven
For other indications

Scientifically Questionable
For most indications, especially to cure any illness

Energy Medicine
In the hands of most practitioners

Further Reading

Botting, Deborah, "Review of Literature on the Effectiveness of Reflexology," *Complementary Therapies in Nursing & Midwifery* 3 (1997): 123–30.

Cassileth, Barrie, *The Alternative Medicine Handbook* (New York: W. W. Norton, 1998), 236–39.

REIKI

What It Is

Reiki comes from the Japanese *rei*, meaning universal, and *ki*, meaning vital force, and is pronounced "RAI-kee." *Ki* is the Japanese term for *prana*, or *chi*, the universal life energy. Proponents claim Reiki was practiced by Buddha and discussed in ancient Sanskrit writings that were lost. Some practitioners believe the therapy was in use in the early part of first-century Rome, and that it was the healing method practiced by Jesus, though there is no biblical or Sanskrit support for this claim.

Modern Reiki was developed out of an experience a Zen Buddhist monk had in the mid-1800s. The monk, Mikao Usui, had been meditating, fasting, and praying on Mount Koriyama in Japan for three weeks when he underwent a psychic experience. He reported that the secret to healing—Reiki—had been revealed to him. Subsequently, others have reported learning more details through channeling, which is the New Age term for a method of consulting spirit guides to obtain information from them.

All Reiki therapies have as their core concept that life energy pervades each person, and that this energy is unconditional, divine, loving, and healing. Illnesses are believed to arise when the energy cannot flow properly through the person, usually due to blockages at the *chakras*, where life energy is converted from one form to another and, ultimately, into physical matter. The practitioner is a channel, allowing the Reiki energy to flow through him or her, directing it toward the patient. Reiki has a number of variations, but the basic methods and beliefs are the same.

Training in Reiki consists of learning to open oneself to the energy so that it can flow freely through the practitioner. The energy itself is believed to know what each patient needs for healing. Reiki training requires involvement of a Reiki Master. Until recently, Reiki was carried out in secret ceremonies, the practitioners entrusted with knowledge they were not to reveal to others. Now Reiki is being openly promoted in popular alternative medicine books and nursing journals.

Practitioners of Reiki must go through various "attunements" during training. A Reiki Master calls upon the help of spirit guides to open students' *chakras* and fill them with life energy. Students report being able to feel the energy flow through them, which often leads to their hands getting hot. Students also intuitively receive special symbols that later become central to their healing practice. At the completion of this ceremony, the first-degree Reiki practitioner can detect and move life energy.

To become a second-degree Reiki, practitioners must learn both to use the symbols received in the first attunement and to send life energy over longer distances. They learn how to contact spirit guides and to use them during healing.

The third level, the Reiki Master, can only be attained through the invitation of a Reiki Master. During this training, practitioners commit their lives to Reiki, come to embody life energy, and give complete control of healing sessions to their spirit guides.

The healing sessions themselves look very much like a Therapeutic Touch session. Practitioners place their hands, palms down, on or above the patient's body. The hands are kept in one place, and the practitioners attune themselves to the life energy. They are taught that they must not try to direct the energy, but let it flow through them. They should initially focus their intention on bringing about harmony and healing, but once the energy starts to flow through them, they do not need to concentrate on what they are doing. The energy flow will cause sensations of hot, cold, tingling, color, or pain, and when these subside (after about five minutes) the practitioner moves to another area. A complete healing session can take an hour or more.

Practitioners also draw or visualize the special symbols to increase the power of the energy being directed. Second- and third-degree Reiki practitioners need not be present with their patients because they claim to be able to send life energy over long distances.

Claims

Most proponents of Reiki claim that it brings about relaxation and relieves pain. However, some proponents claim it can cure and improve almost anything, from schizophrenia to cancer, marital problems to drug addictions. One Reiki Master in India claims he can recharge drained batteries with Reiki.

Study Findings

There have been very few controlled studies of Reiki. The articles in professional journals mostly report case studies (✔), where an individual was said to have recovered or improved after receiving Reiki.

Cautions

Reiki is clearly antithetical to biblical Christianity. Communication with spirits is an integral part of the practice, during both attunements and healing sessions. Contacting spirits is denounced in the Bible as sorcery, mediumship, and spiritism (Leviticus 19:26, 31; 20:6; Deuteronomy 18:9–14; Acts 19:19; Galatians 5:20; Revelation 21:8). Contacting spirit guides is dangerous spiritually, physically, and emotionally. "Be self-controlled and alert. Your enemy the devil prowls around like a roaring lion looking for someone to devour" (1 Peter 5:8). In their literature, Reiki practitioners claim to seek what is called the Kundalini experience, the pinnacle of psychic experiences, which can cause severe emotional and psychological disturbances. (See Yoga, page 285.)

Recommendations

Christians should have nothing to do with Reiki. Those involved with Reiki need protection from demonic spirits. While avoiding the practice of Reiki, we must reach out to its practitioners with the healing power of Jesus.

Treatment Categories

Energy Medicine
Possibly occult   ☹☹☹☹

Further Reading

O'Mathúna, Dónal P., "Reiki as an Adjunctive Therapy for Relaxation and Pain Relief," *Alternative Medicine Alert* 2, no. 12 (December 1999): 136–38.
Stein, Diane, *Essential Reiki* (Freedom, Calif.: Crossing Press, 1995).

SHAMANISM

What It Is

Shamanism, or shamanic medicine, is possibly the oldest form of medicine still practiced today. Most tribal societies have or had their shamans, medicine men, witch doctors, sorcerers, or holy men. The shaman usually was both the healer and priest for the tribe—highly respected. His work often involved lifelong learning. Even today practicing medicine men and shamans frequently combine the rituals specific to their culture with the use of plants that are known to have medicinal properties. Visualization techniques common to some alternative therapies are also included.

Modern-day shamans sometimes include conventional therapies, including various counseling techniques and pharmaceuticals. What is most distinctive about shamanic medicine is not the therapies involved, but the means by which shamans determine what a particular patient needs. This emphasis goes back to the root meaning of the Siberian term "shaman," which is defined as "to know," though with the emphasis on spiritual knowledge.

Shamans go through a long apprenticeship in which they learn how to contact and deal with the spirits of ancestors, animals, or demons. Within shamanism, healing involves becoming more under the influence of these spirits, and allowing them to control more of one's life. To make contact with the spiritual realm, the shaman enters a trance, which can be induced by fasting, hallucinogenic herbs, or rituals that involve dancing, drumming, and chanting. Once the spirits are contacted, the shaman acts as a mediator between the spirits and the patient to find out how the spirits have been offended and why they have sent this illness on the patient. Once this is discovered, the shaman bargains with the spirits to find out what is needed to release the patient from the illness. Then the shaman returns to normal consciousness and carries out the magical practices needed to appease the offended spirits or demons.

Claims

Shamanism is actually a pagan religion in which it is believed that all illnesses are caused by spiritual events. This means that the shaman believes he can cure all illnesses.

With recent interest in alternative medicine, even shamanism is becoming secularized. Some shamans now offer certain practices and therapies to nonbelievers—just for the money they can make or hoping to convert people to their religious beliefs after treatment. While some of these individual therapies (visualization and herbal remedies) may be somewhat effective, each needs to be evaluated on its own merits.

Study Findings

Very little scientific research has been done on the benefits of shamanism. However, study of the Bible reveals very clear advice. Shamanism incorporates occult and magical practices that are clearly forbidden in the Bible (Leviticus 19:26, 31; 20:6; Acts 19:19; Galatians 5:20; Revelation 21:8). In many ways, shamanism is equivalent to sorcery, which is frequently condemned. King Saul used a medium to contact the deceased spirit of Samuel (1 Samuel 28) and was explicitly condemned by God for doing so. "Saul died because he was unfaithful to the LORD; he did not keep the word of the LORD and even consulted a medium for guidance, and did not inquire of the LORD" (1 Chronicles 10:13–14). Occult practitioners (e.g., diviners, dreamers, and mediums) and activities (e.g., sorcery, spells, and astrology) work to misdirect people in their greatest hours of need.

Keep on, then, with your magic spells
    and with your many sorceries,
      which you have labored at since childhood....
All the counsel you have received has only worn you out!
Let your astrologers come forward,
those stargazers who make predictions month by month,
    let them save you from what is coming upon you.
Surely they are like stubble;
    the fire will burn them up.
They cannot even save themselves
    from the power of the flame.
Here are no coals to warm anyone;
    here is no fire to sit by.
That is all they can do for you—
    these you have labored with
    and trafficked with since childhood.
Each of them goes on in his error;
    there is not one that can save you.

Isaiah 47:12–15

While God condemns occult practices (Deuteronomy 18:9–14), he recognizes that we need spiritual guidance. He sent his prophets that we would know the truth about him and aspects of his world. The message of these prophets and of Christ's apostles together give us the Bible, a divinely inspired message, unlike other books. "Above all, you must understand that no prophecy of Scripture came about by the prophet's own interpretation. For prophecy never had its origin in the will of man, but men spoke from God as they were carried along by the Holy Spirit" (2 Peter 1:20–21). However, we must accept that God has revealed only part of what is known in the spiritual world. "The secret things belong to the LORD our God, but the things revealed belong to us and to our children forever, that we may follow all the words of this law" (Deuteronomy 29:29). Shamans use occult practices in attempts to discover things that we have no need to know or should not know because the knowledge may harm us.

Cautions

During their training, shamans are possessed by either their spirit guides or the spirit of their "power animal" (a spirit with the form of an animal). These spirits are responsible for any healing that may occur through the shaman. Involvement with a possessed person may adversely affect others spiritually, or even lead to their possession. Possession is not only spiritually dangerous but can lead to serious mental illness and physical suffering. A significant body of psychological research documents the increased prevalence of psychotic behavior among shamans.

Some shamanic practices can be followed without committing oneself to shamanism, but these practices introduce people to this whole belief system and, therefore, may expose them to demonic oppression—or possession in the case of non-Christians.

Recommendations

Christians should not dabble in the occult or adopt other religions, not even for the sake of health. For this reason, there can be no reason why a Christian should use the services of a shaman. However, Christians should remember that shamans, as with all other non-Christians, deserve and need to hear about the healing which is in Christ. While rejecting the practices and beliefs of shamanism, the shamans themselves should not be rejected.

Treatment Categories

Energy Medicine
Possibly occult ☹☹☹☹

Further Reading

Cassileth, Barrie R., *The Alternative Medicine Handbook* (New York: W. W. Norton, 1998), 314–17.

SHIATSU MASSAGE

What It Is

Shiatsu massage is a Japanese massage therapy strongly influenced by traditional Chinese medicine and developed from acupressure (the word "shiatsu" literally means "finger pressure"). The practice was little known in the West until the early part of the twentieth century when it was revived and combined with some forms of Western medicine. It is believed to have originally been developed as a way to detect and treat problems in the flow of life energy, which, in Japanese, is called *ki*. Practitioners use what is called "*hara* diagnosis" to assess the flow of *ki* along the meridians. *Ki* is believed to be stored in the abdomen, with different regions connected to internal organs via meridians. Practitioners gently press on various parts of a person's abdomen to determine if there are any energy problems. Treatment is carried out to restore a balanced flow of *ki* by applying pressure at various parts of the body, called "acupoints." Pressure is applied by massaging various acupoints using the practitioners' fingers, thumbs, elbows, knees, or feet.

A closely related practice, called *do-in* (or *daoyin*), is basically a self-applied form of Shiatsu.

Claims

In Japan, Shiatsu has been used mostly as a popular means of relieving everyday ailments like headaches, back pain, constipation, and diarrhea. Most commonly it is used as part of a general health maintenance program to "cleanse the body," relieve tension, and promote relaxation. However, practitioners frequently claim to be able to diagnose and treat a far wider variety of ailments.

Study Findings

There are practically no controlled studies on Shiatsu. However, the studies on acupressure and massage would seem to apply to this therapy, indicating that it probably is helpful in relieving stress and tension and may, therefore, help with some chronic pain.

Cautions

When Shiatsu is done with the hands, there is little chance of harm. More care is needed when practitioners use their elbows or feet, as the greater force may cause bruising or other problems. People also report getting cold or flu symptoms after treatments. These are viewed by practitioners as evidence of a "healing crisis," believed to be caused as *ki* is unblocked. This appears highly speculative and should raise concerns about possible spiritual implications.

As with all life energy therapy, these practices are based on a religious belief system alien to Christianity. If a practitioner calls upon spiritual forces to assist in the healing (as is done with Reiki), profound spiritual problems may arise.

Recommendations

Shiatsu massage seems to be effective in bringing about relaxation and relieving stress. However, given that it is a life energy therapy, there seems to be no reason why Christians should use Shiatsu massage when they can enjoy all the same benefits from a regular massage, without the spiritual overtones and dangers.

Treatment Categories

Complementary Therapy
    Relaxation   ☺☺☺☺
    Back pain   ☺☺☺
    Headaches   ☺☺☺
    Chronic pain   ☺☺

Scientifically Unproven
    For other indications

Scientifically Questionable
    To prevent or cure illnesses

Energy Medicine
    In the hands of some practitioners

Further Reading

Woodham, Anne, and David Peters, *Encyclopedia of Healing Therapies* (London and New York: Dorling Kindersley, 1997), 96–97.

TAI CHI

What It Is

Tai Chi, or Tai Chi Chuan, literally means "supreme ultimate power" and is part of traditional Chinese medicine. There are five major styles, with the *yang* form most commonly practiced in the West. As with Qigong, the purpose of the practice is to restore a balanced flow of *chi* and thereby promote health.

Most Westerners are familiar with Tai Chi as a martial art consisting of meditation, breathing exercises, and slow, graceful movements. It comes in short and long versions, lasting around ten or thirty minutes, respectively. Each session is composed of a series of specific postures combined into one long exercise. Practicing outdoors is said to be better because it allows universal *chi* in the earth to rise up through one's feet to replenish the person's own *chi*.

The martial arts aspect of Tai Chi is little understood by practitioners of other forms of karate such as Tae Kwon Do, Kempo, and the like. The movements are so slow and smooth that they are comfortable for the elderly, which is not the case with other forms of martial arts that involve strikes and blocks. However, a skilled Tai Chi practitioner can speed up the movements to serve as a form of self-defense. Many Westerners are also unaware of, or unconcerned with, the spiritual aspects of Tai Chi.

Claims

Practicing Tai Chi is said to bring mental and spiritual clarity. It induces relaxation, benefits posture, and promotes a general sense of well-being (this much is true for more dramatic martial arts as well). It is used more to prevent illness than to help relieve symptoms once someone has become ill. Tai Chi is said to have many general health benefits, such as reducing blood pressure, cholesterol levels, tension, depression, fatigue, and anxiety. Others say it improves a person's circulation, digestion, and appetite.

Study Findings

There have been some studies (✔✔✔) using Tai Chi to help people develop strength and balance so they fall less often. Falling is a significant problem among the elderly. A small number of controlled studies (✔✔✔) found Tai Chi increased flexibility and strength, although some did not. One study (✔✔✔) examined the number of falls people trained in Tai Chi experienced, compared to those taught other balancing programs. The Tai Chi program cut the number of falls in half, a very significant improvement. However, whether these improvements stemmed from the life energy nature of Tai Chi, or the exercise part of the program, was not addressed. Most practitioners would cite the life energy, while most Western students of Tai Chi credit the exercise aspect because it forces them to master balance.

A 1999 study (✔✔✔) of Tai Chi found that while it significantly lowered blood pressure, it produced practically the same improvements as a moderate exercise program. So, while some studies demonstrated benefits from Tai Chi, these benefits appear to be from the general exercise aspects of the program.

Cautions

Tai Chi is a more demanding form of exercise than Qigong. People who are not used to exercising should be particularly cautious and have a general checkup by a physician before starting a Tai Chi program or any exercise program. The studies cited above were all done with healthy volunteers. People who are ill, or weakened by age or disease, should be cautious about starting any exercise program. The benefits from Tai Chi may not be as apparent with unhealthy patients.

The same cautions as expressed with all other life energy therapies apply to Tai Chi. The religious nature and goals of Eastern therapies should not be forgotten. In attempting to introduce people to the universal energy field—and become unified with Universal Consciousness—these practices can be the door to the occult realm.

Recommendations

Tai Chi is frequently offered in the West as both an innocuous exercise regimen and a martial art, often with no religious aspects discussed with students. However, more serious practitioners are often committed followers of Eastern religions and may teach that these beliefs must be embraced to properly learn Tai Chi. Thus, while there may be some general health benefits, Tai Chi may also bring great spiritual harm.

Since exercise programs have been designed for people at every point on the fitness scale, and with a variety of preexisting ailments, there is little reason to adopt one immersed in religious connotations when such nonspiritual alternatives are widely available.

Treatment Categories

Complementary Therapy

Develop strength and balance to prevent falls	☺☺☺☺
Increase flexibility and strength	☺☺☺☺
Cut the numbers of falls in the elderly	☺☺☺
Lower blood pressure or anxiety	☺☺☺

Scientifically Unproven

For other indications

Energy Medicine

In the hands of most practitioners

Further Reading

Udani, Jay K., "Tai Chi to Prevent Falls in the Elderly," *Alternative Medicine Alert* 1, no. 10 (October 1998): 116–18.

Young, Deborah Rohm, et al., "The Effects of Aerobic Exercise and Tai Chi on Blood Pressure in Older People: Results of a Randomized Trial," *Journal of the American Geriatrics Society* 47, no. 3 (March 1999): 277–84.

THERAPEUTIC TOUCH

What It Is

Therapeutic Touch is an alternative therapy that has gained remarkable popularity and acceptability among nurses, though this disturbs some nurses. Close to a hundred nursing colleges teach the practice, and tens of thousands of health care professionals have been trained in it.

Therapeutic Touch is said to be based on a number of ancient healing practices, with some practitioners including biblical laying on of hands in its heritage. Therapeutic Touch first became popular during a period when many members of the health care professions were looking for ways to show greater compassion for patients. Experiments ranged from bringing Navajo and Hopi medicine men into hospitals serving large Native-American populations to having prayer groups request faster healing for heart patients. Many nurses demanded changes in hospital responsibilities so that they could spend more time with their patients.

Therapeutic Touch, as first introduced, seemed like an innocent, loving, and perhaps healing therapy that allowed more contact with patients. What was not always understood was that the therapy is based on the manipulation of nonphysical human energies called *prana,* or *chi.* We therefore believe Christians should avoid this therapy.

Therapeutic Touch practitioners work to sense the nonphysical energies through a form of meditation called "centering." The practitioners gain access to their inner spirits from which they receive guidance for the healing session.

Patients are asked to sit or lie comfortably, and practitioners then pass their hands over the patients. The hands are usually kept two to four inches away from the skin, although practitioners sometimes do make physical contact. The latter is popular with some nurses who feel that it is then a variation of the laying on of hands. They also recognize that touching their patients often yields a relaxation response, especially when the patient is hospitalized and connected to various machines and monitors. An often deeply personal interaction through touch can remind the patient of his or her own humanity and the love of the caregiver. This is another reason why Therapeutic Touch became popular before its more serious ramifications were understood.

The next phase of Therapeutic Touch makes it clear that it is part of that minefield of therapies known as energy medicine. After passing their hands over patients, practitioners assess the patient's energy field for imbalances and disturbances, believed to be the precursors of illness. These are corrected in two ways. One is by "Unruffling," a procedure in which the practitioner uses long sweeps, or passes, of the hands over the body. These are believed to smooth out the energy field. The other method of treatment is to direct energy to specific points of the body. If practitioners "sense" an energy field is "hot," they will send cool energy by visualizing coolness in their minds. If they sense a field is cold, they will visualize hotness, and so on. There is no way to objectively verify these evaluations or treatments.

During all these techniques, practitioners need to remain centered and intent on bringing healing. The patient's energy field is reassessed at the end of a therapeutic session. Then the patient is encouraged to relax for twenty to thirty minutes.

Claims

The most common claims are that Therapeutic Touch elicits relaxation, relieves pain, promotes healing, and boosts the immune system. However, many other claims have also been made. For example, Therapeutic Touch is said to relieve premenstrual syndrome, depression, complications in premature babies, and secondary infections due to HIV, to lower blood pressure, decrease edema, ease abdominal cramps and nausea, resolve fevers, stimulate growth in premature infants, and accelerate the healing of fractures, wounds, and infections. Dolores Krieger, one of the two developers of the practice, also claimed that in "several cases" premature babies who had been declared dead were resuscitated when given Therapeutic Touch. The babies, she claimed, went on to recover completely.

Study Findings

Therapeutic Touch is unique among alternative therapies in having been the subject of much research. However, reviews of this research have generally found it very weak. For example, in the area of wound healing, it is frequently pointed out that two studies (✔✔✔) found that Therapeutic Touch hastened the healing of wounds. Less often cited were more recent studies (✗✗✗✗) that found opposite effects. There are now five studies in this area: two show faster healing with Therapeutic Touch, two show slower healing, and one shows no difference. This adds up to a lack of clear support for its effectiveness in wound healing. Close examination of all the other areas of research relative to Therapeutic Touch reveals similar patterns.

Cautions

Being a therapy based on spiritual life energy means that Christians should avoid this practice. If people feel better as a result of Therapeutic Touch treatments, the most reasonable explanation is that they benefited from the care and attention given by the practitioner. Although frequently derided as "just" a placebo response, these effects are real and reflect the benefits of what used to be called "good bedside manner." However, Christians especially should know that all that feels good is not actually good for us.

The two founders of Therapeutic Touch were Dolores Krieger, a Buddhist, and Dora Kunz, then president of the Theosophical Society in America. The latter organization laid much of the foundation for the New Age movement, and has been a major promoter of Eastern mystical and occult beliefs. *Buckland's Complete Book of Witchcraft* describes a practice that is identical to Therapeutic Touch, but called "*pranic* healing." This has long been practiced within the Wiccan religion. Through involvement with Therapeutic Touch, people can get gradually drawn into these other religious systems. For example, Krieger recommends the use of divination and claims that her students learn to develop psychic means of communicating with trees, birds, and animals.

Therapeutic Touch easily leads into other practices like Reiki or Barbara Brennan's Healing Touch, which involve contacting spirit guides. All of these practices are clearly prohibited in the Bible (Deuteronomy 18:9–14).

While the spiritual implications of Therapeutic Touch must be foremost in our minds, there are other concerns. Krieger has warned that patients can "overload" on Therapeutic Touch, leading to restlessness, irritability, anxiety, hostility, or pain. Others warn that it can make fevers worse, or even stimulate the growth of cancer cells. Some of these effects may be due to the meditative state induced in patients, which has been known to cause problems (see Meditation, page 246).

Placebo effects are benefits arising from therapies that do not physically cause these effects. But adverse effects can be caused in similar nonphysical ways, and are then called "nocebo effects" (see page 30). Even if human life energy does not exist, telling people you are passing energy through them could cause negative effects.

Recommendations

Christians should spend time with those who are ill, praying for them, comforting, massaging, and laying hands on them. But they should connect their practices and motivations directly to Jesus Christ and their belief in his power, not to Therapeutic Touch—or any other therapy tied into Eastern mystical and occult beliefs and practices. While there are superficial similarities between Therapeutic Touch and the Christian laying on of hands, these two ways of approaching spiritual healing are incompatible.

Treatment Categories

Scientifically Unproven
   For any indication   ☹☹☹

Scientifically Questionable

Energy Medicine
   In the hands of most practitioners—possibly occult

Quackery or Fraud
   In the hands of some practitioners

Further Reading

Buckland, Raymond, *Buckland's Complete Book of Witchcraft* (St. Paul, Minn.: Llewellyn, 1987).

Fish, Sharon, "Therapeutic Touch: Healing Science or Mystical Midwife?" *Christian Research Journal* 12 (1995): 28–38.

O'Mathúna, Dónal P., "The Subtle Allure of Therapeutic Touch," *Journal of Christian Nursing* 15 (Winter 1998): 4–13.

TRADITIONAL CHINESE MEDICINE

What It Is

When President Richard Nixon restored relations with China, taking journalists into an ancient culture they knew little about, the land and its traditions seemed both exotic and appealing. Reporters looked superficially at the unfamiliar lifestyles and created an appealing picture that lacked the underlying philosophy. For example, there were images of young and old standing outside in parks, performing ritual movements (usually Tai Chi) that helped them remain supple, keep their balance, and presumably helped them sustain mental and physical alertness. There was discussion of almost miraculous medical concepts such as acupuncture. And there was mention of a society in which moderation, balance, and harmony were the foundations of both medicine and lifestyle.

How uplifting and enlightening this all seemed to people in a culture where self-worth was sometimes determined by acquisitions. While China was in the news, the United States was starting to struggle with the beliefs that led to the bumper sticker: "He who dies with the most toys wins." Some churches were struggling with the idea of prosperity theology that, in its simplest form, stated that God blesses good people with health and wealth. Of course, by this standard, Jesus Christ himself was a failure. People in the United States, Christian and non-Christian, had bought into the belief that the more money and "things" you have, the better you are. Yet many were finding the resulting lifestyle unsatisfying. And now here was a Chinese culture that didn't have all the material benefits, but appeared to have a better grasp on life in general. The attraction was immediate.

Medicine in the United States has since become embroiled in debates over the affordability of medical care, the value of Health Maintenance Organizations, and the competition among hospitals to acquire the latest, ultraexpensive diagnostic technology. How seductively appealing, then, were the concepts of traditional Chinese medicine (TCM) that seemed to focus on wellness and harmony. Soon some of the practices were being introduced into wellness centers throughout the United States and people were talking about the miracles of acupuncture, herbal treatments, and the like.

That first flush of excitement is more than a generation in the past, and we can talk objectively about a subject that has long been misunderstood in the West. Written records about TCM date to between 200 B.C. and A.D. 100 in *The Yellow Emperor's Classic of Internal Medicine.* This book demonstrates that TCM is not just about physical health, but is intertwined with Taoism, the ancient Chinese philosophy and religion. The moderation, balance, and harmony concepts of TCM are part of a very deep spiritual system quite removed from Christianity. To wholly embrace TCM is to accept a religion fundamentally at odds with what most Christians believe to be the Word of God.

Many who were drawn to TCM were not concerned about these inconsistent religious ideas. Many say Christianity is just another expression of Western greed and selfishness and pride. Yet what they rejected was often not an accurate representation of Christian faith. Materialism and selfishness are as erroneous for Christians as they are for those who adhere to Taoism, the underlying faith of TCM. Instead of embracing TCM, those Christians who were appalled by the inequity and materialism of their day should have worked to restore biblical values as given in God's Word. Unfortunately for many, that did not happen.

Just as Christianity was rejected in part due to its misrepresentation, TCM was embraced, to some degree, by accepting some misconceptions about it—some of which have remained to this day. It is important to clarify some of these by looking in detail at how TCM views all life.

The ancient Chinese—and contemporary practitioners of TCM—believe that all of life is made up of opposites called *"yin"* and *"yang."* Each needs the other, and they must always be in balance. Night and day, winter and summer, everything must come into balance with *yin* and *yang.* But just as day must adjust by shortening during the winter months, and night must shorten during the summer months when day is long, so all *yin* and *yang* are constantly making adjustments to maintain harmony.

The body's internal organs are also said to have *yin* and *yang.* As there is stress or relaxation, subtle adaptations take place. So long as the *yin* and *yang* are in proper interrelationship, good health is assured. But when *yin* and *yang* cannot adapt and adjust, illness occurs.

TCM goes further (see Energy Medicine, page 193). It teaches that the body has an invisible vital energy called *chi* or *qi.* This is transported along an elaborate system of energy meridians, also invisible. These link and regulate the organs, and connect to the skin.

There is a great deal more to TCM, too much to describe in any depth here. The major misconception regarding TCM in the West is that it involves the same general approach as conventional medicine except with the addition of acupuncture and some Chinese herbs. That is not the case. TCM is a completely different approach to health and life. Its beliefs are often in conflict with both the science of conventional medicine and the theology of the Bible. A complete shift in world view is needed to fully embrace TCM.

Ironically, even the Chinese people had moved away from TCM until fairly recently. Over the centuries, its practice had waned in many parts of China. After the Cultural Revolution of Mao Tse-tung in 1949, TCM was revived, partly to reestablish Chinese culture and partly to cope with lack of availability of Western medicine during the years when China was closed to the outside world.

Practically, TCM practitioners engage in extensive interviews with patients when they first visit them. In addition to asking questions, TCM practitioners make note of a patient's voice and breathing, as these are believed to be central to the movement of *chi* through the body. A physical exam may include smelling the patient, noting his or her "spirit," and checking the tongue, which is believed to be the surface indicator of internal organ health. Another distinctive diagnostic approach is pulse diagnosis. Conventional medicine uses the pulse to monitor the heart rate, but TCM uses it to monitor the flow of *chi*. Nine different pulses using different pressures are taken, the results believed to provide information about different organs. Iridology is another diagnostic approach where the iris of the eye is examined (see Iridology, page 235).

The primary goal of TCM is to restore or maintain a balanced flow of *chi* through the body. This is accomplished using a variety of therapies, all of which are chosen because of their expected impact on *chi*. Acupuncture is believed to work when needles are inserted into specific acupoints in the meridians, improving the flow of *chi*. The meridians do not correspond to nerves, blood vessels, or any other system known to science. Herbal remedies, moxibustion (the burning of the herb moxa), cupping (placing a cup over the injured area to create suction), acupressure, yoga, Tai Chi, and Qigong are all encouraged with a view to restoring balance between *yin* and *yang*, and promoting the flow of *chi*.

Claims

Traditional Chinese medicine is promoted as a complete health care system able to care for and treat all the health needs of patients. However, Westerners usually use it as a source of complementary therapies for health promotion. While TCM uses all the diagnostic procedures and therapies, Western use often takes various therapies in isolation. Thus, the claims made for acupuncture are usually made in isolation from the rest of TCM, which would not occur in its traditional setting.

Study Findings

Research studies are usually based on one particular therapy or another, not the whole TCM system. Several of these therapies have been discussed separately in this book, with the state of evidence listed. Some aspects of TCM, such as acupuncture for certain types of pain, or Tai Chi as an exercise regimen, are producing beneficial results. Some Chinese herbal remedies, such as red yeast rice, are showing promise. However, much of the system remains untested and unproven. Belief in *chi* is growing, but is based on adoption of some or all of the philosophical and religious world view underlying TCM, not on any demonstration that *chi* actually exists.

Cautions

TCM is based on centuries of folk use, but with little clinical evidence to support its claims. This, in and of itself, should not lead us to reject all of TCM. However, the system promotes many therapies and diagnostic procedures of questionable value.

Promotion of therapies on the basis of traditional widespread use has resulted in much harm throughout human history. When those therapies are all a culture has, their use is tragic, but understandable. When other effective and safe therapies are available, those therapies need not be chosen and should not be promoted. Questionable diagnostic approaches are likely to miss real illnesses and proclaim the presence of problems that may not exist. This will again cause pain and suffering that is avoidable. While some Western practitioners are lauding TCM as a better approach to health care, Chinese practitioners of TCM are adding Western procedures, such as surgery and pharmaceuticals. They retain the underlying religious beliefs of their profession, but when it comes to the delivery of health care, they are recognizing that there are better approaches.

Physical harm can result from herbal remedies that contain toxic instead of beneficial herbs, or from contamination of herbal products. TCM herbal products are unregulated in the United States, making them vulnerable to lax manufacturing and packaging standards. Quality is not consistent. On top of the physical harm, psychological harm can result from involvement in consciousness altering practices like yoga, meditation, and Qigong (see Yoga, page 285; Meditation, page 246; Qigong, page 261). Finally, the spiritual harm that can result from introducing people to a religion other than Christianity cannot be minimized. While some of the underlying beliefs of TCM are compatible with biblical teachings, the central beliefs are different. Many of these therapies introduce practitioners to the occult realm, with all the dangers associated with demonic involvement.

Recommendations

Some of the general approaches to health within TCM are compatible with both Christianity and conventional medicine. The emphasis on balance through diet, exercise, and stress reduction is preferable to the fast-paced, high-stress Western lifestyle. Some particular therapies used for specific conditions have been shown to be of value. However, other TCM therapies recommended for specific ailments are often untested by Western standards, and some that have been tested are ineffective. Since these introduce people to Eastern religious ideas, without evidence of benefit, there seems to be little justification for their use, especially by Christians.

Treatment Categories

Complementary Therapy
  For some indications

Scientifically Unproven
  For most indications

Scientifically Questionable
  For many indications

Energy Medicine
  In the hands of many practitioners

Further Reading

Cassileth, Barrie R., *The Alternative Medicine Handbook* (New York: W. W. Norton, 1998), 28–34.

Woodham, Anne, and David Peters, *Encyclopedia of Healing Therapies* (London and New York: Dorling Kindersley, 1997), 90–91, 140–43, 192–93.

VISUALIZATION

What It Is

Visualization describes a wide range of techniques by which the mind is used to influence the body. People usually sit or lie comfortably, close their eyes, and imagine some relaxing scene or image. By imagining yourself in a more relaxed environment, eventually your body becomes relaxed.

A variation is guided imagery, sometimes experienced in a group setting, where one person describes the image aloud to help you visualize. In both approaches, music is added to enhance the setting.

Visualization can also be more active, as when athletes visualize themselves perfectly running the last lap of a race, or hitting the ball with perfect form. Going through the behavior in one's mind is believed to improve the actions themselves. Some research has found that there can be a muscle reaction that matches what an athlete visualizes. It is believed that the muscle memory from the visualization may help an athlete perform better if competition takes place shortly after the visualization technique.

Visualization in healing is somewhat similar. By imagining the cells and tissues of the body working optimally, some maintain that the cells will start to act this way and thus bring about enhanced healing. The Simonton visualization method, for example, is a popular technique whereby patients visualize their bodies' cells fighting and consuming cancer cells.

A number of alternative therapies incorporate more disturbing forms of visualization. Some incorporate visualization as a way to find guidance from one's inner self or to contact spirit guides. A famous experiment described in a book called *Conjuring Up Philip* started by having people "create" a person named Philip who had certain well-defined characteristics. In séances they visualized contacting this person, and soon were receiving communications from him. This experiment is touted as evidence of the power of visualization, yet few mention the possibility that they may have contacted a spirit who was willing to play their game. Visualization can be an innocent way to relax, or an occult activity.

Claims

Visualization is said to be a way to improve performance, change behavior, and cause relaxation. But it is also said to directly cause healing, send life energy, or contact spirits. The more controversial aspects are tied into the New Age and postmodern belief that people can create reality. Well-known proponents of Eastern healing techniques, Zangpo and Feuerstein, state: "The thoughts and images that we hold in our minds are not just abstract, ineffectual ideas or neurons firing in our brains. They actively shape reality." As such, visualization is believed to demonstrate the power of the mind to change physical reality.

Study Findings

Imagining things in our mind does cause physical responses. If we visualize food, we often feel saliva being produced; if we remember a scary situation, our heart pumps faster. But there is quite a difference between these relatively simple responses and demonstrable proof that visualizing our cells fighting a disease will cause them to be more effective. Lots of anecdotal evidence (✔) backs up these types of claims. However, a number of well-designed, but uncontrolled, studies (✔✔) have found that while relaxation is produced, there is no evidence that visualization lessens any disease or complements other treatments.

Cautions

Clearly, using visualization to call up spirits is prohibited in the Bible. Going deeper into one's own psyche can have adverse effects, just as occur sometimes with meditation. The same authors cited above, who are not Christians, but proponents of visualization and Eastern religions, also claim: "By naively adopting certain visualization practices, we may well endanger our mental and physical health not only in this lifetime *but in future embodiments as well*. . . . Even if a person does not suffer any adverse side effects now, the connection with the lower realms has been made and will take effect in the future" (emphasis in original).

Recommendations

Visualization about neutral images—a peaceful brook, a flower garden, even a relaxing pattern—can be a helpful way to relax. Such visualization may be especially useful in professional counseling. However, there is no evidence to show that visualization itself helps cure any illness or bring about faster healing. Use of visualization to contact our "inner selves" or the spiritual realm is prohibited biblically—and dangerous. If visualization is recommended, ask for a complete description of what will be involved before participating. Avoid attending practitioners likely to involve other New Age therapies or practices.

Treatment Categories

Complementary Therapy
 Relaxation ☺☺☺☺

Scientifically Unproven
 To promote healing

Energy Medicine
 In the hands of most therapists

Further Reading

Owen, Iris M., *Conjuring Up Philip: An Adventure in Psychokinesis* (New York: Harper & Row, 1976).

Zangpo, Shakya, and Georg Feuerstein, "The Risks of Visualization: Growing Roots Can Be Dangerous," *The Quest* (Summer 1995), 26–31, 84.

YOGA

What It Is

Yoga in the United States has frequently been presented as a gentle exercise and relaxation therapy. It is frequently taught through health clubs, senior citizen centers, adult education programs, and similar locations. It is used for stress management and may be recommended to business executives. However, yoga is not an exercise that stands apart from anything else. The word *yoga* literally means "union." As an integral part of Hindu religion, it implies union with the "divine." It is fundamentally a spiritual exercise designed to bring spiritual enlightenment.

Yoga incorporates both *asanas* (physical postures) and *pranayamas* (breathing exercises). The *asanas* are assumed to relax the body and the mind, and bring them into spiritual harmony. The *pranayamas,* while focused on physical breathing, are designed to regulate the flow of *prana,* the Hindu term for life energy. The exercises are to help bring a person into a meditative state from where union with the Great Unconscious occurs, leading to spiritual enlightenment.

Advancement in yoga is expected to bring moral and character changes, with the ultimate goal being the realization of one's divine nature. Given these Eastern roots, yoga is a deeply religious practice.

However, yoga is viewed by many as simply a set of breathing and posture exercises designed to improve strength and flexibility and promote relaxation. The different exercises address breathing, movement, and posture. Certain movements are done while exhaling, others while inhaling. The breathing is coordinated to help maintain various postures.

Different forms of yoga exist, with positions of varying difficulty. The form most commonly practiced in the West is hatha yoga.

Claims

Most commonly, yoga is promoted as a way to reduce stress, increase flexibility, and promote better blood circulation. Other claims have been made that yoga can relieve back and neck pain, and treat epilepsy and asthma.

However, those committed to the spiritual roots of yoga claim it leads to spiritual enlightenment and union with the divine. The pinnacle of such enlightenment is called "Kundalini arousal." In Hindu mythology, Kundalini is the serpent goddess who rests at the base of the spine. When aroused, the serpent travels up the spine, activating a person's *prana* and clearing the person's *chakras* ("energy transformers,") (see Energy Medicine, page 193). The latter releases psychic abilities, including healing powers. Ultimately, Kundalini reaches the head *chakra* that opens practitioners to enlightenment from occult sources and spirit guides.

Study Findings

Clinical research (✔✔✔) shows that yoga exercises can improve physical fitness, Studies (✔✔✔) also have shown it can reduce stress and help relieve chronic pain. Numerous studies have been done with yoga for specific conditions, but many of them have had methodological flaws. However, a number of studies (✔✔) have demonstrated that asthmatic patients show improvements when they add yoga to their overall treatment regimen. Whether these benefits came from the stress reduction and breathing exercises or the life energy and spiritual nature of yoga could not be determined from these studies.

An important point to keep in mind when evaluating these studies is that the benefits came only with sustained, regular practice. The most encouraging study had asthmatic patients practice yoga daily for one hour for six weeks. If yoga is practiced less consistently or for shorter periods of time, there will most likely be less benefit, if any at all.

Cautions

Yoga, it must be remembered, does not cure illness. Using it in place of effective conventional therapies may therefore exacerbate problems. If people believe yoga and meditation can prevent all diseases, they may resist seeking help for serious illnesses until the disease has progressed too far. In addition, some of the postures and the physical exertion may cause physical problems. As with any exercise program, people should ensure they have no underlying health problems and start slowly.

The spiritual dimensions of yoga must also be kept in mind. People who start yoga as a form of exercise will soon find themselves exposed to its religious teachings. Gradually, people may find themselves seeking the spiritual enlightenment that yoga was originally designed to produce. Apart from the spiritual dangers, intense involvement with Eastern spiritual practices is known to cause psychological and emotional problems. People who have progressed to the point of Kundalini experiences have been known to have psychotic breakdowns.

Recommendations

Yoga is an alternative therapy that is difficult to wholeheartedly accept or reject. As a set of physical and breathing exercises, it can improve general well-being. As a deeply religious practice with the goal of union with the divine, it is antithetical to biblical Christianity. In spite of its reputation as a simple calisthenics program, reports of physical and spiritual harm continue to surface. While there may not be clear reasons for Christians to condemn all forms of yoga, Paul gives some helpful advice: "'Everything is permissible for me'—but not everything is beneficial" (1 Corinthians 6:12). Given its origin and risks, the burden rests with the yoga advocate to demonstrate why this form of exercise and relaxation should be chosen when so many other forms exist that have no spiritual underpinnings.

Treatment Categories

Complementary Therapy
Improve physical fitness and flexibility ☺☺☺
Reduce stress ☺☺☺
Relieve chronic pain ☺☺
Asthma ☺☺

Scientifically Unproven
For other indications

Energy Medicine
In the hands of most practitioners

Further Reading

Cassileth, Barrie R., *The Alternative Medicine Handbook* (New York: W. W. Norton, 1998), 248–51.

Greenfield, Russell H., "Yoga as an Adjunct in the Long-Term Relief of Asthma," *Alternative Medicine Alert* 1, no. 11 (November 1998): 127–30.

13

Herbal Remedies, Vitamins, and Dietary Supplements

Herbal medicine is a lot more complicated than just picking some herbs and using them. Herbs are potentially dangerous—some can be fatal. Some interact in negative ways with prescription and over-the-counter medicines. There are many variables involved—in the plants themselves, in their preparation, and in the companies that make and sell them.

The same herb can affect people differently. Age, gender, physical condition, and other factors can influence a person's response to these remedies. The elderly, the chronically ill, and women who are pregnant or breast-feeding should never take herbal remedies without careful coordination with their physician and pharmacist. What might be harmless for some can cause serious health problems, or even death, for others. And children are not little adults, to be given a smaller dose. Any parent considering an herbal remedy for a child should first seek competent medical advice.

The Four Primary Approaches to Herbal Remedies

- Ayurvedic Medicine: In Ayurveda, the traditional medicine of India, the biological reaction of herbs is not a concern. Instead, the herbs fit into a complex system of energy medicine. There are the three *doshas,* or humors, consisting of *vata* (air), *pitta* (fire), and *kapha* (water). These evolve from the five elements of air, fire, water, earth, and ether. In this belief system, herbs are divided by their taste—astringent, bitter, pungent, salty, sour, and sweet. The taste relates to their healing properties. An herbal remedy is always meant to bring balance among the elements, a concept radically different from conventional medicine.
- Traditional Chinese Medicine: A medical system of balance between *yin* and *yang,* traditional Chinese medicine (TCM) categorizes elements similarly to Ayurveda,

though the elements include wood and metal along with earth, fire, and water. TCM practitioners believe there is a direct relationship between an herb and one of the elements. Wood is sour, metal is acrid, fire is bitter, water is salty, and earth is sweet. The herbs are chosen for their taste, their ability to restore balance, and according to an elaborate system in which the herbs are determined to relate to specific medical ills. It is a system that is quite foreign both to scientific understanding and Christian belief systems.

- Herbalism: An herb is viewed in this system either as a means of transmitting life energy or as a way of allowing "nature spirits" to impact people's health. This approach is part of many nature religions, such as shamanism, Native-American religions, and witchcraft (Wicca). While in practice, some herbs containing ingredients that impact the body or mind are used, herbalism teaches that the herbs are spiritually active. Herbs may be chosen because of how the plants resemble the parts of the body that are ill or diseased. Herbalism represents a religious or magical approach to herbs rather than a scientific one.

- Herbal Medicine: Because herbal products are usually slower acting than pharmaceutical equivalents, patients who rely on conventional medicine are more likely to try herbs for conditions that last for years rather than for short-term illnesses. Many modern pharmaceuticals originally were derived from plants, but today are primarily available in synthetic preparations. Of the four approaches to herbal remedies, herbal medicine is considered the most scientific. This approach has led to clinical research which has revealed that some herbs should be considered when treating certain illnesses and conditions.

Similar Names Are Confusing, Can Be Dangerous

One big caution. Look-alike drug names and doctors' bad handwriting have led to medication mix-ups in conventional medicine that have caused complications and even deaths.

The same problem of look-alike names exists with herbal remedies. Plants have both *common* names (e.g., feverfew) and one universally accepted two-part scientific Latin name (feverfew's is *Tanacetum parthenium*). The first word gives the plant's genus; the second its species. Unfortunately, the same species of plant can have numerous common names, and sometimes the same common name refers to several totally different species. For example, the herbal remedy echinacea can be made from a number of different species: *Echinacea purpurea*, *Echinacea pallida*, or *Echinacea angustifolia*. The effect of each species is somewhat different, and no one knows if they have the same strength even when they act in the same way.

Occasionally a scientific name needs to be changed after scientists realize a plant was not classified correctly. As a result, the same plant can be referred to with more than one scientific name. Chamomile is a good example. It is most commonly identified as *Matricaria recutita,* but the same species has also been called *Matricaria chamomilla, Chamomilla recutita,* and a number of other Latin names.

Adding to the confusion on chamomile is the fact that some view chamomile as the same as yarrow. Yarrow *(Achillea millefolium)* is the European variety. And European yarrow was thought to be the same as the American variety, which now turns out to be a separate species *(Achillea lanulosa).* You get the idea.

Vitamins and supplements can have the same problem. For example, vitamin E comes in a variety of forms, known chemically as tocopherols. Some (specifically alpha-tocopherol) have been proven effective for some indications. Yet, there is natural *(d*-alpha-tocopherol) and synthetic *(dl*-alpha-tocopherol). Gamma tocopherol may be the most potent, but is not available in supplement form. Others have not even been studied. Yet they all are called vitamin E.

The supplement glucosamine also comes in different forms—glucosamine hydrochloride and glucosamine sulfate—two completely different chemicals, although in all likelihood they have similar effects on the body.

When referring to herbs, most people use the common English name. But even these common names can vary enormously from country to country—and sometimes even within different parts of the same country.

In our descriptions of herbal remedies, we'll try to make sense of the names by listing all of the most common names for an herb. We want to help you make wise decisions about what you should buy—and *not* buy. We'll let you know which remedies are effective, and which are not. Whenever you're considering an alternative medicine remedy, remember these tips:

1. Know the scientific (Latin) name for any herb or supplement as well as the common name.
2. Know which part of the plant has the best evidence for effectiveness (root, leaves, flowers, stem, or whole plant) and find a brand that specifies which part is used.
3. Don't trust the label on the bottle. The list of ingredients is no guarantee that the product actually contains those ingredients. Find products that state they have been independently tested, and verify those claims.
4. Choose brands on which research has been conducted. Often these are European brands that are now becoming available in the U.S.

A new company, ConsumerLab.com, has begun testing the most popular brands of supplements, herbs, and vitamins. Their initial findings are very troubling. The lab found that a high percentage of products didn't contain the amount of key ingredients that the packages claimed. In some cases, the amount of active ingredient was *much* lower, which is a waste of your money. And some were much too high, which could be dangerous to your health.

To find out which products pass muster, consider subscribing to the ConsumerLab.com Website *(www.consumerlab.com).* Their approach has some limitations, since no one knows the active ingredients in some herbs. So even if the stated amount of an ingredient is in the product, that might not be the compound that makes the herb work. ConsumerLab.com reports on what's *in* a product, not whether that product is effective.

ConsumerLab.com and some other organizations are providing an important first step in evaluating the quality of products. However, tests have been completed on only a small number of products. The product you're considering might not have been tested. What then? Unfortunately, it is hard to know, and you must take a "buyer beware" approach.

The following descriptions of the various alternative herbal remedies, vitamins, and dietary supplements list what is known about each, the claims being made, the data available from high-quality research, the cautions, and our recommendations. Each of the remedies listed is rated on effectiveness and safety. For a full explanation of the criteria used in rating the herbs, vitamins, and supplements, see chapter 11, "How to Use the Rest of This Book."

Here's the key to the symbols used.

EVIDENCE FOR USING REMEDIES:

If the evidence shows a remedy has benefit, we rated the *evidence* (not the benefit) using the following criteria based on how much evidence, and the type of evidence, supports the remedy:

✔✔✔✔ Multiple randomized, controlled trials demonstrate the efficacy and safety of this remedy.

✔✔✔ At least one randomized, controlled trial or nonrandomized trial supports the use of this remedy.

✔✔ Nonrandomized series or numerous case reports in the peer-reviewed medical literature support the use of this remedy.

✔ Anecdotal evidence in humans exists to support the use of this remedy.

EVIDENCE AGAINST USING REMEDIES:

If the evidence shows no benefit, the potential for harm, or actual harm, we rated the *evidence* (not the potential for harm) using the following criteria:

✗✗✗✗ Multiple randomized, controlled trials demonstrate the lack of benefit or potential for harm with this remedy.

✗✗✗ At least one randomized, controlled trial or nonrandomized trial supports the lack of benefit or potential for harm with this remedy.

✗✗ Nonrandomized series or numerous case reports in the peer-reviewed medical literature show the lack of benefit or potential for harm with this remedy.

✗ Anecdotal evidence in humans exists to show the lack of benefit or potential for harm with this remedy.

THE KEY: READER GUIDE

Since the evidence for any particular remedy can include evidence that not only supports its benefits but also shows its potential for harm, we have compiled a single guide that we hope will be useful. This rating is our "best estimate" of the benefit or harm of any particular remedy for any particular indication. Others could (and often do) look at the same evidence and derive different conclusions:

☺☺☺☺   75%–100% confidence that the remedy is potentially beneficial
☺☺☺   50%–74% confidence that the remedy is potentially beneficial
☺☺   25%–49% confidence that the remedy is potentially beneficial
☺   0%–24% confidence that the remedy is potentially beneficial
☹   0%–24% confidence that the remedy is of no benefit or potentially harmful
☹☹   25%–49% confidence that the remedy is of no benefit or potentially harmful
☹☹☹   50%–74% confidence that the remedy is of no benefit or potentially harmful
☹☹☹☹   75%–100% confidence that the remedy is of no benefit or potentially harmful

CATEGORIES OF REMEDIES

Each remedy or herbal remedy also is categorized to define how it can be viewed according to our present knowledge. Some fit in several categories. The categories are:

CATEGORY	CATEGORY NAME
1	Conventional Remedies
2	Complementary Remedies
3	Scientifically Unproven Remedies
4	Scientifically Questionable Remedies
5	Energy Medicine
6	Quackery or Fraud

FURTHER READING

At the end of each remedy's entry, we list recommended further reading. We include here the most significant research studies and the most recent systematic reviews of this research. We found three resources that are particularly thorough in reviewing the clinical evidence regarding effectiveness and safety. The book by Fetrow and Avila is useful for health care professionals with direct patient contact. The Foster and Tyler book is written for a general audience. The third resource, the "Natural Database," by Jellin, Batz, and Hichens, is not only thorough but its Internet version is updated daily—ideal for those with clinical questions regarding remedies. They rate remedies according to increasingly serious side effects as "Likely Safe," "Possibly Safe," "Possibly Unsafe," "Likely Unsafe," "Unsafe," or "Contraindicated."

Fetrow, Charles W., and Juan R. Avila, *Professional's Handbook of Complementary and Alternative Medicine* (Springhouse, Penn.: Springhouse, 1999).

Foster, Steven, and Varro E. Tyler, *Tyler's Honest Herbal: A Sensible Guide to the Use of Herbs and Related Remedies*, 4th ed. (New York: Haworth Herbal Press, 1999).

Jellin, Jeff M., Forrest Batz, and Kathy Hichens, *Pharmacist's Letter/Prescriber's Letter: Natural Medicines Comprehensive Database* (Stockton, Calif.: Therapeutic Research Facility, 1999). Also available by subscription at *www.naturaldatabase.com*.

ALOE

What It Is

Aloe vera is one of the most familiar of all the medicinal herbs. Of the more than 300 species of aloe, only four are believed to have medicinal properties. The most potent medicinal effects are believed to come from *Aloe vera* (also called *Aloe barbadensis*) that is frequently produced in gel form.

Aloe is a drought-resistant succulent (a plant that retains juice in the leaves and stems) found in warm regions. It has been known for its medicinal properties since at least 2100 B.C. Records show it was in use then in Mesopotamia, the region east of ancient Israel.

The aloes mentioned in the Bible (Numbers 24:6; Psalm 45:8; Proverbs 7:17; Song of Songs 4:14, John 19:39) are actually fragrant woods burned as incense—unrelated to what is now called aloe.

Claims

Hand lotions frequently contain aloe. Some razor blades have a thin strip of aloe on them, and aloe is a common ingredient in many shaving creams. One reason: external use of aloe softens the skin. Aloe has been used for centuries in virtually every warm region in the world primarily as a topical preparation for skin cuts and burns, and skin diseases that include acne, eczema, rosacea, psoriasis, and skin ulcers, and for skin hydration. Aloe reduces inflammation, itching, and hives.

Historical records suggest that aloe was an important part of skin health for Egyptian women and, in particular, the Egyptian queens Cleopatra and Nefertiti. Legend has it that Aristotle convinced Alexander the Great to capture the island of Socotra, in the Indian Ocean, in 333 B.C., because of the island's abundant supply of aloe, which then was used to treat wounded soldiers. Many famous ancient healers wrote about aloe, including Dioscorides, Pliny the Elder, Galen, and Celsus. Aloe was first imported to London in 1693. During the eighteenth and nineteenth centuries, aloe was one of the most popular prescribed and over-the-counter medicines.

Aloe has been taken internally for inner cleansing (the gel or juice), for irritable bowel syndrome and a variety of other gastrointestinal disorders (including colic and colitis), asthma, sinus congestion or colds, depression, diabetes, multiple sclerosis, seizures, menstrual complaints, and arthritis. It is used as a laxative (aloe latex), to aid in elimination when a patient suffers from anal fissures or hemorrhoids, and for relief after rectal surgery.

Study Findings

In human and animal studies (✔✔), topical preparations of aloe have been shown to kill a variety of skin bacteria and yeast. Aloe has been shown to inactivate bradykinin, producing anti-inflammatory and analgesic effects. Aloe contains a number of vitamins, including A, C, and E, and has been shown to contain magnesium lactate, which blocks histamine (which can cause pain and itching in the skin). Aloe also contains salicylic acid, the main constituent of aspirin.

Cautions

Aloe is contraindicated for internal use in people with abdominal obstruction, Crohn's disease, ulcerative colitis, gastroenteritis, appendicitis, ulcers, or hemorrhoids. Long-term use of oral aloe has been reported (✗✗) to cause the loss of a number of electrolytes and, in rare cases, has led to heart arrhythmia, edema, neuropathy, or pigmentation of the bowels. You should not use aloe orally in combination with heart or blood pressure medications unless you do so under close medical supervision. The effects of those drugs can be changed by aloe because it affects the way the body handles potassium, and thus can lead to serious health crises.

Aloe should not be taken internally during pregnancy. It has been implicated (✗) in causing miscarriage.

Too large an oral dose of aloe can cause abdominal cramps (✗✗). Though not serious, the person must use a lower dosage in the future.

Note: Aloe gel is not the same as aloe juice. The juice is more likely to cause adverse effects if taken orally.

Recommendations

Aloe appears (✔✔) to be safe and effective as a topical gel for a variety of skin conditions.

Little scientific data is available on oral use of aloe (juice or gel). Information remains largely anecdotal. Aloe is known to be potentially dangerous for people with high blood pressure or heart disease, and should be used under a doctor's close supervision by anyone with such conditions. It should never be ingested by children under twelve years of age or by women who are pregnant or lactating or who could become pregnant. Aloe juice is rated "Likely Unsafe" for long-term oral use by the Natural Database. The gel is rated "Possibly Unsafe," indicating its oral use is not as problematic.

Dosage

Used topically, aloe gel is applied liberally three to five times a day, as needed. Oral use is not recommended.

Treatment Categories

Complementary Therapy
Topical for skin trauma   ☺☺☺
Orally as a stimulant laxative   ☺☺☺☺

Scientifically Unproven

Topical use for acne, eczema, rosacea, psoriasis, and skin ulcers ☹☹☹☹

Internal use for irritable bowel syndrome, asthma, sinus congestion, seizures, diabetes, depression, multiple sclerosis, menstrual complaints, arthritis, and colic ☹☹☹☹

Further Reading

Atherton, Peter, "Aloe Vera Revisited," *British Journal of Phytotherapy* 4, no. 4 (May 1998): 85–92.

Blumenthal, M., J. Gruenwald, T. Hall, C. Riggins, and R. Rister, *German Commission E Monographs: Medicinal Plants for Human Use* (Austin, Tex.: American Botanical Council, 1998).

Foster, H. B., H. Niklas, and S. Lutz, "Antispasmodic Effects of Some Medicinal Plants," *Planta Medica* 40, no. 4 (December 1980): 309–19.

Jellin, Jeff M., Forrest Batz, and Kathy Hichens, *Pharmacist's Letter/Prescriber's Letter: Natural Medicines Comprehensive Database* (Stockton, Calif.: Therapeutic Research Facility, 1999), 30–32.

ANDROSTENEDIONE

What It Is

Androstenedione, also called "andro," became 1998's most famous and controversial dietary supplement in the United States. That's when baseball great Mark McGwire hit more home runs than anyone else ever had in professional baseball. McGwire beat the home run record of Roger Maris. A reporter noticed bottles of androstenedione and other dietary supplements in McGwire's locker. McGwire admitted he was taking the supplements, and said he believed they contributed to his peak fitness.

The use of performance-enhancing drugs by athletes has become an ethical issue. Andro has been banned by many sports organizations (but not by major league baseball). In part due to the criticism McGwire received regarding the example he was setting for younger athletes, McGwire announced the following year that he no longer took andro.

The use of steroids by athletes remains controversial, but popular. Most sporting organizations ban the use of steroids, usually because of their dangerous side effects and the inequity in performance they artificially generate. In 1990, the Anabolic Steroids Control Act made them more difficult to obtain without prescription, and doctors who had been helping some athletes buy them began refusing such nonmedical requests. In response, some athletes have turned to "natural" sources of steroids, commonly known in the gym as "prohormones."

Andro occurs in Mexican yams and Scotch white pine, which means it can be sold almost unrestricted as a dietary supplement in the United States. After it was announced that Mark McGwire used andro, sales of the supplement increased fivefold, including among adolescents. The belief circulated at gyms and workout fields: if you want to hit farther, run faster, or lift more, take andro.

The human body naturally manufactures a variety of steroid hormones. Naturally made androstenedione is converted in the body into other, better known hormones like testosterone and estradiol. Some of these hormones are believed by many to enhance athletic performance.

Claims

Andro is one of several products promoted as a "testosterone booster" to improve sports performance, increase energy, and speed recovery from exercise. Some take it to heighten sexual arousal and function.

Androstenedione is classified as a steroid. Steroids are hormones that have numerous effects throughout the body, including what are called anabolic and androgenic effects. Athletes look for the anabolic effects of increased muscle mass, decreased body fat, and physical aggressiveness. They hope to avoid any of the androgenic effects, which deal with the development of male organs and male characteristics. Some men do report (✘) undesirable androgenic side effects—such as acne, breast soreness and swelling, abnormal cholesterol levels, shrinking of the testicles, behavioral changes, decreased levels of the male hormone testosterone, and an increased risk of pancreatic and prostate cancer. In women, these steroids might cause masculinization with deepening of the voice, facial hair growth, acne, genital enlargement, abnormal bleeding, male-pattern baldness, and coarsening of the skin. Female athletes from behind the Iron Curtain of communism were regularly suspected of using steroids because of how masculine some of them appeared.

Pharmaceutical researchers have made hundreds of steroids, hoping to find anabolic products without androgenic effects, but have not been completely successful.

Study Findings

In spite of andro's popularity, there is little research to support its use. The earliest use of andro was with the former East German sports establishment. They developed a short-lasting nasal spray that could be used without detection when athletes were tested for drugs at competitions.

After the Berlin Wall fell, other countries gained access to the East German research and practices, leading one group of Germans to seek a patent for androstenedione. The patent application claimed (✔) andro led to higher blood testosterone levels, but gave hardly any details.

The first randomized controlled trial of oral androstenedione was reported in 1999. In the first part, ten men were given either andro or a placebo. Over the next six hours, the blood androstenedione levels of those given the steroid first increased and then returned to normal. No other steroid blood level, when compared to those taking the placebo, changed.

In the second part of the study (✗✗✗), twenty men started a weight-training program, with half taking andro, the other half taking a placebo. After eight weeks, everyone's overall body composition, muscle strength, and muscle fiber analysis showed they had made important gains. However, there were no significant differences between those who took andro and those who took the placebo, nor did they differ in testosterone levels. However, those taking andro had much higher levels of estrogen (an important *female* steroid) and lower HDL cholesterol levels. HDL is the "good" form of cholesterol, with lower levels being associated with heart disease. These findings have recently been repeated in two more studies (✗✗✗✗).

Cautions

Although no visible adverse effects were reported in the above studies, elevated estrogen levels have been associated with some forms of heart disease and cancer. People who naturally produce larger amounts of androstenedione have been found in some (though not all) studies (✗✗) to have a higher risk of certain cancers. The long-term effects of taking andro have not been studied. Another study found several androstenedione products contaminated with another banned steroid, raising concerns about product quality.

Also of great concern is the extent to which people will go to achieve athletic success. As former competitive athletes, both of us understand the desire to win and the lure of accomplishment and approval athletically. But for Christians, the costs of pursuing fame and wealth must be evaluated in light of God's values. This is especially important when considering the lengths to which we will go as parents to help our children achieve sports success.

A gifted athlete may gain a competitive advantage from some drugs, although not from andro. However, the cost will be high in terms of what it teaches about the importance of winning no matter what. The moral, ethical, and physical toll can be extremely destructive. Spiritually, the hoped-for medal and other honors easily become false gods.

Recommendations

Both authors of this book and almost all major sports and sports medicine organizations see no reason for using androstenedione, and a number of significant reasons to avoid it. The information available (✗✗) on androstenedione lends no support to its alleged value as a performance-enhancing agent, but does raise concerns about its potential side effects, especially when taken long-term. Dangerous side effects are a risk with long-term use of most performance-enhancing drugs. Young athletes, who will not benefit from taking andro, are actually buying into false values. Andro should not be used by women who are pregnant or lactating. The Natural Database rates andro as "Possibly Unsafe."

Dosage

Athletes usually take 50 to 100 mg of androstenedione twice a day about an hour before exercise or first thing in the morning.

Treatment Categories

Scientifically Unproven
Improve sports performance, increase energy, speed recovery
from exercise, or heighten sexual arousal or function   ☹☹☹

Further Reading

Jellin, Jeff M., Forrest Batz, and Kathy Hichens, *Pharmacist's Letter/Prescriber's Letter: Natural Medicines Comprehensive Database* (Stockton, Calif.: Therapeutic Research Facility, 1999), 52–53.

O'Mathúna, Dónal P., "Androstenedione for Performance Enhancement: Hard-Hitting Hormone or Harmful Hype?" *Alternative Medicine Alert* 2, no. 9 (September 1999): 97–100.

Yesalis III, Charles E., "Medical, Legal, and Societal Implications of Androstenedione Use," *Journal of the American Medical Association* 281, no. 21 (June 1999): 2043–44.

ANTIOXIDANTS

What It Is

Antioxidants are a diverse group of compounds that carry out the same chemical reaction—they prevent or delay oxidation. Oxidation is a chemical reaction where, most commonly, oxygen atoms are added onto other compounds. A familiar example of oxidation is the rusting of iron. Oxidation reactions, which are required for life, occur in every cell of the body.

The process by which food is broken down to release its energy involves numerous oxidation reactions, which is partly why we continually need to breathe in oxygen. Many biological compounds can undergo oxidation, but this is sometimes not desired in the body. Particularly sensitive to oxidation are proteins, lipids (fatty substances which make up all cell membranes), and DNA, the chemical of our genes. While we want to oxidize our food, we don't want to oxidize these other compounds. Inappropriate oxidation can destabilize healthy molecules, leading to what is known as oxidative stress that can cause such serious problems as brain damage and may contribute to the aging process.

When oxygen reacts with other compounds in our body, it sometimes produces what are known as "free radicals." A free radical is a chemical that contains an unpaired electron. Normally, electrons in compounds exist in pairs and are therefore chemically stable. When an atom or group of atoms contains an unpaired electron, it seeks out another chemical so that it can pair up that electron and become more stable.

Free radicals often exist for but a fraction of a second before they react in one of two ways. They are either safely disposed of by the body's natural defense mechanisms or they may react and form other free radicals. The latter chemical reaction can cause irreversible damage. For example, free radicals are able to oxidize LDL cholesterol, the "bad" variety that allows cholesterol to adhere to artery walls, possibly clogging the arteries and hindering blood flow. Oxidized LDL is more easily taken into blood vessel walls, leading to heart disease because of the way this narrows the blood vessels. Other damage caused by free radicals is involved in the development of other chronic diseases, and plays a part in the aging process in general.

At the most extreme, there is a free radical chain reaction that continues to destroy needed compounds in the body until the free radicals are eliminated by what are called "free radical scavengers." Among those scavengers are antioxidants. More important, the antioxidants can both slow production of free radicals and repair damage caused by oxidation.

A number of vitamins work as antioxidants in the body. These include vitamin C, vitamin E, and beta-carotene (which is related to vitamin A). These are also the vitamins found in many of the fruits and vegetables promoted for good health—carrots, tomatoes, citrus fruits, potatoes, green peppers, cabbage, spinach, carrots, sweet potatoes, kale, broccoli, and pumpkins, among others. A number of other compounds found in the body act as antioxidants. Some of the alternative therapies we discuss elsewhere in detail are believed to work, at least in part, by being antioxidants. These include chelation therapy, grape seed extract, and selenium.

Claims

Free radicals are continually produced by the body and continually scavenged by the body's natural antioxidants. We also have enzymes that eliminate free radicals and other enzymes that can repair some of the damage they cause. However, parts of the body will still experience some free radical damage despite these natural defenses. This problem is increased for people who smoke or work in smoke-filled environments.

Some believe that aging is caused or accelerated, at least to some extent, by the gradual accumulation of damage from free radicals. This is why antioxidants are being promoted to prevent general deterioration that occurs with aging. Other, more specific, benefits are also being promoted.

Probably the area of biggest interest for antioxidant use is prevention of heart diseases, especially atherosclerosis (clogging of the arteries), which can lead to heart attacks. Other age-related diseases involving oxidative damage for which antioxidants are being recommended include strokes, cancer, cataracts, and Alzheimer's disease.

Study Findings

The role of antioxidants in the prevention of heart disease has been studied for decades. One of the underlying causes of heart disease is the buildup of plaque in the arteries. This begins when cholesterol is deposited on the inside of vessels. Cholesterol-transporting molecules (LDLs) are oxidized, causing them to release their cholesterol into the blood vessel walls. This hardens the vessels, restricts blood flow, and sometimes leads to blockage of the arteries. While a number of surgical treatments are now available to correct this, prevention is preferable. Antioxidants prevent oxidation of LDLs in lab experiments, and now they are being studied to see if they prevent heart disease in people.

Epidemiological studies are complex surveys where people are asked about many factors related to their health. These (✔✔) have shown, for example, that increasing the amount of vitamin E or beta-carotene in the diet is associated with a lower risk of death from heart disease. Since both are antioxidants, some view this as evidence that antioxidants protect against heart disease. However, the connection is not as clear-cut as it seems. The studies are epidemiological in nature—a little like surveys taken after the fact. Both of these compounds do a variety of things in the body, and any one of these might protect the heart. It might also be that people who consume vitamin E supplements are actually doing something else that is providing the real heart protection. For example, they might eat more fruits and vegetables, or they might exercise more regularly. It could be these other activities, or the combination of vitamin E supplements and all these other factors, are providing the protection.

For these reasons, controlled clinical studies are needed before definite conclusions can be reached. Studies (✘✘✘) with beta-carotene showed that no cardiac protection was provided with these supplements. Early results with vitamin E looked more promising in two studies (✔✔✔), but not in two other large studies (✘✘✘). The first American study (✘✘✘✘), published early in 2000, examined the effects of conventional drugs, vitamin E supplements, or placebo in almost 10,000 patients with heart disease. Those taking conventional drugs cut their risk of further negative effects by 20 to 25 percent; those taking vitamin E did no better than those taking placebo.

The Institute of Medicine is the body charged with setting the recommended levels of various nutrients in the diet. It is part of the National Academy of Sciences, which is a private, nonprofit society of distinguished scientists with a congressional charter to advise the federal government on scientific issues. In April 2000, a new set of Dietary Reference Intakes (DRIs) for antioxidants was published by the institute, which expanded and changed what were previously called Recommended Dietary Allowances (RDAs). The RDA is now one of four types of DRIs, with nutrients being assigned a particular DRI depending on the quality of scientific evidence available for that nutrient. For the antioxidant report, U.S. and Canadian experts reviewed all of the clinical research on vitamin C, vitamin E, selenium, and the carotenoids (such as beta-carotene). Their report concluded that "it has not been possible to establish that dietary antioxidants or other nutrients that can alter the levels of these [oxidative stress] biomarkers are themselves causally related to the development or prevention of chronic diseases."

The report recommended new daily adult RDAs for vitamin C (75 mg for women and 90 mg for men—with an additional 35 mg per day recommended for smokers), vitamin E (15 mg alpha-tocopherol), and selenium (55 micrograms). The RDA is the average daily dietary intake that will meet the nutritional needs of almost all healthy individuals. Vitamin E recommendations are made more complicated because the vitamin has eight natural forms. The active form in humans is alpha-tocopherol. Only small proportions of other forms are converted into alpha-tocopherol. Many products do not clearly state which form they contain, making it difficult to know the amount of active material in the product. Regarding carotenoids, no recommendations were issued because there was insufficient data upon which to base conclusions. These RDAs affect both the United States and Canada.

Cautions

Early studies seemed to indicate that beta-carotene reduced the incidence of some cancers, but later results raised important concerns. Studies (✗✗✗) began showing that smokers and people exposed to other cancer-causing agents like asbestos who took beta-carotene supplements had even higher rates of cancer than people with the same risk who did not take the supplements. High doses of beta-carotene caused changes in enzyme levels in animals that made other cancer-causing agents more dangerous. Some studies suggest that too much vitamin C may have a pro-oxidative effect for some people—causing harm or disease.

For these and other reasons, some researchers urge caution in the number of antioxidant supplements people add to their diet. As with most good things, too much can have a detrimental effect. The Institute of Medicine report on antioxidants contained a new feature establishing a Tolerable Upper Intake Level (UL) for supplements. The UL is the highest level likely to have *no* risk of adverse health effects for almost everyone. People taking more than the UL expose themselves to greater risks of having adverse effects. The UL for vitamin C was set at 2000 mg per day based on the risk of serious diarrhea. The UL for vitamin E is 1000 mg per day based on the increased risk of bleeding because vitamin E can prevent blood from clotting. The UL for selenium is 400 micrograms per day based on the risk of selenosis, a condition associated with hair loss and nail sloughing. No UL was set for the carotenoids, but again this was due to a lack of information, not because there is no risk of negative effects.

The Institute of Medicine has recommended that people not take over 2000 mg of vitamin C per day. Other studies have shown that several grams of vitamin C per day may be appropriate for reducing or eliminating the side effects of such high physical stress treatments as cancer chemotherapy. The problem is that what is appropriate varies with many factors, including the height, weight, age, and general health of the patient.

All these risks are associated with large amounts of antioxidant supplements. A diet rich in foods that contain antioxidants has not been associated with these risks. The only known risks of eating large quantities of these foods are those that come with overeating in general.

Recommendations

A diet rich in fruits and vegetables will provide significant amounts of antioxidants. However, some recommendations made by people promoting the health significance of antioxidants require you to either take supplements or consume many pounds of certain fruits and vegetables, which is not a practical solution. The effects of consuming large quantities of antioxidant supplements over long periods of time are not known. In contrast to the complex mixture of antioxidants found in natural foods, antioxidant supplements are highly purified and concentrated. Alternative therapists recommending supplements apparently do not realize this contradicts their recommendations for a return to the natural mixtures present in herbal remedies.

The best advice is to meet most of your antioxidant needs through a healthy diet supplemented by a single multivitamin. However, ConsumerLab.com published results on its subscription-based Website in 2001 regarding twenty-seven multivitamin products. The alarming results are summarized on page 406. There may be particular people, such as those at high risk for cancer or heart disease, or pregnant women, who need supplementation. This should be monitored by a health care professional. Until more is known about these supplements, prudence demands caution.

Treatment Categories

Conventional Therapy
   Specific need for some level of antioxidants   ☺☺☺

Scientifically Unproven
   Massive supplements to prevent and treat chronic diseases   ☹☹

Quackery or Fraud
   In the hands of some practitioners

Further Reading

Institute of Medicine, *Dietary Reference Intakes for Vitamin C, Vitamin E, Selenium, and Carotenoids* (Washington, D.C.: National Academy Press, 2000).

Smaglik, Paul, "Food as Medicine," *The Scientist* (May 24, 1999), 14.

BACH FLOWER REMEDIES

What It Is

Edward Bach (1880–1936) was a thoroughly unconventional yet intensely compassionate man who began his career as a medical physician, then switched to homeopathy when he felt conventional medicine was not adequately helping his patients. However, homeopathy also was not the answer in Bach's mind. He left his job in a London homeopathic hospital to find better treatments than either pharmaceuticals or homeopathic preparations. Increasingly, he had come to believe that all illness was caused by emotional problems—"our fears, our anxieties, our greed, our likes and dislikes." He thought that if he could find a way to change a patient's emotions, good health would follow.

Bach moved to Wales and enjoyed walking through the woods. He appreciated the wildflowers and noticed his reaction when seeing a new blossom. He came to the conclusion that different flowers elicit different emotional responses.

The doctor was convinced that he was highly intuitive. He is said to have used his psychic ability to determine which plants affect which emotions. For example, if he was feeling worried when he started his walk, he would hold his hand over the different plants he passed, sensing which one alleviated his concerns. If he was angry, he would use the same approach to find the plant that eased his tension. Over time he isolated thirty-eight different plants that he said consistently affected his emotions. These formed the basis for his healing formulas.

Bach assumed that what affected him would work with others. He analyzed how best to obtain the healing power of the plant and settled on the collection of dew accumulating on flower petals just before dawn. He believed the early rays of sunlight transferred the flowers' healing power into the dew.

Dew collection was slow and limited. When Bach's practice began to grow, he needed a way to treat more patients. He settled on the idea of suspending flowers in clear springwater and exposing them to direct sunlight. This approach is in use to this day.

Remedies are supplied in concentrated solutions preserved with alcohol. These are diluted, and four drops of the appropriate flower remedy needed for emotional change are applied four times a day to the tongue.

Over time, other delivery methods were developed. Some flowers are boiled in a saucepan with two pints of springwater. The liquid is decanted, filtered through three layers of blotting paper, and mixed 1:1 with brandy. The final liquid can be dropped on the tongue or diluted and drunk in a partial glass of juice or water. It can also be rubbed on the knees or wrists, behind the ears, on the temples, or even sprayed into the mouth with an atomizer. All are said to work equally well.

Bach's psychic abilities were also used in determining the emotional problems underlying a person's illness. He would intuitively decide that loneliness or anger or grief or some other emotion caused a patient's illness. Then he would choose the flower remedy accordingly, providing the drops and advising the patient to imagine that a healing light was penetrating his or her whole being, relieving the emotional problem. Bach felt that the flower remedies worked because the sun caused the transfer of healing energy from the flowers to the dew or water solution in which they were soaked. These energies, he believed, helped to restore the imbalances in people's "life energy" that he said were behind all emotional disorders.

Claims

Proponents have long lists of testimonials (✔) as to the benefits of the remedies. Bach flower remedies are believed to cure all illnesses since these are all caused by emotional problems. Particular flower remedies are said to alleviate specific problems. For example, talkative people are obsessed with their own troubles and experiences. They need heather blossoms to feel better. Someone who is going through a major life change—either biochemical, such as puberty or menopause, or psychological, such as divorce or going to a new home—will want walnut blossoms. Someone who is impatient with others will benefit from the impatiens plant. Someone with vague fears that constantly trouble them should use aspen, though those with extreme terrors will require rock rose. If you are overwhelmed by your work, perhaps becoming depressed by all you have to do, you will be helped by elm.

There is even a five-flower combination remedy (Rescue Remedy®) meant to be used as an emergency stress formula, such as following an accident or sudden loss of a loved one. The formula is available in the traditional form and as a cream, the latter to be used for stiff muscles, headaches, burns, insect bites, bruises, cuts, and sprains.

Study Findings

No research evidence supports the use of Bach flower remedies to cure illness or resolve emotional problems. Very few clinical tests have examined Bach flower remedies. The largest was a 1999 randomized, double-blind trial (✗✗✗). One hundred healthy university students were given either Rescue Remedy or placebo, and their anxiety levels before examinations were measured using standard testing procedures. No significant differences were found between those taking the flower remedy and those taking placebo.

Chemical analysis of the remedies reveals only springwater and alcohol. Bach recognized the important role of mind-body influences in health that account for much of alternative medicine's current popularity. Taking the time to acknowledge and deal with one's emotional issues can benefit many people, regardless of whether or not they use these remedies.

Cautions

From a medical perspective, a real danger with these remedies is that people might use them in place of seeking effective medical or psychological help. From a theological perspective, the remedies seem to be steeped in psychic mysticism. Using these may expose the patient to teachings and practices that are contradictory to Christianity. Certainly if you have inadvertently used Bach flower remedies in the past, you need not fear that you have contaminated yourself with evil spirits. Paul's response to questions about whether Christians should eat meat sacrificed to idols applies here: "Eat anything sold in the meat market without raising questions of conscience, for, 'The earth is the Lord's, and everything in it'" (1 Corinthians 10:25–26). Nevertheless, we can envision no reason why a Christian should knowingly use Bach flower remedies.

Recommendations

Unresolved emotional issues may play a role in some people's illnesses. These issues should be addressed in appropriate ways. Some will be able to address these issues informally on their own or with family and friends, while others will need more formal help from trained professionals.

Christians should be building deep relationships within the body of Christ so that we can help one another with these emotional and relational issues. Since these often involve areas of spiritual growth, we should acknowledge God's desire to help us mature in these areas. There should be no reason for us to turn to flower remedies to accomplish what the Spirit of God promises to do. Paul gave thanks for his Christians friends, "being confident of this, that he [God] who began a good work in you will carry it on to completion until the day of Christ Jesus" (Philippians 1:6).

Treatment Categories

Scientifically Questionable
> For any indications   ☹☹☹☹

Energy Medicine

Quackery or Fraud
    In the hands of some practitioners

Further Reading

Ankerberg, John, and John Weldon, *Can You Trust Your Doctor?* (Brentwood, Tenn.: Wolgemuth & Hyatt, 1991), 260–61.

Armstrong, N. C., and E. Ernst, "A Randomised, Double-Blind, Placebo-Controlled Trial of a Bach Flower Remedy," *Perfusion* 12 (1999): 440–46.

Cassileth, Barrie, "Flower Remedies," (New York: W. W. Norton, 1998), 82–85.

BILBERRY

What It Is

Bilberries, also called European blueberries *(Vaccinium myrtillus),* have long been a popular fruit for eating and cooking. The berries, which grow on a shrub closely related to the cranberry bush, are found most commonly in northern and central Europe as well as in the Rocky Mountains. They have great nutritional value, and it was as a result of their regular use in preserves that claims of medicinal qualities were made. Today bilberry fruit extract has become one of the most popular herbal remedies sold in the United States. The extract is also considered one of the standard medical tools among European physicians faced with treating a variety of eye disorders.

Claims

Bilberry has become popular primarily for its alleged ability to improve vision. During World War II, pilots in the British Royal Air Force enjoyed bilberry preserves with their meals. Those who ate the preserves felt they had better vision when flying night bombing runs. Since nothing else seemed to explain the changes in their night vision, they concluded that the bilberries must have been enhancing their ability to see.

Today bilberry extract is used to treat a host of vision problems, including glaucoma, cataracts, diabetic retinopathy, night vision, and macular degeneration. Others recommend it for angina, heart disease, venous insufficiency, varicose veins, and atherosclerosis. Bilberry leaf taken orally is used to treat diabetes, arthritis, and gout. It is also used for the treatment of either diarrhea or diabetes. The latter two conditions have long been treated in Europe with bilberries, but it is their impact on vision that has given the extract its American popularity.

Study Findings

The active ingredients in bilberry that seem to impact health are compounds called "anthocyanins." These are a type of compound called "flavonoids," which are known to have antioxidant properties. Bilberry leaves also contain high levels of chromium, which may lower blood sugar in some individuals (see Chromium, page 323).

Studies with animals have shown that anthocyanins stabilize collagen, make blood capillaries less porous after injury, and reduce swelling. They have also been found to improve circulation through the smallest blood vessels.

Bilberry fruit extracts have been tested in a number of studies (✔✔) on people with a variety of vision problems. However, almost all of these studies had few patients, no controls, and were of very short duration, making any firm conclusions difficult.

In the two controlled studies on night vision (✗✗✗), small improvements were noted within the first couple of hours of taking the extract, but one week later those taking the extract had no better night vision than those taking the placebo. The World War II use was not scientific, and the impact of bilberries is known only through anecdotes (✔), not controlled studies. Given the superstitious nature of some men in high-risk wartime activities, it is also possible that the bilberry preserve eating became almost a talisman for good luck.

Commission E in Germany concluded that bilberry is possibly effective for acute diarrhea, circulatory problems, and when used for mild inflammation of the mouth or throat.

Cautions

Although adverse effects from taking the extract have not been reported, some animals given bilberry fruit extract for prolonged periods developed anemia, acute excitatory states, and problems with muscle tone. Large doses were fatal to the animals. Considering the extract's effect on blood flow, interactions with anticoagulant therapy could occur.

As with all dietary supplements sold in the United States, their quality varies enormously. A study was done of the anthocyanin concentration in fifteen bilberry extracts. The product with the most had over 100 times as much anthocyanins as the product with the least, and the others had every level in between. Another study estimated that people need 50 mg of anthocyanins daily to see some benefit. Of the fifteen bilberry products tested, only five would give this amount of anthocyanins if taken as recommended. However, the latest recommendations regarding the intake of antioxidants include a new reference, the Tolerable Upper Intake Level. This recognizes that taking too many antioxidants can cause adverse effects. This can be a real problem, given the great variation in antioxidant concentrations in bilberry extracts.

Recommendations

There is very little clear evidence to support the use of bilberry fruit extract for the treatment of eye problems. Its popularity in Europe does not mean that it is valid, nor does it mean that it should be a treatment of first choice. Given that many other proven effective treatments are available, standard therapy should not be avoided or delayed. Given the toxic effects found in animals, bilberry extract use should be limited to only short periods.

Dosage

The dose varies considerably, with little known about how much is needed. Researchers have used 60 to 120 mg of bilberry extract twice a day for eye problems.

Treatment Categories

Complementary Therapy

Acute diarrhea	☺☺
Circulatory problems	☺
Sore throat	☺☺
Diabetes	☺

Scientifically Unproven

Any other indication, including glaucoma, cataracts, night vision, angina, arthritis, gout, heart disease, atherosclerosis, venous insufficiency, or varicose veins	☹☹

Further Reading

Barrette, Ernie-Paul, "Bilberry Fruit Extract for Night Vision," *Alternative Medicine Alert* 2, no. 2 (February 1999): 20–21.

Fetrow, Charles W., and Juan R. Avila, *Professional's Handbook of Complementary and Alternative Medicine* (Springhouse, Penn.: Springhouse, 1999), 65–67.

Jellin, Jeff M., Forrest Batz, and Kathy Hichens, *Pharmacist's Letter/Prescriber's Letter: Natural Medicines Comprehensive Database* (Stockton, Calif.: Therapeutic Research Facility, 1999), 99–101.

Prior, Ronald L., and Guohua Cao, "Variability in Dietary Antioxidant Related Natural Product Supplements: The Need for Methods of Standardization," *Journal of the American Nutraceutical Association* 2, no. 2 (Summer 1999): 46–56.

BLACK COHOSH

What It Is

For centuries, Native Americans knew the herbal remedy black cohosh as "squaw-root." It was used almost exclusively for the treatment of both menstrual cramps and to ease the pain of childbirth. The former use is still popular. The latter has fallen into disfavor because of possible risks to the fetus.

Black cohosh, also known as black snakeroot, rattleroot, and bugwort, is an herbal remedy made from the underground parts (roots and rhizome) of a North American plant called *Cimicifuga racemosa.* Be aware that blue cohosh is a completely unrelated plant *(Caulophyllum thalictroides),* although both are called squawroot and used similarly.

Claims

Black cohosh was used by Native Americans for a variety of ailments including rheumatism, sore throats, and menstrual problems. It continues to be popular as a way of decreasing hot flashes and as an alternative to hormone replacement therapy. Other uses are for premenstrual cramping, dysmenorrhea, indigestion, and as an insect repellent.

Study Findings

During the 1960s, extensive animal studies were carried out to identify any estrogen-like compounds in black cohosh on the theory that these would explain the anecdotal reports. No estrogen-like compounds were found, but later studies revealed that the extract lowered levels of luteinizing hormone, which is involved in menstruation.

Five clinical studies in Germany used a commercial product available there called Remifemin®. This is a standardized extract designed to deliver consistent amounts of triterpene glycosides (although whether these are the active ingredients is not clear). The first three studies were not blinded, but the second two were (✔✔✔). Good relief of menopausal symptoms was reported by many of the women given the extract, compared to those who received a placebo. In one study, women taking black cohosh reported the same degree of relief as those taking hormone replacement therapy, while those given a placebo reported no improvements.

Cautions

Because black cohosh has some effect on menstruation and female sex hormones, it should not be used during pregnancy or breast-feeding. It increases the risk of miscarriage. (This advice is standard for virtually all herbs. The effect of most herbs on developing fetuses remains unknown. When herbs are deemed appropriate, their use should be monitored by a medical physician who is knowledgeable about herbal remedies.) The most common side effects of black cohosh are intestinal problems, although little is known about its toxicity. For this reason, those who prescribe the remedy in Germany recommend that it be taken for no more than three to six months.

Recommendations

Black cohosh appears to bring relief from some menstrual and menopausal symptoms, although very little is known about how it might do this. All the clinical data available tested only one German product, Remifemin®, which is now available in the U.S. There is no guarantee that other products will give the same results. Because of the general lack of information, especially on its toxicity, the use of black cohosh cannot be wholeheartedly recommended, although it certainly warrants further research. It has been rated "Unsafe" in pregnancy and lactation by the Natural Database and should not be used by women who are pregnant or breast-feeding. For those women who cannot, or would prefer not to, use hormone replacement therapy during menopause, black cohosh may offer some benefit. Care should be taken not to confuse black cohosh with blue cohosh, the latter being much more toxic.

Dosage

Dosage recommendations vary widely from 8 to 2400 mg of the dried rhizome or root three times daily. The German Commission E recommended 40–80 mg/day of Remifemin. Do not confuse black cohosh with two unrelated plants, blue cohosh and white cohosh.

Treatment Categories

Complementary Therapy
　　Managing symptoms of menopause, especially hot flashes　　☺☺☺
　　Managing premenstrual symptoms and menstrual cramps　　☺☺

Scientifically Unproven
　　Stimulating menstruation　　☹☹
　　Indigestion
　　Rheumatism
　　Any other indication

Further Reading

Foster, Steven, and Varro E. Tyler, *Tyler's Honest Herbal: A Sensible Guide to the Use of Herbs and Related Remedies*, 4th ed. (New York: Haworth Herbal Press, 1999), 51–53.

Jellin, Jeff M., Forrest Batz, and Kathy Hichens, *Pharmacist's Letter/Prescriber's Letter: Natural Medicines Comprehensive Database* (Stockton, Calif.: Therapeutic Research Facility, 1999), 112–13.

Tillem, Joya, "Black Cohosh for the Treatment of Perimenopausal and Menopausal Symptoms," *Alternative Medicine Alert* 3, no. 2 (February 2000): 17–19.

BURDOCK

What It Is

Burdock is arguably the most cursed of herbs used for medicinal purposes. This is not because it has been condemned, but rather because of the nature of the plant itself. The burdock, which is native to Europe and grows widely in the United States, has hooked burs. Anyone who, while walking in the woods, brushes the plant will carry away one or more burs in their clothing or on their skin. Shakespeare's England had so many burdock plants dotting the countryside that the playwright used it in one of his productions as a symbol of an annoyance that will not go away. The audience of his day understood well what he meant.

The herbal medicine made from burdock is usually made from the dried roots of two separate types of burdock plants—*Arctium lappa* (great burdock) and *Arctium minus* (common burdock). Both are used interchangeably. Its best-known use has been as a tonic to purify the blood. This use remains popular in Eastern Europe, which still is the main source of this herbal remedy.

Claims

Dried burdock is used as a "blood purifier" when made into a tea. However it is also used to treat chronic skin conditions, like acne, eczema, dry skin, and psoriasis. Other claims have been made that dried burdock root eliminates excess fluid (acts as a diuretic), and is useful for treating infections and fever. Others use it for anorexia nervosa, rheumatism, gout, colds, and cystitis. In Asia, fresh roots and leaves are eaten as food. It tends to lower blood sugar levels and so is believed to prevent diabetes.

Study Findings

Numerous studies have examined burdock extracts and found a wide variety of ingredients. Although tested in animal studies, few of these ingredients have been tested in humans. About half the weight of the plant consists of a carbohydrate called "inulin," which makes the fresh material nutritious. Some evidence (✔✔) supports the claim that burdock lowers blood sugar levels. Overall, however, there is little evidence to support the many other claims made for burdock.

Cautions

Theoretically, burdock's effects on blood sugar may be helpful. However, for people whose diabetes is otherwise stabilized, taking burdock may lower blood sugar too much. Allergic reactions have also been reported (✘) by some people using burdock for skin conditions. The most serious problem with burdock arises from contamination. Burdock roots look similar to those of belladonna, or deadly nightshade *(Atropa belladonna)*. A number of cases of atropine poisoning have been reported (✖) by those taking burdock preparations that were later shown to have been contaminated with belladonna root. The symptoms of atropine poisoning include blurred vision, headache, slurred speech, dry mouth, and restlessness, but can deteriorate to hallucinations and seizures. If these begin after taking burdock, immediately call your physician or poison control center and inform them what you have taken. This again demonstrates why anyone considering using any herbal remedy should make sure they use only products prepared by knowledgeable, reputable providers.

Recommendations

Fresh burdock may add variety to salads and provide some mildly beneficial health effects for those who are not diabetic. However, the drying process eliminates many of these benefits. There is little clinical evidence to support the many medicinal claims of burdock. It should not be used by women who are pregnant or breast-feeding, and has been rated "Likely Unsafe" in pregnancy by the Natural Database. It should not be used during lactation due to lack of reliable information. If you decide to purchase the dried root, make sure you use a reputable brand.

Dosage

People usually take 2 to 6 grams of the dried root three times daily, or use the root to make a tea.

Treatment Categories

Complementary Therapy
Nutritious plant food ☺☺
Diabetes ☺

Scientifically Unproven
Acne, eczema, dry skin, psoriasis, rheumatism, gout, colds, cystitis, or any other indication

Further Reading

Fetrow, Charles W., and Juan R. Avila, *Professional's Handbook of Complementary and Alternative Medicine* (Springhouse, Penn.: Springhouse, 1999), 110–13.

Foster, Steven, and Varro E. Tyler, *Tyler's Honest Herbal: A Sensible Guide to the Use of Herbs and Related Remedies*, 4th ed. (New York: Haworth Herbal Press, 1999), 71–72.

Jellin, Jeff M., Forrest Batz, and Kathy Hichens, *Pharmacist's Letter/Prescriber's Letter: Natural Medicines Comprehensive Database* (Stockton, Calif.: Therapeutic Research Facility, 1999), 169–70.

CAPSAICIN

What It Is

Capsaicin is the active ingredient in cayenne or chili peppers, also known as capsicum and hot pepper extract. Hot peppers have been cultivated for centuries, resulting in many varieties of the most common species, *Capsicum frutescens* and *Capsicum annum*.

Claims

Hot peppers have been used primarily as a spice in cooking, but also have a long tradition of medicinal use. Capsaicin is used both orally and topically. Orally it has been used for gastrointestinal problems (to stimulate digestion and for gas, colic, diarrhea, cramps) and for circulation, high cholesterol, seasickness, fever, atherosclerosis, and heart disease. Topically it is used to relieve the pain of osteoarthritis, rheumatoid arthritis, and neuralgia (a sharp or burning pain that originates in nerves).

Capsaicin (like mustard plasters) was known as a "counterirritant," a substance placed on a painful area to cause further irritation, which somehow relieved the original pain. Others claim that capsaicin taken orally can reduce blood cholesterol and decrease the tendency of the blood to clot.

In the early 1970s, nutrition experts at the University of Arizona in Tucson studied the health value of the typical Mexican peasant diet, which included jalapeño peppers so hot that the eater's face would flush. At the time it was believed that the pepper's ability to elevate body temperature helped keep the peasants healthy when much of their food led to severe intestinal problems. While chili peppers are different, they, too, can elevate body temperature and thus are suspected of being able to have some of the same effects. This would also account for the relative safety of the food we call chili. Chili, which includes chili peppers and other ingredients, was originally developed in the nineteenth century in the American Southwest as a way to avoid wasting meat that had started to spoil. Allegedly those who ate the meat prepared as chili did not get sick.

Study Findings

The counterirritant effects of capsaicin have been extensively researched (✔✔✔✔), leading to FDA approval of capsaicin as an external analgesic. It is available in a number of over-the-counter creams and works well when used appropriately. Capsaicin causes depletion of Substance P, which is how peripheral nerves transmit painful stimuli back to the spinal cord. Capsaicin therefore prevents the brain from perceiving the pain. However, it takes a few days to use up the Substance P already in the painful area. Capsaicin is therefore only effective when used repeatedly for chronic pain such as is seen in arthritis and neuropathy. It should be applied four to five times daily for at least four weeks. Evidence to support the internal use of capsaicin is insubstantial, with the possible exception (✔✔) of its use as a digestive stimulant.

Cautions

Ironically, if all the Substance P in an area is not depleted, the intensity of the pain may increase. It is therefore very important that enough capsaicin cream be used. This can be a problem when people make their own creams, as the amount of capsaicin varies extensively between varieties of peppers. Capsaicin is extremely irritating to eyes, open wounds, and mucous membranes. After applying the cream to the skin, residual capsaicin is practically insoluble in cold water and only slightly soluble in hot water. It can be removed from the hands using vinegar. The cream may be helpful for shingles or psoriasis, but the skin should be monitored carefully for signs of excessive irritation.

Recommendations

Capsaicin is an effective analgesic for certain types of arthritis and chronic pain in the nerves of the arms or legs. It has few side effects so long as it is kept away from the eyes and open wounds. It has been rated "Likely Safe" in pregnancy and lactation by the Natural Database, but only when taken as a food or used topically. Capsaicin may be unsafe when taken orally in amounts larger than in food, especially for children and women who are pregnant or breast-feeding. As those who have eaten hot peppers know, there is great variability in people's taste for peppers. These differences apply to skin tolerance as well as taste buds.

Dosage

Capsaicin is very potent, so topical preparations often contain between 0.025 and 0.075 percent capsaicin, which should be applied no more than three or four times a day.

Treatment Categories

Conventional Therapy
Topically for chronic peripheral nerve pain (neuropathy) ☺☺☺☺
Some forms of arthritis ☺☺☺☺

Complementary Therapy
Orally as a digestive stimulant ☺☺
Shingles and psoriasis ☺

Scientifically Unproven
Most gastrointestinal problems, circulation, high cholesterol, seasickness, fever, atherosclerosis, heart disease, or any other medical indication

Further Reading

Foster, Steven, and Varro E. Tyler, *Tyler's Honest Herbal: A Sensible Guide to the Use of Herbs and Related Remedies*, 4th ed. (New York: Haworth Herbal, 1999), 89–91.

Jellin, Jeff M., Forrest Batz, and Kathy Hichens, *Pharmacist's Letter/Prescriber's Letter: Natural Medicines Comprehensive Database* (Stockton, Calif.: Therapeutic Research Facility, 1999), 197–98.

Schiedermayer, David, "Capsaicin (Hot Pepper Extract) for Neuropathic Pain," *Alternative Medicine Alert* 1, no. 1 (January 1998): 7–9.

CHAMOMILE

What It Is

Sometimes it seems that in the history of the Western world, there have been two consistent "Mom Medicines." The first is chicken soup, lovingly, though not always tastefully, prepared. It might be greasy or water thin. It might have dumplings or noodles, meat or vegetables, or just come as a clear broth. Whatever the case, you always felt better after sipping it because, in many a home, it represented all the love and concern you needed when you were afflicted with everything from colds and fevers to influenza and general malaise.

The second "Mom Medicine" is chamomile tea; a drink made from the daisylike, apple-scented flower cultivated worldwide. Most Americans should be familiar with the form known as German, or genuine chamomile; botanists have about a dozen different Latin names for it, with the most common ones being *Matricaria recutita* and *Matricaria chamomilla*. Roman, or English, chamomile *(Anthemis nobilis)* is a completely different plant. But no matter what the variety, one use has always been the same. It is the beverage served when you are tossing and turning in bed or anxiously pacing the floor, unable to sleep.

The pagan Anglo-Saxons were so delighted with the herb that they became convinced it was one of nine sacred herbs given to humans by the god Woden. What makes chamomile different from other Mom remedies is that after thousands of years of use, anecdotal evidence has been scientifically evaluated and somewhat validated—though not for every use. Roman chamomile, though widely used, contains ingredients that are similar, but not identical, to German chamomile. There is very little clinical information on the herb. Most of the existing information concerns German chamomile, but is quite often also applied to Roman chamomile.

German chamomile is an important example of how an herb's preparation affects its activity. The flower heads contain numerous compounds; some are soluble in water, others are not. A tea made from the flower heads will contain mostly the water-soluble compounds. Making the tea in a closed container is said to capture more of the volatile essential oils, which are not very water soluble. Other remedies are made by soaking the flower heads in alcohol to obtain an extract that contains significantly more of the compounds that are not water soluble. These alcohol extracts, or tinctures, have very different effects in the body and should only be used externally.

Claims

In contemporary German culture, chamomile is considered a cure-all and is used orally as a sedative and spasmolytic (for treating intestinal and menstrual cramps), and topically as an anti-inflammatory and wound-healing agent. The tea, made from the tiny flower heads, may suppress muscle spasms and reduce inflammation in the digestive tract. It's used for menstrual cramps, flatulence, and seasickness. Topically, chamomile oil or ointment may be applied as an anti-inflammatory for skin and mucous membrane problems, hemorrhoids, and leg ulcers. As an inhalant it has been used to treat respiratory difficulties. A volatile oil is mainly responsible, so the tea must be made from fresh herb. When fresh, it is said to smell like apples; when old, it is said to smell like hay. It must be steeped long enough to release the oil, generally at least ten minutes in a closed container.

Study Findings

Animal studies support chamomile's traditional use as a wound healer and as an anti-inflammatory, antispasmodic, and antianxiety agent. One component, apigenin, binds the same receptors as antianxiety prescription drugs like Valium®, and exerts anxiolytic and mild sedative effects in mice and relaxes intestinal spasms. The essential oil acts as an antioxidant and kills some skin bacteria *(Staphylococcus)* and yeast *(Candida* species).

However, very few human studies have evaluated these traditional uses. A number of studies (✔✔) have been done on a German product called Kamillosan®, but those involved in these studies were often not blinded. Given this limitation, the preparation consistently brought improvements to a variety of skin disorders. However, other controlled trials have had less conclusive results. A recent controlled trial (✘✘✘) found no difference between chamomile and placebo in preventing inflammation of the mouth in patients receiving chemotherapy. In another randomized, placebo-controlled trial (✘✘✘), radiation-induced skin reactions were less frequent and appeared later in chamomile-treated areas, but the differences were not statistically significant.

Cautions

The FDA considers chamomile safe, with no known adverse effects in pregnancy, lactation, or childhood. However, some experts believe German and Roman chamomile may damage the developing child before birth and stimulate the uterus, and both have been rated "Likely Unsafe" in pregnancy by the Natural Database. Since there is virtually no information on chamomile's use during lactation, it should not be used while breast-feeding. However, chamomile caused no adverse reactions in any of the human trials discussed earlier. Patients with severe allergies to ragweed should be warned about possible cross-reactivity to chamomile and other members of the aster family (e.g., echinacea, feverfew, and milk thistle). Roman chamomile causes more allergic problems than German chamomile.

Recommendations

While chamomile's therapeutic effects and safety remain to be definitively proven in human trials, its beneficial effects seen in animals, and its good safety record in wide-spread traditional use by humans, make it an acceptable home remedy for soothing mild skin irritation, intestinal cramps, and for agitated nerves. In the United States, it is commonly consumed as a tea or applied as a compress. The tea must be steeped for at least ten minutes in a closed container in order to have the maximum medicinal impact. It should not be taken in conjunction with other sedatives, such as benzodiazepines or alcohol. People allergic to ragweed or flowers in the daisy family could suffer allergic reactions. Alcohol extracts should only be used externally.

Dosage

When taken orally, about 3 grams of the dried flower heads are used to make a tea which can be taken up to three or four times a day. For topical use, ointments with 3 to 10 percent extracts can be used three times a day.

Treatment Categories

Conventional Therapy

Soothing mildly agitated nerves	☺☺
Soothing intestinal cramps	☺
Soothing colic	☺
Inducing sleep	☺☺

Complementary Therapy

Topically:

Soothing skin irritation	☺☺
Mucous membrane inflammation	☺☺☺
Mouthwash for mild oral cavity mucosal infections	☺☺
Bath additive for ano-genital inflammation	☺☺

Orally:

Protecting against gastric ulcers	☺
Antioxidant	☺
Inhalant for respiratory inflammation or irritation	☺

Scientifically Unproven

Other indications

Further Reading

Foster, Steven, and Varro E. Tyler, *Tyler's Honest Herbal: A Sensible Guide to the Use of Herbs and Related Remedies*, 4th ed. (New York: Haworth Herbal Press, 1999), 105–8.

Jellin, Jeff M., Forrest Batz, and Kathy Hichens, *Pharmacist's Letter/Prescriber's Letter: Natural Medicines Comprehensive Database* (Stockton, Calif.: Therapeutic Research Facility, 1999), 411–13, 1196–97.

Maiche, A. G., P. Gröhn, and H. Mäki-Hokkonen, "Effect of Chamomile Cream and Almond Ointment on Acute Radiation Skin Reaction," *Acta Oncoogica* 30, no. 3 (1991): 395–96.

Schulz, Volker, Rudolf Hänsel, and Varro Tyler, *Rational Phytotherapy: A Physician's Guide to Herbal Medicine*, 3d ed. (Berlin, Germany: Springer-Verlag, 1998), 253–56.

CHAPARRAL

What It Is

Chaparral is the favorite scenery of old cowboy movies. The term refers in general to an area dense in shrubs and small trees. However, when we speak of herbal remedies, we are referring to the creosote bush, the most common shrub found in the desert areas of the southwestern United States and Mexico. The botanical name of the bush is *Larrea tridentata,* although *Larrea divaricata* and *Larrea mexicana* also refer to either the same shrub or one that is very similar. The bush is a source of creosote, which has led to much interest in finding uses, especially medicinal uses, for the other plant material.

Claims

Native Americans have made a tea from the leaves and twigs and used it for a wide variety of conditions, including arthritis, cancer, venereal disease, tuberculosis, colds, and as a hair tonic. During the 1960s, interest focused on its anticancer properties, in particular the principal ingredient in the tea, nordihydroguaiaretic acid (NDGA). More recently, claims have focused on its antifungal, antibacterial, and antiviral properties. Because of these claims, chaparral has become a popular herbal remedy among those infected with HIV.

Study Findings

Rats given NDGA did show slower growth in their cancers, but when chaparral tea was studied in humans, the results were extremely variable. NDGA is a potent antioxidant, which may explain why it affects various living systems. However, no clinical studies support any of the alleged benefits of using chaparral.

Although anecdotal reports of an "anticancer" effect (✔) may justify very careful and controlled studies, readers should also be aware that chaparral use has been shown to stimulate the growth of certain tumors.

Cautions

When the studies with rats were continued for longer periods of time, those given chaparral developed problems in their lymph nodes and kidneys. Thirteen cases of liver damage have also been reported (✗✗) in people taking chaparral. Two of these people required liver transplants. In 1992, the FDA issued a warning of the potential link between chaparral and liver toxicity. In addition, several cases of kidney failure have been reported (✗✗) after ingestion of chaparral. This led to removal of many products from stores, although these have been reappearing in recent years. For example, one dietary supplement containing chaparral is being marketed for fever blisters. The manufacturer states that a patented manufacturing process renders the product nontoxic; however, to our knowledge, this claim has not been confirmed by others.

Recommendations

Since chaparral has not been demonstrated to be effective, and because it can have serious toxic effects, taking it in any form cannot be recommended. Chaparral should be avoided. Anyone already suffering from liver damage or jaundice should certainly avoid this remedy completely.

Dosage

No dose is safe.

Treatment Categories

Scientifically Unproven
    For any indication   ☹☹☹☹

Scientifically Questionable
    For any indication   ☹☹☹☹

Quackery and Fraud
    In the hands of some practitioners

Further Reading

Foster, Steven, and Varro E. Tyler, *Tyler's Honest Herbal: A Sensible Guide to the Use of Herbs and Related Remedies*, 4th ed. (New York: Haworth Herbal Press, 1999), 109–11.

Jellin, Jeff M., Forrest Batz, and Kathy Hichens, *Pharmacist's Letter/Prescriber's Letter: Natural Medicines Comprehensive Database* (Stockton, Calif.: Therapeutic Research Facility, 1999), 229–30.

Sheikh, Nasreen M., Rosanne M. Philen, and Lori A. Love, "Chaparral-Associated Hepatotoxicity," *Archives of Internal Medicine* 157, no. 8 (April 1997): 913–19.

CHONDROITIN SULFATE

What It Is

Chondroitin sulfate naturally occurs in the cartilage of human and other organisms, including sea cucumber and shark cartilage. It is a very large molecule made from modified carbohydrates. Chondroitin sulfate is one of a number of compounds called "proteoglycans" (formerly known as mucopolysaccharides) which act as lubricants within joints. Preparations are made by extracting chondroitin from animal cartilage, most commonly from bovine trachea.

Claims

Public interest in chondroitin sulfate skyrocketed after publication of the immensely popular book *The Arthritis Cure* (New York: St. Martin's Press, 1997). Osteoarthritis is a degenerative disease in which cartilage and, eventually, bone, are broken down, leading to pain, stiffness, joint swelling, and deformity. Treatment has primarily been limited to exercise and pain relievers. However, chondroitin sulfate, usually in combination with glucosamine sulfate, is now being touted by some as an actual "cure" for arthritis, although their literature shows they really mean just osteoarthritis. It is also said to be able to reverse some of the damage to the cartilage that has already occurred. In some countries it is used as an intramuscular injection.

Chondroitin sulfate is also used for ischemic heart disease, osteoporosis, and elevated cholesterol levels. Topically, it is used for dry eyes and as a medium for cornea transplantation.

Study Findings

Loss of proteoglycans and changes in the structure of chondroitin sulfate have been shown to occur during the development of osteoarthritis. During the 1990s, controlled clinical trials (✔✔✔) were reported on the use of chondroitin sulfate for osteoarthritis. A 1998 study (✔✔✔) showed, with X-rays, what appeared to be the preservation of cartilage in the knees of patients with moderate to severe osteoarthritis who took chondroitin sulfate for more than one year. Another 1998 study (✔✔✔) using X-rays showed that chondroitin protected patients from severe finger joint damage. A review of research in this area found several studies showing benefits, but the higher the quality of the study, the lower the amount of benefit found. Nevertheless, these studies consistently showed that patients taking chondroitin sulfate had reduced pain, used less pain medication, and had improved mobility, compared to those taking placebo. The subjects in all of these studies continued to use their usual analgesics.

One controlled trial in humans (✔✔✔) compared a product (Cosamine DS®) containing chondroitin sulfate, glucosamine sulfate, and manganese ascorbate to placebo. Those taking the Cosamine DS reported significantly less osteoarthritic knee pain. However, since the trial compared only the combination to placebo, we have no way of knowing which component in the Cosamine was the most helpful.

Chondroitin is a very large molecule and studies show that only 8 to 18 percent of an orally ingested dose is absorbed into the bloodstream. However, it has been theorized, due to the studies showing its effectiveness, that it may be broken down in the digestive tract into smaller, more easily digested, and medically active compounds.

Many chondroitin products sold in America may be inferior. In December 1999 and January 2000, ConsumerLab.com purchased brands of chondroitin and combined glucosamine and chondroitin products. These products were then tested to determine whether they possessed the labeled amounts of the claimed glucosamine and chondroitin. Nearly one-third of all the products did not pass testing. Among the glucosamine and chondroitin combination products, almost half (six out of thirteen) did not pass— all due to low chondroitin levels. The two chondroitin-only products also did not pass. In contrast, all ten of the glucosamine-only products passed the testing. One possible explanation for the low pass rate for chondroitin-containing products is economic— chondroitin costs manufacturers approximately four times as much as glucosamine. The brand names of products that passed testing can be viewed at the subscription-based ConsumerLab.com Website (*www.consumerlab.com*).

Studies have shown that the benefits from chondroitin are usually delayed. They may take up to three months to appear after the product is started. However, there is also a lingering effect of up to three months of benefit after the product is stopped.

Cautions

Side effects were infrequent in the studies (✘✘✘) that have been conducted. Some nausea and stomach and intestinal disturbances have been reported.

Chondroitin sulfate when given by injection can be painful. Some have raised concerns about bleeding because chondroitin sulfate is similar in structure to heparin, which prevents blood clotting. This has not been reported as a problem in clinical trials.

In January 2001, the Institute of Medicine issued a new Tolerable Upper Intake Level (UL) for manganese, which is contained in the Cosamine DS product mentioned above. The manufacturer quickly adjusted its formulation to bring it into compliance with the new UL. But adults taking Cosamine DS manufactured before that adjustment was made would exceed the new manganese UL of 11 mg per day. This points to the importance of examining the list of all ingredients in a remedy, and checking the date of manufacture. Older batches of Cosamine DS have too much manganese. Vegetarians should be particularly cautious as their diet likely includes more manganese, present mostly in nuts, legumes, tea, and whole grains.

Recommendations

Although research with chondroitin sulfate is relatively new, the early results are promising. McAlindor's review in 2000 concluded that although the positive effects of chondroitis are "exaggerated," that "some degree of efficacy appears probable." Arthritis is a common and painful condition affecting millions of Americans. The most common treatments for osteoarthritis usually involve pain relievers that are prone to serious adverse effects. A safe and effective remedy directed at the underlying cause of the disease would be a welcome addition.

Long-term studies are needed to ensure that the benefits from chondroitin sulfate that have been seen over a few months will last into years. This research also would help to determine whether there are any harmful effects from taking chondroitin for prolonged periods of time.

Glucosamine, along with chondroitin sulfate, is widely recommended, but this combination has not been well studied in clinical trials. Since chondroitin sulfate is sold as a dietary supplement, products of different quality will remain available. Choose only reputable brands.

Dosage

The dose depends on the person's weight and is usually given along with glucosamine. An average daily dose would be 1200 mg chondroitin and 1500 mg glucosamine. This is usually divided into two to four doses, taken with food.

Treatment Categories

Complementary Therapy
Osteoarthritis   ☺☺☺☺
Topical for dry eyes   ☺☺

Scientifically Unproven
Heart disease, high cholesterol, osteoporosis, use with glucosamine
Any other indication

Further Reading

Jellin, Jeff M., Forrest Batz, and Kathy Hichens, *Pharmacist's Letter/Prescriber's Letter: Natural Medicines Comprehensive Database* (Stockton, Calif.: Therapeutic Research Facility, 1999), 251–52.

Leeb, Burkhard F., Harald Schweitzer, Karin Montag, and Josef S. Smolen, "A Meta-analysis of Chondroitin Sulfate in the Treatment of Osteoarthritis," *Journal of Rheumatology* 27, no. 1 (January 2000): 205–11.

McAlindon, Timothy E., Michael P. LaValley, Juan P. Gulin, and David T. Felson, "Glucosamine and Chondroitin for Treatment of Osteoarthritis: A Systematic Quality Assessment and Meta-analysis," *Journal of the American Medical Association* 283, no. 11 (March 2000): 1469–75.

CHROMIUM

What It Is

Chromium is the mineral that few people appreciated or understood for many, many years. It is known as a trace element, which means that little is needed by our bodies. In fact, so little of the mineral is needed that it was not recognized as being essential until 1959. Even now that it is better understood, much remains unclear. Many do not get the USDA estimated safe and adequate daily dietary allowance, but this appears to have no ill effects for most. The Institute of Medicine adequate daily intake level is 25 micrograms for women, 35 micrograms for men (one microgram equals one millionth of a gram). A number of studies found no detrimental effects in people consuming diets with less than 20 micrograms chromium daily.

Fortunately, if there remains enough "kid" in you to eat peanut butter on a regular basis, you will get as much chromium as you need. Chromium is present in peanuts as well as in wheat grain, dried yeast, and other whole grains. Foods such as liver, American cheese, cereals, and wheat germ also contain the mineral. These natural sources contain tiny amounts of chromium, and only 1 to 2 percent of that is absorbed into our bodies, but that appears to be enough for almost everyone. In spite of the tiny amounts needed, a growing number of proponents are recommending chromium, and many are buying more and more supplements containing the mineral.

Claims

According to Barbara Stoecker, a researcher specializing in chromium, the top two selling mineral supplements in the United States are calcium and chromium. This is because the most popular uses for chromium relate to two areas of serious concern—to treat diabetes and to help people lose weight. In addition, chromium is said to increase people's energy, improve sports performance, reduce cravings, cure acne, assist with sleep, relieve depression, reduce high blood pressure, and even increase how long people live. Is it any wonder that chromium is in such demand?

Chromium is usually sold as a complex called "chromium picolinate" because this form of chromium is said to be better absorbed from most people's intestinal tracts. It is often added to herbal combinations, especially those sold to help with weight loss, including the very popular Metabolife 356®.

Study Findings

Research on chromium as a treatment for diabetes must be considered separately from all the other claims. Laboratory research has shown that chromium plays an important role in the way insulin works to regulate blood sugar. A number of clinical studies on the health effects of chromium were published in 1999 from an international conference sponsored in part by the U.S. Department of Agriculture. Foremost among these were several studies (✔✔✔) showing that chromium supplements did help a certain group of people with type 2 diabetes mellitus. This form of diabetes, formerly called "adult-onset diabetes," is linked to overweight, and can usually be controlled without insulin therapy (which is needed in type 1 diabetes). In the clinical studies, some patients taking supplemental chromium were able to reduce the amount of prescription diabetic medications they took, but others showed no improvements. Most researchers believe that chromium benefits only those patients who lack chromium in their diet. They believe that if you already absorb enough chromium from your food, you will have no added benefit from a supplement. Unfortunately this knowledge is not as practical as it seems. There is currently no test available to reliably determine if someone is chromium deficient.

While chromium may be helpful for some people with diabetes, there is very little evidence that it helps with weight loss. Furthermore, at least one study (✘✘✘) found that chromium picolinate caused weight gain in young, obese women who did not exercise. A few studies have found it effective in reducing body fat, but many more (✘✘✘✘) have found it ineffective. The studies focused on chromium for diabetes reported no weight loss among the patients. The U.S. Navy conducted one of the larger studies in this area (✘✘✘) and found the chromium supplements no better than a placebo for fat loss or weight loss. However, taken orally, chromium has been found (✔✔✔) to reduce levels of cholesterol and triglycerides.

Cautions

One of the ongoing controversies in this area relates to the safety of taking chromium supplements. During the clinical research studies, no adverse reactions were reported. The United States EPA safe exposure dose is 350 times the recommended daily intake, and animal studies have found it very safe. The Institute of Medicine was unable to set a Tolerable Upper Intake Level because of insufficient data. However, case reports (✘✘) of toxicity, especially involving kidney damage, have started to appear in the medical literature. At doses of 200 to 400 micrograms per day, chromium has been reported to cause mental and muscle disturbances. At doses of 1.2 to 2.4 grams per day, anemia and other blood system problems have been reported.

The Natural Database rates chromium as "Likely Safe" in pregnancy and lactation even when used to treat diabetes in pregnancy (gestational diabetes). Chromium when taken as a supplement does not increase the normal chromium level of normal breast milk.

Two studies using tissues grown experimentally found that chromium picolinate can cause genetic damage, which could lead to cancer. Some experts believe this is due to the chromium picolinate combination, not chromium itself, and are looking for other ways to administer chromium. Very little study has been conducted in this area, which should signal caution in using chromium for extended periods of time.

Recommendations

Chromium is an essential part of the diet, not a drug with a similar effect in everyone. A deficiency of chromium can cause problems.

The strongest evidence for the effective use of chromium supplements exists for treating diabetes in those patients who are chromium deficient. Since there is no reliable way to test for such a deficiency, someone with type 2 diabetes might want to discuss a trial of chromium with his or her physician. Close monitoring of the blood glucose levels is essential. If the chromium helps, other medications may need to be reduced. If it doesn't, other medications would need to be maintained.

More importantly, exercise, diet, and weight-control play a very large role in managing diabetes and should not be neglected. If chromium supplements are beneficial, continued monitoring is important, especially of the kidneys, since the diabetes itself may lead to some renal problems which chromium might make worse.

Although chromium may be worth trying for patients with high cholesterol or triglyceride levels, there are much more effective options available.

Dosage

The recommended adequate intake of chromium is 25 micrograms for women and 35 micrograms for men. Many products contain chromium picolinate and recommend taking 200 micrograms three times a day.

Treatment Categories

Complementary Therapy

Type 2 diabetes in those who are chromium deficient	☺☺☺
Type 2 diabetes in those who are not chromium deficient	☹☹☹
High cholesterol and triglycerides	☺

Scientifically Unproven

Losing weight	☹☹☹☹
Improving athletic performance	☹☹☹

Increasing energy   ☹☹

Assisting with sleep

Relieving depression

Reducing high blood pressure

For any other indication

Further Reading

Jellin, Jeff M., Forrest Batz, and Kathy Hichens, *Pharmacist's Letter/Prescriber's Letter: Natural Medicines Comprehensive Database* (Stockton, Calif.: Therapeutic Research Facility, 1999), 252–53.

O'Mathúna, Dónal P., "Chromium Supplementation in the Treatment of Diabetes Mellitus, Type II," *Alternative Medicine Alert* 3, no. 4 (April 2000).

Porter, David J., Lawrence W. Raymond, and Geraldine D. Anastasio, "Chromium: Friend or Foe?" *Archives of Family Medicine* 8 (September/October 1999): 386–90.

Stoecker, Barbara J., "Chromium," in *Modern Nutrition in Health and Disease*, 9th ed. (Baltimore, Md.: Williams & Wilkins, 1999), 277–82.

COENZYME Q$_{10}$

What It Is

Coenzyme Q$_{10}$, also called "Co-Q$_{10}$" or "ubiquinone," is an antioxidant found in many foods, especially meat and seafood. Co-Q$_{10}$ is a fat-soluble compound chemically similar to the fat-soluble vitamins E and K. Co-Q$_{10}$ works like a vitamin in many ways, but is not classified as one because it is produced in the human body (and vitamins are not). It is needed to allow the production of energy by the body's cells, and to prevent oxidation within membranes. It is most widely used in Japan where the government, in 1974, approved Co-Q$_{10}$ for treatment of heart failure. It is reported to be extensively used in Europe and Russia. Most Co-Q$_{10}$ is made by fermenting beets or sugarcane with a special strain of yeast.

Claims

A number of years ago, Co-Q$_{10}$ was an extremely popular dietary supplement said to prevent aging, cure cancer, and raise energy levels. The reasons for this were largely theoretical and anecdotal. For example, it was found that Co-Q$_{10}$ is present in greater levels among the young and vigorous than among the elderly and infirm. The theory was that perhaps a reduction in the antioxidant caused some of the ravages of aging. Taking this idea a step further, it was postulated that if people began taking the antioxidant, they could actually reverse aging by restoring the same chemical balance in their bodies that they had when young.

This type of postulating is the basis for much scientific research. However, it is nothing more than an idea. But that was enough for some who touted the theory in the popular press as "fact," reporting that scientists had unlocked the secret to reversing aging. Even though the theory had *not yet been tested,* the implication was that the discovery was being confirmed.

Next came advertisements with headlines along the lines of "Scientists Have Discovered the Fountain of Youth" and "The Miracle Pill That Can Add Years to Your Life."

Co-Q_{10} is expensive, and its popularity has dropped off. Today, Co-Q_{10} is primarily promoted to prevent a variety of heart conditions, including congestive heart failure and angina. It is also used for diabetes, high blood pressure, Huntington's disease, muscular dystrophy, chronic fatigue, AIDS, and male infertility. Some use it topically for periodontal disease and to prevent wrinkles.

Study Findings

One of the original theories about Co-Q_{10} was shattered in the early part of March 2000 when test results (✗✗✗) found the antiaging properties to be meaningless. Yes, the antioxidant decreases with age. No, there seemed to be no direct cause and effect that could be countered by taking the supplements.

The issue of heart disease is less clear. A number of studies (✔✔) have shown that people with certain types of heart disease have a lower level of Co-Q_{10}. However, most studies (✔✔✔) show that long-term treatment of patients with congestive heart failure (up to 100 mg) only slightly improves maximal exercise capacity and quality of life. In some clinical trials, the proportion of patients who showed improvements was similar to the proportion who benefited from conventional drugs like ACE inhibitors and digoxin. The review by Overvad and colleagues concluded that double-blind trials (✔✔✔✔) show positive cardiac effects from taking Co-Q_{10} supplements, especially in chronic heart failure. They emphasized that these effects need to be researched further because all of the studies had problems in their designs. An April 2000 study of Co-Q_{10} (✗✗✗) found no added benefit from supplements for patients with congestive heart failure receiving standard medical therapy.

Some of these cardiac studies (✔✔✔) have shown positive effects on angina and high blood pressure. There are reports (✔✔) of Co-Q_{10} reducing the cardiotoxicity of chemotherapy (with Adriamycin®). Case reports (✔✔) exist of improved function in Huntington's disease and muscular dystrophy after use of Co-Q_{10}, but the first unblinded trial (✗✗) in Huntington's patients found no benefits. It may (✔) improve immune system function in patients with AIDS. Small studies (✗✗) have shown no effect on blood sugar in diabetics. Studies (✗✗✗) have shown no improvement in athletic performance with Co-Q$_{10}$ or, when applied topically, for periodontal disease. No studies have determined whether long-term improvements result with Co-Q$_{10}$, nor have they compared it directly to conventional medicines.

Concerns about the quality and purity of Co-Q$_{10}$ sold in the United States were addressed by ConsumerLab.com, an independent testing company that permits promoters to use its flask-shaped seal of approval on products that pass its criteria—usually meeting German testing standards concerning the quantity of active ingredients in the preparation. Of twenty-nine products tested, all but one contained the amount of Co-Q$_{10}$ listed on the label (the one product that failed contained only 17 percent of what the label claimed). The results of these and other tests can be viewed by subscribing to their Website.

Cautions

In the clinical studies involving Co-Q$_{10}$, no significant adverse effects have been reported from taking 200 mg daily for six to twelve months, or 100 mg daily for up to six years. Some people did report (✗) short-term nausea. Furthermore, statins (drugs which reduce cholesterol levels) and some oral diabetes drugs (Micronase®, Dymelor®, and Tolinase®) reduce levels of Co-Q$_{10}$. The clinical significance of this is not known.

Recommendations

Overall, early enthusiasm for Co-Q$_{10}$ as a cardiac supplement is diminishing as more high-quality research is being reported. There is no proof that it reduces death rates from heart disease. The benefits that have been reported may be due to its being an antioxidant. However, it is a very expensive antioxidant, given that fruits and vegetables provide large quantities of these compounds. In addition, much remains uncertain about how Co-Q$_{10}$ might work and how well it works over the many years someone could be taking it. Furthermore, there are a number of well-established, conventional drugs that are relatively inexpensive and reduce the risk of death in patients with heart failure. People at risk for cardiac problems may want to consider using Co-Q$_{10}$, but should consult their physicians, especially if they are already taking another heart medication, a cholesterol-lowering drug, or an oral agent for diabetes—as Co-Q$_{10}$ could potentially react with each of these medications.

The Natural Database recommends that Co-Q$_{10}$ not be taken during pregnancy or lactation as there is insufficient information about its use in either condition.

Dosage

Most studies have used 50 to 200 mg divided into two or three doses during the day.

Treatment Categories

Complementary Therapy

Congestive heart failure   ☺☺

Angina   ☺☺

High blood pressure   ☺

Reducing risk of harm to the heart
(cardiotoxicity) in patients receiving
chemotherapy agent Adriamycin   ☺☺

Scientifically Unproven

Antiaging   ☹☹☹

Improving sports performance   ☹☹

Improving function in people
with Huntington's disease   ☹

Diabetes   ☹

Muscular dystrophy

Chronic fatigue

Male infertility

Preventing atherosclerosis

Periodontal disease

Any other indication

Further Reading

Jellin, Jeff M., Forrest Batz, and Kathy Hichens, *Pharmacist's Letter/Prescriber's Letter: Natural Medicines Comprehensive Database* (Stockton, Calif.: Therapeutic Research Facility, 1999), 271–73.

Khatta, Meenakshi, Barbara S. Alexander, Cathy M. Krichten, Michael L. Fisher, Ronald Freudenberger, Shawn W. Robinson, and Stephen S. Gottlieb, "The Effect of Coenzyme Q$_{10}$ in Patients with Congestive Heart Failure," *Annals of Internal Medicine* 132, no. 8 (April 2000): 636–40.

Overvad, K., B. Diamant, L. Holm, G. Holmer, S. A. Mortensen, and S. Stender, "Coenzyme Q$_{10}$ in Health and Disease," *European Journal of Clinical Nutrition* 53, no. 10 (October 1999): 764–70.

COMFREY

What It Is

Comfrey is a very popular herb used both alone and in combination with many other herbs. The leaves, roots, and rhizome (a rootlike stem) of a number of *Symphytum* species are used in these preparations. The plant grows widely throughout North America, also going by the common names of blackwort, knitbone, and slippery root.

Claims

Comfrey has been lauded by some as a wonder herb and cure-all. The most common use was in a cream that was believed to promote healing of cuts, bruises, burns, and wounds. It has been used as a gargle for periodontal disease and sore throats. For internal consumption, it was usually made into a tea (or a blended extract known as "green drink"). It was said to heal stomach ulcers, cleanse the blood, and relieve bronchial congestion. Some have recommended comfrey for excessive menstrual flow, diarrhea, persistent cough, rheumatism, bronchitis, cancer, and angina.

Study Findings

Analysis of the compounds contained in comfrey shows that about one-third of the root consists of a carbohydrate called "mucilage." This type of compound could form a thin film over the skin, providing some protection and soothing irritation. Another compound called "allantoin" is found in the roots and this is known to stimulate cell proliferation, which would be useful in wound healing. Studies (✔✔) have shown effectiveness when comfrey is used topically for treating bruises and sprains. However, no other beneficial ingredients have been found in extracts of comfrey, while several compounds known to have serious toxic effects have been found.

Cautions

All comfrey species contain a variety of compounds called pyrrolizidine alkaloids, with the roots containing about ten times as much of these materials as the leaves. All of these compounds are known to be toxic to the liver and may cause liver and lung cancer.

In animals given comfrey, liver and bladder tumors developed within six months, and other liver damage was clearly visible. Numerous cases of veno-occlusive liver disease (blood vessels in the liver become blocked, leading to death of liver tissue) have been reported after people ingested comfrey. One article in the British journal *Lancet* suggested that the most common cause of this particular disease is ingestion of plants containing pyrrolizidine alkaloids. For this reason, most medical authorities recommend that comfrey not be taken internally for any reason. The American Herbal Products

Association has recommended that all products with toxic pyrrolizidine alkaloids (like comfrey) be labeled with the statement, "For external use only. Do not apply to broken or abraded skin. Do not use while nursing."

Recommendations

Comfrey may have some value when applied externally for the treatment of mild bruises or sprains. Since there are numerous other pharmaceutical and natural remedies available for these conditions, we cannot think of any good reason to choose comfrey. If anyone insists on using comfrey, it should be used cautiously and for short periods since active ingredients in topical medications can be absorbed through the skin. Comfrey preparations should never be used on cuts or where the skin is broken. The risks of toxicity make any internal use of comfrey unwarranted and external use unwise. The Natural Database states that comfrey should not be used even topically during pregnancy as there is no information to show it is safe. It is rated "Unsafe."

Dosage

No oral dose of comfrey is safe, and few would recommend using it topically. Do not use comfrey ointment on broken skin or for longer than ten days.

Treatment Categories

Complementary Therapy
Topically on unbroken skin, for bruises or sprains—yet because of its
potential toxicity, we do not recommend its use ☹

Scientifically Questionable
Gargle for periodontal disease and sore throats ☹☹☹
Oral use for stomach ulcers, bronchial congestion, persistent cough,
bronchitis, excessive menstrual flow, diarrhea, rheumatism,
cancer, angina, or any other medical indication ☹☹☹☹

Scientifically Unproven
Topically to promote healing of cuts or abrasions ☹☹

Further Reading

DerMarderosian, Ara, ed., "Comfrey," in *The Review of Natural Products* (St. Louis, Mo.: Facts and Comparisons, October 1995).

Foster, Steven, and Varro E. Tyler, *Tyler's Honest Herbal: A Sensible Guide to the Use of Herbs and Related Remedies*, 4th ed. (New York: Haworth Herbal Press, 1999), 121–25.

Jellin, Jeff M., Forrest Batz, and Kathy Hichens, *Pharmacist's Letter/Prescriber's Letter: Natural Medicines Comprehensive Database* (Stockton, Calif.: Therapeutic Research Facility, 1999), 283–84.

CRANBERRY

What It Is

Mention cranberries, and the first thought most Americans have is of the smooth or whole berry sauces served most frequently during holiday gatherings. Cranberry juice is also popular as a nonalcoholic drink of choice. Adding to its popularity is that many have heard that the juice can protect them from urinary tract infections (UTI). As an herbal remedy, apart from the juice and the sauce, cranberry has been one of the top ten best-selling herbal remedies for a number of years in the United States. The berries are widely available, growing throughout the United States on a small shrub *(Vaccinium macrocarpon)*, also called the "trailing swamp cranberry."

Claims

In a study published in 1923, one healthy volunteer ate cooked cranberries and soon afterward had urine that was more acidic. Since bacteria causing UTIs do not grow as well in more acidic environments, cranberry products quickly gained a reputation for preventing and treating UTIs. This reputation continues to this day.

Additionally, cranberry juice is said to lessen the odor of stale urine. Odor is an especially problematic and embarrassing aspect of incontinence. Cranberry juice has also been used as a diuretic, as an antiseptic, and to treat cancer and fever.

Study Findings

After the earliest report (✔) found cranberry juice lowered urine acidity, other studies (✘✘) found contradictory results. By the 1980s it became clear that cranberry juice did not consistently lower urine acidity. However, it was found (✔✔) to produce compounds that can prevent bacteria from adhering to the lining of the urinary tract. This action prevents bacteria from replicating and growing.

The first controlled study (✔✔✔) of cranberry juice was published in the *Journal of the American Medical Association* in 1994. Elderly women drinking 10 oz. of cranberry juice per day had fewer UTIs than those drinking a similar-tasting red drink. However, a 1999 controlled study (✘✘✘) with children at high risk for developing UTIs found that drinking cranberry juice did not change the frequency of their infections.

Cautions

No toxicity or adverse effects have been reported with cranberry juice until large quantities are consumed; drinking more than a gallon of the juice causes diarrhea. However, many cranberry drinks contain lots of sugar, thereby adding many calories if consumed frequently.

Particular caution is needed with juice made from any other cranberries than the common North American variety *(Vaccinium macrocarpon)*. Alpine cranberry *(Vaccinium vitis-ideae)*, high-bush cranberry *(Viburnum opulus*, or cramp bark), and mountain cranberry *(Arctostaphylos uva-ursi*, or uva-ursi) are similar-looking bushes whose fruit is made into juices recommended for UTIs. These all contain compounds called hydroquinolones that can cause liver toxicity. These juices should not be used for extended periods by anyone, and should never be given to children under twelve years of age. Women who are pregnant or breast-feeding should also avoid these forms of cranberries.

Recommendations

Cranberry juice and extracts may provide some protection against UTI, although there is very little clinical evidence to support this. Since the juice is readily available and relatively inexpensive, it could easily be added to one's diet, especially for people who are prone to UTI. The berries may also provide some benefit from their antioxidants, although they contain a small amount compared to other sources like bilberry and grape seed. However, once symptoms of a UTI develop, consult a physician about starting a course of antibiotics.

Dosage

Most studies use 10 to 16 oz. of juice a day, although little is known about how much is needed to prevent or treat urinary tract infections.

Treatment Categories

Complementary Therapy
    Treatment or prevention of UTIs   ☺☺
    Urinary deodorizer for incontinent patients   ☺☺

Scientifically Unproven
    Other indications

Further Reading

DerMarderosian, Ara, ed., "Cranberry," in *The Review of Natural Products* (St. Louis, Mo.: Facts and Comparisons, July 1994).

Fetrow, Charles W., and Juan R. Avila, *Professional's Handbook of Complementary and Alternative Medicine* (Springhouse, Penn.: Springhouse, 1999), 201–4.

Jellin, Jeff M., Forrest Batz, and Kathy Hichens, *Pharmacist's Letter/Prescriber's Letter: Natural Medicines Comprehensive Database* (Stockton, Calif.: Therapeutic Research Facility, 1999), 306–7.

Lee, Yee-Lean, John Owens, Lauri Thrupp, and Thomas C. Cesario, "Does Cranberry Juice Have Antibacterial Activity?" *Journal of the American Medical Association* 283, no. 13 (April 2000): 1691.

CREATINE

What It Is

Creatine is a commonly used sports supplement that has become very popular with weight lifters and football players. Unlike steroids and stimulants, creatine is a normal component in the diet, found in meat and fish. Even vegetarians can usually make enough creatine within their own bodies as it is made in the liver from other proteins. The importance of creatine in exercise was noted as far back as 1847 when the meat obtained from wild foxes killed after foxhunts was compared with that of foxes raised in captivity. The wild fox meat had more than ten times the amount of creatine. In spite of this early information, it wasn't until the 1990s that creatine burst onto the athletic scene when British sprinters claimed it gave them a significant, and legal, boost in energy. The International Olympic Committee and the National Collegiate Athletic Association do not ban creatine, as it is a normal constituent in people's diet. Creatine has since been mass-marketed to such an extent that in 1999 in the United States, 2.5 million kilograms were used as a supplement.

Claims

Many high school and college football programs openly or quietly support the use of creatine. When Mark McGwire broke Roger Maris's home run record in 1998, creatine was one of the supplements he admitted he was taking. Some products claim creatine will make a well-trained athlete 5 percent stronger or faster. While that may not seem like a whole lot, it could turn a good athlete into a great athlete—if it is true! For the recreational runner, or the person who lifts weights on occasion, creatine is said to provide more energy and delay the onset of fatigue. That would certainly be welcome—if it is true!

Study Findings

Creatine does play an important role in providing energy for muscles during exercise. The actual energy-molecule in muscle cells is a substance called ATP. When we first start to exercise, ATP provides the energy, but it is almost completely used up within a couple seconds. To get us through the next few seconds, ATP stores are replenished using a substance made from creatine called "creatine phosphate" (CP). Therefore, creatine does play an important role in fueling muscles, but only for high-intensity exercise that lasts less than half a minute. Theoretically, then, by increasing the amount of creatine in the body, an athlete might be able to perform at high intensity for slightly longer periods of time. Also, since creatine is vital to replenishing ATP levels, more creatine in the body might allow the muscles to recover more quickly for the next bout of exercise.

Studies (✔✔) have found that creatine supplementation does increase the amount of creatine and CP stored in muscle cells. Athletes taking 20 grams of creatine daily for three days increased their levels by 17 percent, but more than half the creatine was excreted unchanged in their urine. There were also large differences in the way people responded. Those whose levels started the lowest (usually vegetarians) changed the most. This variability is thought to have influenced the results of the studies that looked at whether supplementation improved people's athletic performance.

Since the 1990s, more than thirty randomized clinical trials have been conducted using creatine for performance enhancement. However, all of these studies were relatively small, with the largest having only forty subjects, and the average, twelve subjects. Given the variability of how people respond to creatine, this makes it very difficult to draw firm conclusions about the effectiveness of creatine. These studies have used mostly healthy male athletes, and have tested them running, swimming, bicycling, kayaking, and weight lifting. Overall, the results have been very variable. A 1999 review of this research found eleven studies (✔✔✔✔) with positive results, six (✗✗✗✗) with mixed results, and eleven (✗✗✗✗) with negative results. A meta-analysis of thirty-two studies (✗✗✗✗) presented at the American College of Sports Medicine's meeting in 2000 showed no overall effect of creatine supplementation on high-intensity performance.

When the studies are examined a little closer, some patterns start to emerge. For recreational and aerobic exercise (✗✗✗✗), there is clearly no improvement in performance. The creatine-CP system plays very little role in this sort of exercise. For one-time anaerobic exercise (i.e., full-out exertion like sprinting or power lifting) (✗✗✗✗), there is no benefit. This type of exercise depends mostly on stored ATP, not CP. However, when athletes do repeated bouts of high-intensity, short duration exercise, with rests under a few minutes long (✔✔✔), creatine supplementation does appear to provide some limited benefits. This sort of exercise is important in training, where athletes may do an all-out sprint, rest, and go again. Similarly, weight lifters may do an all-out lift, rest, and go again. It appears that creatine may allow athletes to perform this sort of exercise at higher intensities and for more repetitions. This more intense training might better prepare the athlete for competition. However, almost all the studies have been done in controlled environments, and it is not known if creatine leads to improved performance when it matters most—in competition. There is also the danger that the more intense training could lead to injury or leave the athlete burned out.

Cautions

Many anecdotal reports (✗) of muscle cramps, gastrointestinal problems, and kidney problems have been reported. However, studies have recorded no adverse effects. Theoretically, long-term supplementation makes kidney problems likely, but we found only one study examining this issue. It monitored a small number of athletes (✔✔) taking 10 grams of creatine daily for up to five years, and found no kidney problems.

However, two case reports (✗) of kidney problems after creatine supplementation have been reported. These patients may have had kidney disease before taking the supplements, which would warrant people with kidney disease, or at high risk for it, being particularly cautious about taking creatine. Anyone taking other medication that might interfere with the kidneys should also be careful.

The only other established side effect of creatine (✗) is that it leads to weight gain of two to six pounds due to increased water retention in the muscles. This may be a problem for athletes competing in weight categories and might lead to unhealthy ways to reduce their weight for competition. Given the huge interest among high school athletes in creatine, it is disappointing that no information is available on the safety of this practice. For this reason, the American College of Sports Medicine recommends against creatine supplementation for those under eighteen years of age. Very little information is available on the effects of long-term supplementation for any age group. In addition, creatine should be avoided by women who are pregnant or lactating as there is insufficient reliable information about its use in these situations.

There is some concern that creatine products sold in the United States may be of variable quality. ConsumerLab.com, an independent testing company that uses German testing standards to test herbs, vitamins, and supplements sold in the United States, tested thirteen creatine products purchased in 2000. Most of the products met the standards. One failed because it contained less of the ingredients listed on the label, and a significant amount of impurities was found (see *www.consumerlab.com*).

Note: Creatine is broken down in the body to creatinine and excreted in the urine. Creatinine levels are regularly checked by physicians as a way to spot certain problems, such as kidney diseases. Creatine supplementation leads to elevated creatinine levels, mimicking kidney disease, even though the kidney function may be normal.

Recommendations

For athletes whose training involves high-intensity repetitions, creatine supplementation may provide some benefits. But people vary a lot in how much they respond, and the improvements are not large. For example, in one study with power lifters, those who took creatine lifted 7.8 kg more after supplementation, but those who took a placebo were able to lift 7.0 kg more. The difference was statistically significant, but may not really be significant from a practical standpoint, especially with the unknown potential for adverse effects.

As Christians, we must also be concerned about how far we go in promoting athletic achievement. Both of us were competitive athletes and have been blessed in many ways from our experiences in sports. But the desire to win must be balanced against other important values. Taking supplements of uncertain benefit and safety is not warranted. It too easily communicates to others, especially youngsters, that winning is all-important, no matter what the cost.

For recreational athletes and those who exercise aerobically, creatine supplementation will be of no benefit. Given the lack of data on long-term safety, it would be advisable not to take the supplements for extended periods of time. Creatine is readily available in meat and fish, so these foods will provide adequate amounts for almost everyone.

Dosage

Athletes usually start with a "loading" dose of 20 grams per day for four to six days (usually taken in 5-gram portions four times a day, often mixed in sugary drinks). Following this, a 2-gram daily dose is taken to maintain the elevated levels. However, researchers have found that the same amount of creatine can be stored in the muscles after taking 3 grams per day for 30 days. This second regimen is considered to be easier on the kidneys.

Treatment Categories

Complementary Therapy

Enhancing muscle performance during
brief, high-intensity, anaerobic exercise ☺☺☺

Possibly increasing muscle mass ☺

Scientifically Unproven

Recreational or aerobic exercise ☹☹☹

Increasing endurance or improving
performance in most highly
trained athletes ☹☹☹

Further Reading

Demant, T. W., and E. C. Rhodes, "Effects of Creatine Supplementation on Exercise Performance," *Sports Medicine* 28, no. 1 (July 1999): 49–60.

Jellin, Jeff M., Forrest Batz, and Kathy Hichens, *Pharmacist's Letter/Prescriber's Letter: Natural Medicines Comprehensive Database* (Stockton, Calif.: Therapeutic Research Facility, 1999), 307–8.

Terjung, Ronald L., et al., for the American College of Sports Medicine, "The Physiological and Health Effects of Oral Creatine Supplementation," *Medicine & Science in Sports & Exercise* 32, no. 3 (March 2000): 706–17.

DHEA

What It Is

Dehydroepiandrosterone (DHEA) is a steroid hormone, meaning it is a chemical messenger carrying information around the body. It is found in high concentrations in the brain. Our bodies produce it in particularly high quantities during two periods of our lives. The first is during fetal development, with the production almost stopping at birth. The second period begins around the age of seven and rises to a maximum in the mid-twenties before gradually dropping off. By the time you are in your sixties, you will typically have only 10 to 20 percent of your youthful peak values of the hormone.

This drop-off rate has led people to speculate that DHEA may be the elusive fountain of youth! Yet the actual function of DHEA is unknown. All that is certain is that our bodies normally use it to make many of the other hormones we need.

Claims

Daily DHEA supplements are supposed to slow aging, burn fat and build muscle mass, strengthen the immune system, treat lupus, and help prevent heart disease, cancer, diabetes, Alzheimer's, and Parkinson's diseases. They allegedly will also boost libido, alleviate depression, and increase general feelings of strength, stamina, and well-being. The latest claim is that it will be a natural alternative to hormone replacement therapy in postmenopausal women and will treat vaginal dryness and increase bone strength.

Other alternative medicine providers promote DHEA supplements for conditions such as chronic fatigue and immune dysfunction syndrome and fibromyalgia syndrome. Most of these providers will first check either serum or salivary levels of DHEA and then supplement with small amounts of DHEA (10 to 50 mg per day) and monitor DHEA levels.

Study Findings

The last couple of decades have produced studies suggesting that DHEA may actually play a role in many of the conditions listed in the above claims. However, most of these studies were done on animals. In general, animal studies are an important step to developing safe and effective treatments for human. However, there is a very significant caution needed with animal studies—and those with DHEA in particular. Humans and a few primates are the only species known to produce DHEA naturally and to have such high blood levels. This means that the results of these animal studies are not directly applicable to humans. They help move research along, but should not be used to make confident claims about the effect of DHEA in humans.

Unfortunately, because marketers have seized on the results of early studies that may or may not turn out to be correct, abundant unfounded claims circulate about the benefits of DHEA. Since 1994 it has been widely advertised and freely available as a dietary supplement, which has helped to promote widespread use before its effectiveness and safety have been fully investigated.

These early, positive studies stimulated research into DHEA in humans, the results of which are just starting to appear. Some studies (✔✔) in older people have shown preliminary evidence that DHEA can enhance people's mood and can have antidepressant effects. Improvements in memory or attention were not found (✘✘). Several studies (✘✘✘) have shown that decline in DHEA levels is independent of the mental status and decline of aging men. A man with a very high DHEA level is as likely to have worsening mental ability with age as a man with a very low level. Research results released in 2000 (✔✔) showed that low DHEA levels are associated with an increased risk of ischemic heart disease in middle-aged men. Men with the lowest DHEA levels had a 59 percent increased risk of heart disease. However, these data do not answer the question whether taking DHEA will bring up these levels or reduce cardiovascular risk in men.

Some athletes who use DHEA claim it increases testosterone levels to allow muscle building and more vigorous training. Very few studies have examined these claims, but a 1999 study (✘✘✘) with young, healthy men given DHEA found that it neither increased testosterone levels nor gave the men any more muscle or strength gains than when they took a placebo.

The forms of DHEA sold in Europe have been judged by experts there as possibly safe and effective when taken as an adjunct for the treatment of systemic lupus erythematosis (SLE) and when taken for depression. Similar results were found for erectile dysfunction in men and when women used DHEA vaginally to treat vaginal atrophy or to increase bone density (osteoporosis or osteopenia). Furthermore, it is felt safe and effective as a replacement therapy for women with documented adrenal gland insufficiency. In these cases (✔✔) it has been found to improve well-being and sexuality.

As of this writing, it remains too early to tell whether DHEA will become a useful and safe therapeutic agent. More research is needed to confirm whether any particular problems can be treated by DHEA, although it does seem to improve a person's sense of well-being. Research into its potential adverse effects is needed, especially with long-term use.

Cautions

One of the biggest concerns about DHEA arises from it being a natural steroid. These compounds are powerful, with a wide range of actions. High blood levels of DHEA have been linked (✘✘) to a number of cancers, especially breast cancer in women and prostate cancer in men. DHEA can be converted in the body into testosterone, estrogen, and other sex hormones. This leads to fears that high doses will have negative effects on the many functions influenced by these other hormones. High levels of these hormones have also been implicated in a number of cancers and heart disease.

In addition, DHEA use is associated (✘✘) with acne, increased facial hair, loss of scalp hair, deepening of the voice, weight gain, decreased HDL cholesterol (healthy cholesterol), abnormal liver tests, insulin resistance, and mild insomnia.

Another problem with DHEA arises from its availability since 1994 under the Dietary Supplement Health and Education Act. These products are no longer regulated by the FDA or any other federal agency. So, for example, a 1998 study of DHEA products found that fewer than half of them contained the amount of DHEA stated on the label; some contained none at all! Other products claim to contain plant steroids that can be converted into DHEA. However, this chemical conversion process does not occur within the human body!

The Natural Database rates DHEA as "Possibly Unsafe" when used long-term, in high doses, or during pregnancy or lactation.

Recommendations

At this point, research does not conclusively support the use of DHEA supplements for most of the purposes for which they are marketed. Although it may not be unreasonable for a health care provider to use this supplement while monitoring blood or salivary levels, there is still virtually no compelling evidence that this type of intervention is effective—and there are significant theoretical risks from DHEA since it is a steroid hormone that can impact numerous biochemical processes in humans and may stimulate cancer. Therefore, some researchers have commented that use of DHEA outside of a carefully monitored clinical trial is unwarranted. Those interested in eternal youth should look elsewhere (Revelation 21:4).

Dosage

Most studies use 50 mg a day for DHEA treatment. Higher doses have been used for specific conditions.

Treatment Categories

Complementary Therapy

Documented DHEA deficiency	☺☺☺
Adjunct for treatment of systemic lupus erythematosis	☹
Depression	☹
Erectile dysfunction	☹
Vaginally for vaginal atrophy	☹
Increase bone density (osteoporosis or osteopenia)	☹

Note: At this time potential risks in most cases appear to outweigh potential benefits.

Scientifically Unproven

    Antiaging or sports performance   ☹☹

    Any other indication

Further Reading

Brown, Gregory A., Matthew D. Vukovich, Rick L. Sharp, Tracy A. Reifenrath, Kerry A. Parsons, and Douglas S. King, "Effect of Oral DHEA on Serum Testosterone and Adaptations to Resistance Training in Young Men," *Journal of Applied Physiology* 87, no. 6 (December 1999): 2274–83.

Jellin, Jeff M., Forrest Batz, and Kathy Hichens, *Pharmacist's Letter/Prescriber's Letter: Natural Medicines Comprehensive Database* (Stockton, Calif.: Therapeutic Research Facility, 1999), 326–27.

Parasrampuria, J., K. Schwartz, and R. Petesch, "Quality Control of Dehydroepiandrosterone Dietary Supplement Products," *Journal of the American Medical Association* 280, no. 18 (November 1998): 1565.

Ricchini, William, "Cutting Through the Hype: Hormone Replacement Therapy with DHEA," *Advance for Nurse Practitioners* 6, no. 11 (November 1998): 73–74.

ECHINACEA

What It Is

Echinacea was a primary medicine for the various Native-American tribes living in the central plains where the plant grows wild. The type known as purple coneflower *(Echinacea purpurea)* was the treatment of choice for insect bites, snakebites, colds, sores, toothaches, and a variety of infections.

Today there are three varieties of this herb in use, and it has become one of the top ten best-selling herbs in the United States. *Prevention Magazine* reported that in 1999, it was the fifth most common herb taken on a regular basis in America (after garlic, ginseng, ginkgo, and St. John's wort). *Echinacea purpurea* is the most popular echinacea species used in herbal remedies. However, *Echinacea angustifolia* and *Echinacea pallida* are also used, sometimes interchangeably, even though they have somewhat different effects in the body, and no one really knows if they are equally effective. All species grow naturally in central and eastern United States.

Claims

The knowledge and use of *Echinacea purpurea* was passed from Native Americans to Europeans gradually settling farther and farther west. However, its use dropped off after the development of antibiotics in the middle of the twentieth century.

Interest in echinacea was revived after reports emerged from Germany that a number of clinical trials found it helped prevent and treat colds and flu. Today, echinacea is marketed as a natural cure for the common cold. Historically it has been used for many problems, including, but not limited to, pyorrhea, tonsillitis, boils, rheumatism, migraines, dyspepsia, wounds, eczema, bee stings, hemorrhoids, psoriasis, and varicose ulcers.

Study Findings

From a standpoint of evidence, the expressed juice from the tops of *E. purpurea* and the roots of *E. pallida* and *E. angustifolia* are the best tested preparations, and those most likely to be efficacious (*E.* is short for *Echinacea)*. The other parts of the various species of *Echinacea* may be helpful, but we are not aware of any research to support their use.

Early interest in echinacea was generated by a small number of clinical trials in Germany (✔✔✔) that found people taking echinacea got about one-third fewer colds than those taking a placebo. Those taking echinacea in these studies also reported less severe symptoms when they did get a cold, and that the symptoms went away sooner. Laboratory tests have found that echinacea stimulates the immune system to help people fight off infections. However, all these results were from a relatively small number of studies that, while being randomized and controlled, were not designed as rigorously as possible.

Two recent larger randomized, double-blind trials (✘✘✘) have not produced the same sorts of positive results. Melchart's 1998 study used extracts of *E. purpurea* and *E. angustifolia* and found that those subjects who took either had a slightly lower incidence of colds (though not a statistically significant reduction). Based on this and other studies, they estimated that taking echinacea might reduce someone's chance of getting a cold by 10 to 20 percent. Grimm's study (✘✘✘) reported that an extract of *E. purpurea* did not significantly reduce the incidence of colds, nor did it decrease their duration or severity.

A review in *The Cochrane Library* of all the echinacea studies up to 1998 found sixteen controlled studies (✔✔✔). Overall they concluded that there seems to be a consistent, though small, benefit from taking echinacea. At this writing there is better evidence that echinacea helps alleviate and shorten the cold or flu (a viral upper respiratory infection, or URI) than there is evidence that it prevents those illnesses. For example, Brinkeborn's study in Sweden found that three *E. purpurea* preparations were similarly effective in reducing cold symptoms by 50 to 60 percent. This was significantly different from the placebo, which alleviated symptoms by 30 percent.

Much uncertainty remains about echinacea, in particular because of the many different plants and preparations that are on the market. Furthermore, in the United States poor product quality may explain poor consumer satisfaction with echinacea. While more than 14 million Americans regularly use echinacea, a *Consumer Reports* survey in May 2000 found that only 18 percent said it helped their allergies and only 21 percent said it helped with upper respiratory infections.

Concerns about the quality and purity of echinacea sold in the United States are being addressed. ConsumerLab.com, an independent testing company that permits promoters to use its flask-shaped seal of approval on products which pass its criteria—usually meeting German testing standards concerning the quantity of active ingredients in the preparation—is planning to test echinacea products in 2001. Results, when available, can be viewed on the subscription based Website (*www.consumerlab.com*).

Cautions

Taken in reasonable doses, side effects from echinacea have been relatively mild. In clinical trials, some people have reported nausea or constipation. The most common negative reaction is to echinacea's unpleasant taste. *Echinacea* species are members of the daisy family, so people with ragweed allergies should be cautious when taking these preparations.

Some people take echinacea throughout the winter months to prevent colds and flu. No studies have been done on the safety of long-term echinacea use. There is some evidence (✗✗) that taking it for more than eight to ten weeks may weaken the immune system, leaving the person more susceptible to infections. Those who already have diseases of the immune system (such as multiple sclerosis, AIDS, or tuberculosis) could have further deterioration if echinacea is taken for more than a month or two. Echinacea should be avoided during pregnancy and lactation as there is no reliable information on its safety for this use.

Recommendations

Echinacea may provide some help in relieving the symptoms of colds and flu. Most German studies with positive results were conducted with a product called Echincin®, now available in the U.S. as Echinoguard®. There is less evidence that echinacea prevents infections. Given its apparent safety, it may be a helpful option when a cold or flu begins, but should not be used for extended periods of time. It should not be used by pregnant or breast-feeding women.

Dosage

The juice is sometimes used (6 to 9 ml a day), but in tablet form up to about 1 gram of dried material is taken three times a day. There is great variability in the types of preparations used.

Treatment Categories

Complementary Therapy
    Orally:
        Immune stimulant for shortening duration of the common cold   ☺☺☺
        Supportive treatment of flu-like symptoms that accompany many colds   ☺☺

Topical:
Minor skin trauma   ☺☺☺

Scientifically Unproven
Prevention of colds and flu   ☹☹
Any other indications

Further Reading

Brinkeborn, R. M., D. V. Shah, and F. H. Degenring, "Echinaforce® and other *Echinacea* Fresh Plant Preparations in the Treatment of the Common Cold," *Phytomedicine* 6, no. 1 (March 1999): 1–5.

Grimm, Wolfram, and Hans-Helge Müller, "A Randomized Controlled Trial of the Effect of Fluid Extract of *Echinacea Purpurea* on the Incidence and Severity of Colds and Respiratory Infections," *American Journal of Medicine* 106, no. 2 (February 1999): 138–43.

Jellin, Jeff M., Forrest Batz, and Kathy Hichens, *Pharmacist's Letter/Prescriber's Letter: Natural Medicines Comprehensive Database* (Stockton, Calif.: Therapeutic Research Facility, 1999), 342–44.

Melchart, Dieter, Ellen Walther, Klaus Linde, Roland Brandmaier, and Christian Lersch, "Echinacea Root Extracts for the Prevention of Upper Respiratory Tract Infections," *Archives of Family Medicine* 7 (November/December 1998): 541–45.

Melchart, Dieter, K. Linde, P. Fischer, and J. Kaesmayr, "Echinacea for Preventing and Treating the Common Cold (Cochrane Review)," in *The Cochrane Library*, no. 1 (Oxford: Update Software, 2000).

ELDERBERRY

What It Is

Elderberries have long been the subject of both myth and medicine. Archaeologists have traced the cultivation of the shrub back at least to the Stone Age, and there have been stories throughout Europe concerning the connection of the bush with spirits and witches. It was even used as the vehicle for arsenic when the notorious Brewster sisters dispatched lonely bachelors with elderberry wine adulterated with poison in the play and movie *Arsenic and Old Lace*.

Quite apart from the fantasies and theatrical use, the berries, grown on a variety of elder shrubs from the *Sambucus* genus, have been enjoyed in pies, preserves, and, of course, wine. (The edible berries have to be cooked or there is a risk of nausea, vomiting, and diarrhea when eaten.) The most popular species used in herbal medicine include the flowers and cooked fruit of the American elder *(Sambucus canadensis)* and the cooked berry of the European elder *(Sambucus nigra)*.

Claims

Ripe elderberries have been used for centuries as flavorings and to makes juices and elderberry wine. The medicinal remedies have primarily been made from extracts of the flowers.

Traditionally, elderberries have been used most commonly for their diuretic and laxative effects. Many other uses have been reported, ranging from treatment of measles, cancer, and toothache to repelling insects. Another use has been to treat diabetes. Others recommend American elderberries for epilepsy, gout, headaches, neuralgia, psoriasis, rheumatism, sore throats, and constipation. European elder flowers have been used for coughs, colds, laryngitis, flu, and sinusitis. European elderberries have been used for the flu, constipation, sciatica, neuralgia, and cancer.

Elder flowers, usually mixed with yarrow and peppermint leaves, are often brewed into a tea to act as a mild stimulant.

Study Findings

Very little clinical support for the vast majority of the uses of elderberry extract exists. However, very recent research on animals did find that the extract lowered blood glucose levels through insulin-like activity. In addition, one human trial (✔✔✔) showed that a product containing the European elderberry juice (Sambucol®) may shorten the duration of influenza and relieve some of the symptoms of the flu in adults and children. The specific compounds causing this, or any of the other alleged effects, have not been identified. This anecdotal evidence and promising early studies need to be explored in greater depth.

Cautions

All parts of the American elderberry contain cyanogenic glycosides that can release cyanide. These compounds are more prevalent in the leaves, stems, and unripe fruit, and should therefore not be used in preparing elderberry juice. The flowers and ripe fruit usually are free of these compounds. Children using the stems as peashooters (✘) have suffered cyanide poisoning. Other adverse reactions, which may also be related to the cyanide, include diarrhea and vomiting. The European elder is not reported to contain cyanogenic compounds. The Natural Database claims that elderberries in an amount greater than that found in food should not be used during pregnancy or lactation. However, one elderberry product, Sambucol, has been used safely in children.

Recommendations

Elderberries have been used to make juice and wine for centuries. This may provide some health benefits, but these are very mild. Medicinal use of many of these products seems unwarranted, at least with the American elder, given the risk of cyanide poisoning and the availability of other pharmaceutical and natural remedies to effectively treat the conditions for which elderberries are recommended. However, other than nausea, vomiting, and diarrhea if the fruit is not cooked sufficiently, a clinical trial of European elderberry syrup reported no adverse effects in adults or children.

Dosage

No consensus exists.

Treatment Categories

Complementary Therapy
Flu   ☹

Scientifically Unproven
Any other medical indication   ☹☹

Further Reading

DerMarderosian, Ara, ed., "Elderberry," in *The Review of Natural Products* (St. Louis, Mo.: Facts and Comparisons, July 1992).

Fetrow, Charles W., and Juan R. Avila, *Professional's Handbook of Complementary and Alternative Medicine* (Springhouse, Penn.: Springhouse, 1999), 235–37.

Jellin, Jeff M., Forrest Batz, and Kathy Hichens, *Pharmacist's Letter/Prescriber's Letter: Natural Medicines Comprehensive Database* (Stockton, Calif.: Therapeutic Research Facility, 1999), 44–45, 363–65.

EPHEDRA

What It Is

Ephedra is one of those herbal remedies that seems to be on the "must use" list of everyone from young adults seeking to maximize their work, school, and intimate lives with minimal sleep, to sleep-deprived parents of new babies, to older individuals hoping to regain their youthful vigor. If the stories are to be believed, the herb will serve as a stimulant, increase sexual pleasure, and even help you lose weight. Of greater interest to those with breathing problems is the fact that ephedra has long been connected to treatment for asthma, bronchitis, and even the common cold. Some users claim that it also eases suffering from arthritis.

Ephedra is also known as "herbal ecstasy" because of its stimulant ability, "herbal fen-phen" for its alleged ability to help people shed unwanted weight, and by the Chinese names Ma Huang and Ma Huanggen. Ma Huanggen, made from the rhizome and root of Chinese ephedra *(Ephedra sinica),* is rarely used except for someone troubled by night sweats. Ma Huang, made from the stem and branches of this same plant, has been the source of most of ephedra's alleged benefits.

The genus *Ephedra* contains more than forty different plant species, each with its own specific mixture of compounds called alkaloids. The most common alkaloid is ephedrine. Other than Chinese ephedra, the most common medicinal species of ephedra include intermediate ephedra *(Ephedra intermedia)* and Mongolian ephedra *(Ephedra equisetta).*

Claims

Ephedra has been used traditionally in China for more than 5000 years, primarily for the treatment of asthma. Just the stems and branches were used, not the entire plant. Later in China, Ma Huang was used to treat bronchitis, hay fever, the common cold, and other ailments.

The alkaloid ephedrine is widely used in conventional medicine as a decongestant and asthma remedy. Other ephedra alkaloids commonly prescribed by physicians include pseudoephedrine and norephedrine. The *Ephedra* species native to North America *(Ephedra nevadensis),* often called American ephedra or Mormon tea, contains none of these alkaloids—therefore it lacks both the therapeutic benefits and the risks of other *Ephedra* species.

All the ephedra preparations are said to provide natural ways to control asthma, lose weight, boost energy levels, and increase sexual pleasure. Some claim it can be used for a natural, legal high. Many ephedra manufacturers add caffeine to their products to enhance the effects. Some herbalists recommend it as an appetite suppressant, cardiovascular stimulant, and central nervous system stimulant.

Study Findings

Decades of research have shown that ephedrine and pseudoephedrine are effective nasal decongestants and relieve bronchial asthma. They also increase blood pressure, heart rate, constriction of blood vessels, bronchial dilation, and central nervous system stimulation. They can suppress coughing and are anti-inflammatory in animal studies. They have been available in a number of over-the-counter pharmaceutical preparations since the 1930s. These drugs act by stimulating the central nervous system, which explains why they simultaneously affect numerous body systems. This also means they must be carefully monitored to ensure the correct dose is taken.

However, positive results with ephedrine do not necessarily mean ephedra products are as effective. Since alkaloid content in the various *Ephedra* species varies, the amount of ephedrine in any herbal remedy will vary, making careful dosing impossible with herbal remedies. Very few clinical studies with ephedra could be found, and none were found that supported a beneficial role. One study (✗✗) reported it increased heart rate and blood pressure, but with much variability between subjects. Another study (✗✗✗) found none of the biochemical changes that would be expected, given the claims made for ephedra as a weight-loss product. Ten of eleven other herbs commonly advertised as natural weight-loss products failed this same test.

Cautions

Ephedra products contain drugs that have been demonstrated (✗✗✗✗) to have a wide range of effects in the body. Their side effects include high blood pressure, increased heart rate, heart palpitations, anxiety, restlessness, headache, psychoses, stroke, heart attack, cardiac arrhythmias, and death. For this reason, ephedra products are likely to interact with other drugs taken to influence these systems. As of 1998, forty-four deaths had been reported to the FDA (✗✗), along with hundreds of other adverse effects, involving ephedra products. Many of these occurred in teenagers using the products to get high, lose weight, or enhance athletic performance. Ephedrine is notorious for causing kidney stones, which have also been reported (✗✗) after taking herbal ephedra.

Of concern also is the great variability in ephedra products. A 1997 study examined nine products labeled "Ephedra extract." Two contained no ephedrine. If people followed the directions on the labels of the other products they would have consumed anything from 5 mg to 89 mg of ephedrine alkaloids daily. Anyone who had been taking one brand who switched to another could easily take too much.

Another problem was discovered when four of the products showed a pattern of alkaloids that does not occur in any known *Ephedra* species. The most likely explanation is that these products were spiked with synthetic drugs. Similar studies published in 1998 (with nine Ma Huang products) and in 2000 (with twenty ephedra products) found the same problems. In half the products tested in the 2000 study, researchers found at least a 20 percent discrepancy between the alkaloid quantity in the product and the amount listed on the label. One product contained no ephedrine alkaloids at all.

The Natural Database rates ephedra as "Likely Unsafe" when the typical dose is exceeded, when used long term, when used in children under age six, and in breast-feeding mothers. It is rated as "Contraindicated" during pregnancy, as it may induce uterine contractions.

Recommendations

The active ingredients in ephedra are powerful drugs with a broad range of effects throughout the body. These drugs are readily available in standardized pharmaceutical preparations. Using herbal remedies to obtain these compounds "naturally" only adds uncertainty and danger. There is no reason to use these remedies.

Dosage

The FDA recommends doses should not exceed 8 mg total ephedrine alkaloids every six hours or 24 mg a day. Some products recommend much higher quantities. In most cases it seems impossible to know how much herbal material contains this amount of drug. Great care should be taken with these products.

Treatment Categories

Conventional Therapy

In the form of ephedrine made to pharmaceutical standards, for short-term therapy:

Acute bronchospasm	☺☺☺☺
Asthma	☺☺☺☺
Nasal congestion	☺☺☺☺

Complementary Therapy

In the form of ephedra or Ma Huang

Weight loss	☹☹☹☹
Sports performance	☹☹☹☹
Euphoria	☹☹☹☹

Scientifically Unproven

Weight loss or sports performance	☹☹☹☹
Other indications	☹☹☹☹

Further Reading

Betz, Joseph M., Martha L. Gay, Magdi M. Mossoba, Sarah Adams, and Barbara S. Portz, "Chiral Gas Chromatographic Determination of Ephedrine-Type Alkaloids in Dietary Supplements Containing Má Huáng," *Journal of AOAC International* 80, no. 2 (March–April 1997): 303–15.

Fetrow, Charles W., and Juan R. Avila, *Professional's Handbook of Complementary and Alternative Medicine* (Springhouse, Penn.: Springhouse, 1999), 239–42.

Gurley, B. J., S. F. Gardner, and M. A. Hubbard, "Content Versus Label Claims in Ephedra-Containing Dietary Supplements," *American Journal of Health System Pharmacy* 57, no. 10 (May 2000): 963–69.

Jellin, Jeff M., Forrest Batz, and Kathy Hichens, *Pharmacist's Letter/Prescriber's Letter: Natural Medicines Comprehensive Database* (Stockton, Calif.: Therapeutic Research Facility, 1999), 44–45, 352–54.

EVENING PRIMROSE

What It Is

The evening primrose is a North American wildflower *(Oenothera biennis)* whose fragrant yellow blooms, lasting just one night, have long delighted hikers and lovers out for an evening stroll. The fruit pods contain many small seeds from which an oil is extracted.

Evening primrose oil (EPO) contains a relatively high proportion of essential fatty acids (EFA). EPO from commercial strains of the flower contains about 72 percent of one particular EFA called "cis-linolenic acid" (LA), and 9 percent of gamma-linolenic acid (GLA). EPO is one of the richest plant sources of GLA. Only borage oil (24 percent GLA) and black currant seed oil (16 percent GLA) contain more. These two compounds (GLA and LA) play an essential role in the inflammatory and immune responses of the body.

Claims

EPO has been called the King's Cure-All in England, where it is enormously popular, and for good reason. In the United Kingdom it is approved, "prescription only," for allergy-related eczema. It is recommended there, and in the United States, by herbal medicine practitioners for everything from calming hyperactive children to speeding wound healing and curing cancer. In Canada it is approved as a dietary supplement to increase essential fatty acid intake. In the Great Lakes region, Native-American tribes used the entire plant both as a painkiller and to make a sleeping medication.

What has made it one of the most popular herbal remedies in the United States has been the connection established between GLA and inflammatory diseases. Thus, EPO is recommended for the treatment of rheumatoid arthritis, dermatitis, eczema, psoriasis, and asthma. It is also commonly promoted for cardiovascular disease, premenstrual syndrome, fibrocystic breast disease, and multiple sclerosis. Others recommend it for breast pain, high cholesterol, Raynaud's phenomena, Sjogren's syndrome, post-viral fatigue syndrome, diabetic neuropathy, neurodermatitis, and some pregnancy-related problems.

Study Findings

Research into the role of EFAs in inflammation is proceeding at a rapid rate and producing interesting results. Studies have shown that supplementing the diet with sources high in the omega-9 and omega-3 EFAs can result in increased levels of anti-inflammatory EFAs and improvements in people's health. However, many of these studies were small and of poorer quality, and their results must be interpreted cautiously.

The EFA with the most promising anti-inflammatory effect is eicosapentenoic acid (EPA). High levels of EPA are found in cold-water fish (like salmon, sardines, cod, and halibut) and the oils extracted from them (like cod liver oil). The EFA that best promotes normal (and abnormal) inflammatory reactions is arachidonic acid (AA). It is found in animal fat, dairy fat, shellfish, and mollusks.

The important role of GLA in the diet has been clearly demonstrated. Certain diseases are caused, or made worse, by low dietary EFA or impairments in the body's ability to make GLA (e.g., depression, arthritis, cardiovascular disease, inflammatory bowel disease, and insulin resistance). In studies of these sorts of conditions, EPO theoretically could be expected to bring some relief.

At this writing, there have been very few high-quality studies of the use of EPO in humans. A few studies (✔✔✔) involving people with rheumatoid arthritis and osteoarthritis have found that patients used less pain medication when taking EPO compared to those taking placebo. However, the EPO did not cause changes in the severity of the disease itself.

Studies of people's diets in a number of different cultures have demonstrated that the more fish people consume, the lower the incidence of depression. There is also a correlation (✘✘) between depression and the type of EFA people consume. As the ratio of AA to EPA increases, the incidence of depression also increases. While these types of studies (called epidemiological studies) are intriguing, and very important for suggesting future research projects, they do not demonstrate that depression can be treated effectively by changing the EFAs in your diet. To our knowledge, no studies have been done where EPO has been given to humans with depression.

Patients with allergy-related dermatitis and eczema showed improvements in some studies (✔✔✔✔), but not in others (✘✘✘✘), including the largest, best-designed one. Usually in these studies, the EPO is applied topically, but oral EPO has also been shown to be effective. Although EPO seems to help allergy-related dermatitis, it appears to have no effect on allergic asthma or psoriasis. GLA and AA have been shown (✔✔) to significantly reduce blood cholesterol levels, and would thus be expected to be beneficial in patients concerned about developing heart disease. However, to our knowledge, studies on EPO's effect on heart disease itself have not been reported. EPO has been reported in at least one randomized controlled trial (✔✔✔) to have some mild benefits in patients with ulcerative colitis. Multiple randomized controlled trials (✘✘✘✘) have shown EPO to be no better than placebo for the treatment of premenstrual syndrome.

European trials have looked at EPO for a number of medical indications. Human trials (✔✔✔) have shown effectiveness when taken for breast pain. Effectiveness also was found (✔✔) for a variety of chronic, painful conditions, including Sjogren's syndrome, diabetic neuropathy, rheumatoid arthritis, and irritable bowel syndrome exacerbated by PMS. Reports (✔) also have been made of its effectiveness for Alzheimer's disease. It has been found ineffective in four human trials (✘✘✘✘) for preventing preeclampsia. It has also been found ineffective (✘✘✘) in shortening the length of labor.

Cautions

Overall, EPO (and other sources of the "good" EFAs such as nuts, cold-water fish oil, and black currant oil) appears to be safe and well tolerated. EPO can sometimes cause indigestion, nausea, soft stools, abdominal pain, and headache. However, the effects of long-term use, as would be required for many of the conditions for which it is recommended, have not been examined. Studies of this aspect of use are especially important since 4 to 8 grams daily are often suggested. This amount of oil is also relatively expensive and has led to efforts to find other sources of GLA. There is also some concern about product quality.

Although borage oil contains a higher percentage of GLA than EPO, it can also contain toxic pyrrolizidine alkaloids. It should not be used in place of EPO.

The Natural Database rates EPO "Possibly Unsafe" in pregnancy and "Possibly Safe" during lactation.

Recommendations

While certain people can clearly benefit from supplementing their diet with GLA, this does not mean that everyone needs to take evening primrose oil. By analogy, your car won't run any better on a full tank of gas than it will on a half tank. But if you're out of gas, or the gas cap is locked, you need some other way to get the gas in the gas tank. In the same way, if your body doesn't make enough GLA, or you're getting very little in your diet, evening primrose supplements would be a good option to try if you suffer from any of the inflammatory diseases we mentioned.

Dosage

Doses in the range of 2 to 4 grams daily are commonly used, though much higher doses are sometimes recommended.

Treatment Categories

Conventional Therapy

In the United Kingdom: allergy-related eczema	☺☺
In Canada: increasing essential fatty acid intake	☺☺☺

Complementary Therapy

Pain of cyclic and noncyclic breast pain (mastalgia)	☺☺☺
Pain associated with osteoarthritis and rheumatoid arthritis	☺☺☺
Elevated blood cholesterol	☺
Adjunct to treating inflammatory bowel disease (ulcerative colitis)	☺
Sjogren's syndrome	☺
Diabetic neuropathy	☺
Irritable bowel syndrome exacerbated by PMS	☺☺
Alzheimer's disease	☺
Decreasing insulin resistance in Type 2 diabetes	☺

Scientifically Unproven

Allergic asthma	☹☹☹
Psoriasis	☹☹☹
Depression	☹
Preventing heart disease	☹
PMS symptoms	☹☹☹
Preventing preeclampsia	☹☹☹☹
Shortening labor duration	☹☹☹☹
Any other medical indication	

Further Reading

Belch, Jill J. F., and Alexander Hill, "Evening Primrose Oil and Borage Oil in Rheumatologic Conditions," *American Journal of Clinical Nutrition* 71, suppl. (January 2000): 352S–356S.

DerMarderosian, Ara, ed., "Oil of Evening Primrose (OEP) (EPO)," in *The Review of Natural Products* (St. Louis, Mo.: Facts and Comparisons, August 1997).

Fetrow, Charles W., and Juan R. Avila, *Professional's Handbook of Complementary and Alternative Medicine* (Springhouse, Penn.: Springhouse, 1999), 524–27.

Jellin, Jeff M., Forrest Batz, and Kathy Hichens, *Pharmacist's Letter/Prescriber's Letter: Natural Medicines Comprehensive Database* (Stockton, Calif.: Therapeutic Research Facility, 1999), 368–70.

FENNEL

What It Is

Fennel was once one of the most important herbs for people terrified of witches. Just as garlic developed the reputation for being a defense against vampires, so fennel could be used to protect you from any spell being cast. Hippocrates, the famous physician in ancient Greece, liked fennel, noting through his anecdotal research that it seemed to help lactating women increase milk production. Over the centuries fennel has been known as a culinary herb used widely in foods, especially in stews, soups, salads, beverages, and condiments. It is also used as a fragrance in some cosmetics.

The herb's Latin name, *Foeniculum vulgare,* literally means fragrant hay, reflecting the plant's feathery leaves growing at the end of a tall stalk. The parts used medicinally are the fruit, which are so small they are often referred to as seeds. The fruit contains oils that are either isolated and purified or used as part of the whole dried fruit.

Claims

Fennel fruit and oil are used to relieve a variety of digestive problems. It is most commonly used as a carminative, which is an agent used to relieve flatulence. Other uses include appetite suppression, as a purgative, and cough suppressant. Fennel water is commonly used in Europe to relieve colic and calm babies. Herbalists recommend it to increase lactation, promote menstruation, increase libido, and treat bronchitis, back-ache, bedwetting, snakebites, and to improve appetite.

Study Findings

Very few studies have been conducted on the clinical effects of fennel. Studies reported by the German Commission E were mostly on animals and tissues, but did indicate (✔✔) that fennel is possibly effective for treating mild gastrointestinal spasm, abdominal fullness, gas, and upper respiratory tract mucous membrane inflammation. Fennel honey syrup is used in Europe (✔) for upper respiratory infections in children. Animal studies have found that extracts of the seeds have estrogen-like activity, and fennel was studied extensively during the 1930s as a potential source of synthetic estrogens when this area of research first began. These studies did not yield viable products.

Cautions

Fennel used in cooking or teas has not produced problems, except for an occasional allergic reaction. However, use of larger quantities of fennel "seeds," or the very concentrated volatile oil made from them, may have serious side effects. Ingesting the oil (✘✘) can lead to nausea, vomiting, seizures, and respiratory problems. In animals, the oil has caused liver damage. Other allergic problems include dermatitis and cross-reactivity with related species like celery, carrots, and mugwort.

One component of fennel fruit, estragole, is called a procarcinogen. This means it may be a precursor of cancer-causing substances. Therefore, most experts recommend that use in amounts larger than found in food should be limited to short periods of time.

Another problem was found with fennel samples examined in Italy. Investigators found that many samples were contaminated with bacteria known to cause infectious gastrointestinal diseases. The fennel plant is very similar to hemlock, which causes vomiting, paralysis, and death in very small amounts. For this reason, make sure any fennel you use, even for cooking, comes from a reliable source.

The Natural Database rates fennel in amounts larger than found in foods as "Possibly Unsafe" when used orally for prolonged periods of time and "Likely Unsafe" for use in pregnancy or lactation. They consider it "contraindicated" in pregnancy.

Recommendations

Fennel has a long tradition of use in adding flavor and fragrance to food. It may also have some value as a digestive aid. There is little other evidence to support its use in quantities larger than used in condiments. The risks associated with ingesting large amounts of the oil argue against any of its potential medicinal uses.

Dosage

A dose of 5 to 7 grams daily of dried fennel fruit or seed is recommended, or 0.1 to 0.6 ml of fennel oil.

Treatment Categories

Complementary Therapy
Short-term therapy for mild spastic disorders of the GI tract ☺☺
Abdominal fullness and gas ☺☺
Cough and bronchitis ☺

Scientifically Unproven
Any other indication ☹

Further Reading

DerMarderosian, Ara, ed., "Fennel," in *The Review of Natural Products* (St. Louis, Mo.: Facts and Comparisons, August 1994).

Foster, Steven, and Varro E. Tyler, *Tyler's Honest Herbal: A Sensible Guide to the Use of Herbs and Related Remedies*, 4th ed. (New York: Haworth Herbal Press, 1999), 157–58.

Jellin, Jeff M., Forrest Batz, and Kathy Hichens, *Pharmacist's Letter/Prescriber's Letter: Natural Medicines Comprehensive Database* (Stockton, Calif.: Therapeutic Research Facility, 1999), 44–45, 372–74.

FEVERFEW

What It Is

If you lived in Greece during the time of Jesus, you would have encountered feverfew as a medicine for hot inflammations and hot swellings. Historians believe that these terms refer to what today we would call arthritis joint discomfort. Thus this is a plant with a lengthy history of use.

Over the years, feverfew has had numerous botanical names, including *Tanacetum parthenium* and *Chrysanthemum parthenium*. It is a member of the daisy family, a perennial seen in fields and along roadsides. The flowers have yellow disks and ten to twenty white-toothed rays. The leaf, either fresh or freeze-dried, is generally used in herbal preparations.

Claims

Feverfew has been grown in gardens in Europe for centuries. Currently feverfew is a popular herbal remedy for the prevention and treatment of migraine. In traditional and folk use, feverfew is touted as helping to treat fever, arthritis, menstrual difficulties, cough, chest colds, "melancholy," "sadness of spirit," vertigo, headache, colic, flatulence, indigestion, worms, hysteria, and difficulty urinating. It has also been promoted as a topical treatment for insect bites and as an insect repellent when planted around a house or garden. By far the most common use is for migraine headache prophylaxis and treatment.

Study Findings

The systematic review by Pittler and colleagues located four randomized, placebo-controlled trials of feverfew for prevention of migraine. In one, patients were randomized to receive 50 mg of dried feverfew or placebo for six periods of four weeks each. The contents of both active and placebo bottles were sprinkled with a small amount of feverfew powder so that opening both types of capsules gave identical smells. In this study (✔✔✔), the group taking placebo showed significantly more migraine attacks. In another study (✔✔✔), the treatment group of migraine sufferers received standardized feverfew powdered leaves. There was a 24 percent reduction in the number of attacks during feverfew treatment, but no significant change in the duration of individual attacks. There was a significant reduction in associated nausea and vomiting and a nonsignificant trend toward reduction in attack severity. A third study (✔✔✔) also found more benefit for those taking feverfew than placebo. However, the fourth trial (✘✘✘) was both the largest and best controlled, and showed no benefit to using feverfew to prevent migraine headaches. Another trial (✘✘✘), not included in the above review, also found no benefit from feverfew. Given the variability in results, the reviewers concluded that while feverfew has shown benefit, its benefit "has not been established beyond reasonable doubt." The United States Headache Consortium, formed from numerous professional medical organizations, in its 2000 guidelines rated feverfew as a second-line agent for the prevention of migraine headaches.

It should be noted that these studies are at times cited as support for feverfew treatment of migraine. However, none of these studies was primarily concerned with treatment of acute attacks. They were studies solely of feverfew's ability to reduce the number of attacks endured by migraine sufferers. Even those using feverfew occasionally experienced a migraine, and though it was less often than when not using feverfew, once it struck, it lasted as long as usual for the test subject. The Headache Consortium guidelines did not include feverfew in the list of agents for treatment of migraines.

Apart from these clinical studies, there has also been one randomized control trial (✘✘✘) showing that feverfew was not helpful for rheumatoid arthritis.

Cautions

Occasional mouth ulcerations and gastric irritation (in 5 to 15 percent of users) have been reported (✘✘) with the use of fresh feverfew leaves, but have not been reported with the use of dried leaves in capsules. Other reported adverse effects include skin rashes, rapid heart rate, indigestion, colic, and weight gain. Feverfew is a member of the daisy family, and should not be used by people with known allergies or sensitivity to other members like ragweed, chamomile, or yarrow. Other adverse effects reported include dizziness, light-headedness, slightly heavier periods, heartburn, skin rash, and diarrhea.

Those who had used feverfew for several years and then abruptly stopped taking the herb, experienced the recurrence of incapacitating migraines (what are called "rebound headaches").

Feverfew has been said (✖) to cause miscarriage, to increase menstrual flow, and to cause uterine contractions in pregnant women at term. Therefore, feverfew is contraindicated during pregnancy. However, there is no information on feverfew excretion in breast milk. There is no data concerning the use of feverfew in children, but some experts say it should not be used in children twelve or younger. The Natural Database rates feverfew as "Contraindicated" in prenancy and recommends avoiding it when breast-feeding.

Feverfew has been reported (✖✖) to decrease the blood's ability to clot, so it is prudent for patients on aspirin to avoid feverfew until safety studies are available.

As with all herbal remedies, products vary widely in their quality. One study examined three feverfew products *(Tanacetum parthenium)* and found that only one contained the active ingredient of feverfew—parthenolide. This chemical may be the major antimigraine constituent, but even if it is not, its absence indicates there was no feverfew in these two products.

Recommendations

Evidence from clinical trials suggests that feverfew, taken daily for from three to eight months, can be effective and safe in reducing the incidence of migraine headaches. However, it has not been compared to standard prescription medications used to prevent migraine headaches, nor has it been tested for the treatment of migraine headaches.

Dosage

Studies have used daily doses of 50 to 100 mg of feverfew extract.

Treatment Categories

Conventional Therapy
Second-line agent for prevention of migraine headache   ☺☺☺

Complementary Therapy
Treatment of migraine headache   ☹

Scientifically Unproven
Rheumatoid arthritis   ☹☹
Other indications

Further Reading

Awang, D., "Prescribing Therapeutic Feverfew," *Internal Medicine* 1 (1998): 11–13.

DerMarderosian, Ara, ed., "Feverfew," in *The Review of Natural Products* (St. Louis, Mo.: Facts and Comparisons, September 1994).

Jellin, Jeff M., Forrest Batz, and Kathy Hichens, *Pharmacist's Letter/Prescriber's Letter: Natural Medicines Comprehensive Database* (Stockton, Calif.: Therapeutic Research Facility, 1999), 377–78.

Pittler, M. H., B. K. Vogler, and E. Ernst, "Feverfew for Preventing Migraine (Cochrane Review)," in *The Cochrane Library* (Oxford: Update Software, 2000), Issue 4.

GARLIC

What It Is

Garlic is the herb most commonly taken by Americans. *Prevention Magazine* reports that more than 24 million Americans regularly take garlic supplements. It has been credited with many things, both real and imagined, yet its uses are occasionally at cross-purposes with one another. For example, everyone who has ever gone on a dinner date and wanted to maintain kissing-fresh breath has heard the warning not to eat anything with garlic. The lingering odor puts an instant damper on romance. Yet garlic is also said to increase sexual prowess.

Lovers of horror stories and low-budget drive-in movies know the importance of keeping garlic hanging around the neck if you have to venture out during a full moon. This may be folklore's only protection against vampires, though whether it has magical properties when confronting the undead or simply offends their sense of smell is unclear.

Apart from myth, garlic, whether slivered, minced, used as whole cloves, or crushed, is one of the most common aromatics used in cooking. *Allium sativum,* also known as poor man's treacle or clove garlic, is said to have originated in Central Asia. Eventually, it was introduced into the Mediterranean area. It is now cultivated worldwide.

The medicinal parts of garlic are the whole fresh clove, the dried clove, and the oil prepared from the clove. It is a member of the allium plant family, which includes onions, shallots, and leeks. These plants contain sulfur-rich derivatives of the amino acid cysteine, which are thought to have medicinal benefits.

When raw garlic is cut or crushed, the enzyme alliinase interacts with the cysteine compound alliin, inside the clove, to produce allicin. Allicin gives garlic its typical aroma and taste, but is fairly volatile and usually breaks down either in a few hours at room temperature or after twenty minutes of cooking. More stable compounds such as ajoene and dithiins are formed when garlic is macerated with oil. These compounds may be stable for more than a year.

Allicin is also thought to be one of the most important medicinal substances in garlic, although little or no allicin is present in the intact garlic clove. The garlic plant produces allicin as a natural defense against bacteria and other organisms. Allicin is highly irritating and has been shown to kill bacteria in laboratory studies.

The instability of allicin makes it difficult to study its clinical effects and those of its derivatives. Numerous investigators are studying allicin's blood-thinning activity, antibacterial or antifungal properties, and antioxidant potential. Most clinical studies have used dried garlic powder tablets, and that is the preparation that we will discuss.

Claims

The ancient Egyptians, Greeks, Romans, Babylonians, and Chinese all wrote about the healing properties of garlic. In Egypt, the *Codex Ebers Papyrus* (1550 B.C.) mentioned the healing power of garlic. Pliny the Elder and Herodotus mentioned the medicinal use of garlic. Chinese healers used garlic as a treatment to lower blood pressure. Hippocrates is said to have used garlic in the fifth century B.C. to treat leprosy. In 1722, French citizens reported protection from the plague if they drank garlic vinegar. In 1858, Louis Pasteur reported the antibacterial activity of garlic. Garlic was administered as an antiseptic poultice during World War I.

Garlic is said to aid in the lowering of serum lipids and to prevent age-dependent vascular changes. Garlic has long been thought to be effective in the prevention of heart disease by lowering cholesterol and acting as a mild blood thinner. Herbalists use garlic for high blood pressure, diarrhea, ringworm, hypersensitive teeth, colds, flu, cough, headache, athlete's foot, gout, rheumatism, cancer, snakebites, and as an aphrodisiac.

Study Findings

Studies in isolated hepatocytes (liver cells) indicate that key enzymes in the body's natural process for making cholesterol, particularly one enzyme called "HMG-CoA reductase," may be inhibited by the sulfur-containing substances in garlic. This is the same enzyme that is affected by prescription medications called "statins" that reduce cholesterol levels.

Many clinical trials (✔✔✔) have reported that garlic lowers cholesterol, but most of these have had only a small number of patients. A meta-analysis of five selected trials in 1993 included a total of 410 individuals. Three trials used dried garlic powder tablets, one trial used garlic powder, and another used a garlic extract. The dose of garlic was equivalent to approximately one-half to one clove of garlic per day. Overall (✔✔✔), there was a 9 percent reduction in cholesterol levels in the garlic-treated subjects.

Another meta-analysis was published at the end of 2000 and included thirteen studies. The authors concluded there was evidence that garlic lowered cholesterol levels more than placebo (✔✔✔), but only to a very small extent. They questioned whether this would make any difference to patients' health. Additionally, when only the six studies of highest quality were examined (✗✗✗✗), garlic did not produce statistically significant reduction in cholesterol levels. The most recent study we examined, published in January 2001 (✗✗✗), also found no cholesterol-lowering benefit from garlic.

Animal studies indicated that the sulfur-containing compounds in garlic may inhibit the development of atherosclerosis (hardening of the arteries). Garlic seems to also indirectly affect atherosclerosis-related diseases by reducing elevated blood pressure and lipid levels, and probably by preventing the formation of blood clots. Studies with animals found that garlic could both prevent the formation of atherosclerotic plaques that narrow the arteries and reduce their size. Garlic's direct effect on atherosclerosis is thought to be due to its ability to reduce lipid content in arterial cells and to prevent the accumulation of lipids between the cells. A systematic review of these later clinical trials (✔✔✔) with garlic led to the conclusion that garlic has potential in the prevention and control of cardiovascular disorders. A large number of additional clinical trials are now under way which should make possible more definite statements about the use of garlic for prevention and treatment of atherosclerosis-related diseases.

A meta-analysis of eighteen epidemiological studies (✔✔) revealed that eating raw garlic cloves may have a beneficial effect in preventing stomach and colorectal cancer. However, epidemiological studies are not controlled studies, and there was much variability between the studies, with some of very low quality. Most of the studies were conducted in China, where garlic cloves release significantly more allicin than garlic from anywhere else in the world (three times as much as garlic grown in the United States). The authors were cautious in their conclusions, but this is likely to be an area of great interest in the future.

Even though garlic is taken more often than any other herb, a *Consumer Reports* survey of nearly 47,000 Americans (✗✗) found that only 18 percent said it helped their high cholesterol, only 15 percent said it helped their arthritis, and only 12 percent said it helped their back pain. This poor consumer satisfaction, in spite of the slightly positive research results, could be explained by the lack of regulation of these products in the United States, which can result in poor product quality. In addition, there are significant manufacturing differences among the garlic preparations.

Fresh garlic may be the only preparation that achieves a significant amount of allicin in the diet. The odor and stomach upset that may be caused by chewing raw garlic, however, make it a poor choice for a cholesterol-lowering agent. Cooked garlic may be better tolerated, but prolonged cooking will also inactivate the sulfur-containing compounds thought to be beneficial. No well-designed long-term studies using raw or cooked garlic are available.

Because of the variability among products, manufacturers currently usually show the allicin content or allicin potential as a description of their potency. There are significant technical difficulties in the commercial preparation of garlic supplements, however, because of the rapid breakdown of the volatile sulfur compounds.

Manufacturers have devised methods to attempt to preserve allicin. Garlic powder tablets are coated and contain freeze-dried fresh garlic. In fact, according to the Natural Database, most of the clinical studies that have shown benefit from garlic have tested the brand name product Kwai®. Once ingested, the surface coating of the tablet dissolves in the stomach, allowing the enzyme alliinase to convert inactive alliin to the active allicin. The tablet is odorless since digestion of the capsule is supposed to occur sufficiently far along in the digestive tract to avoid a garlic odor.

Another method uses rapid drying of cut garlic, presumably before allicin is produced. The rapid degradation of these compounds following drying minimizes the allicin content in standard garlic powder. Yet another method involves inactivating alliinase and adding the enzyme back to the final dried product. Unfortunately, alliinase is easily denatured by stomach acid. Products using distilled garlic oil or garlic powder have shown conflicting results in humans and cannot be recommended at this time.

One study in Germany reported that only about 25 percent of the garlic products available had an amount of allicin equivalent to one clove of fresh garlic. Some odorless products did not contain any active compound. Concerns about the quality and purity of garlic sold in the United States are being addressed. ConsumerLab.com, an independent testing company that permits promoters to use its flask-shaped seal of approval on products that pass its criteria—usually meeting German testing standards concerning the quantity of active ingredients in the preparation—is planning to test garlic products in 2001. Results, when available, can be viewed by subscribing to their Website.

Cautions

Garlic is generally considered safe. The most common problems are an undesirable garlic taste and smell, something that unfortunately can also occur with the so-called "odorless" preparations on the market.

Raw garlic can cause stomach upset, reflux, and gas symptoms and may also be caustic to the skin. Garlic may have some blood-thinning activity, so it is not recommended for patients taking blood thinners or aspirin. Garlic may enhance the effects of the blood thinner warfarin (Coumadin®) and may increase the effects of other antiplatelet drugs, oral diabetic drugs, or insulin.

The Natural Database rates garlic as "Possibly Unsafe" when used orally or topically in large amounts, especially in children. It is rated "Likely Safe" in pregnancy and lactation, when ingested in the amounts commonly found in foods, but "Possibly Unsafe" during pregnancy and lactation in amounts greater than those found in foods.

Recommendations

Evidence from a number of studies suggests that garlic may have a mild cholesterol-lowering and blood-pressure-lowering effect. This effect seems to be more evident in individuals with elevated cholesterol or blood pressure levels. The beneficial German studies used Kwai, while Japanese researchers used Kyolic®. Both products are now available in the U.S. A number of well-designed trials, however, have failed to show any significant benefit from garlic supplements. High-dose garlic may prevent or stimulate the regression of the cholesterol plaques that cause atherosclerosis. The varying quality of garlic preparations may account for some of the different results among studies.

Fresh garlic can certainly be recommended as a component of a plant-centered diet and as part of an overall strategy of lifestyle modification to lower cholesterol levels. The powdered garlic products may be used as well; however, there are concerns about limited shelf life for these products as well as a lack of knowledge about consistency in the manufacturing process.

Garlic may be lightly cooked to avoid the side effects of raw cloves, but too much cooking will deactivate the sulfur-containing compounds that may be the active agents.

For patients with hypercholesterolemia, the cholesterol-lowering effect of garlic is modest and garlic does not substitute for medical drug therapy if greater reductions in cholesterol are desired.

Eating a clove of garlic every day may have some benefits in preventing cancer, although this finding is relatively new.

Dosage

For effects related to heart disease, most studies use 600 to 900 mg a day, usually divided into three doses. The cancer prevention effects were seen from eating the equivalent of one clove of garlic a day. There is great variability in garlic product strengths.

Treatment Categories

Complementary Therapy
Hypercholesterolemia, high blood pressure, atherosclerosis   ☺
Prevention of stomach and colorectal cancer
Prevention of age-related vascular changes

Scientifically Unproven
Other indications, including topical applications

Further Reading

Barrett, B., D. Kiefer, and D. Rabago, "Assessing the Risks and Benefits of Herbal Medicine: An Overview of Scientific Evidence," *Alternative Therapies in Health and Medicine* 5, no. 4 (July 1999): 40–49.

Fleischauer, Aaron T., Charles Poole, and Lenore Arab, "Garlic Consumption and Cancer Prevention: Meta-Analyses of Colorectal and Stomach Cancers" *American Journal of Clinical Nutrition* 72, no. 4 (October 2000): 1047–52.

Jellin, Jeff M., Forrest Batz, and Kathy Hichens, *Pharmacist's Letter/Prescriber's Letter: Natural Medicines Comprehensive Database* (Stockton, Calif.: Therapeutic Research Facility, 1999), 407–9.

Koscielny, J., D. Klüssendorf, R. Latza, R. Schmitt, H. Radtke, G. Siegel, and H. Kiesewetter, "The Antiatherosclerotic Effect of *Allium sativum*," *Atherosclerosis* 144, no. 1 (May 1999): 237–49.

Schulz, Volker, Rudolf Hänsel, and Varro Tyler, *Rational Phytotherapy: A Physician's Guide to Herbal Medicine*, 3d ed. (Berlin, Germany: Springer-Verlag, 1998), 112.

Stevinson, Clare, Max H. Pittler, and Edzard Ernst, "Garlic for Treating Hypercholesterolemia. A Meta-Analysis of Randomized Clinical Trials," *Annals of Internal Medicine* 133, no. 6 (September 2000): 420–29.

Warshafsky, Stephen, Russell S. Kamer, and Steven L. Sivak, "Effect of Garlic on Total Serum Cholesterol: A Meta-Analysis," *Annals of Internal Medicine* 119, no. 7 (October 1993): 599–605.

GINGER

What It Is

Ginger *(Zingiber officinale)* is a perennial plant with thick, underground lateral stems called "rhizomes" that are used for medical and culinary purposes. The aboveground stem can grow to heights of twenty-four feet. Ginger is native to southern Asia, but is now cultivated extensively throughout the tropics. The very best quality ginger is said to be grown in Jamaica, but more than 80 percent of the ginger imported to the United States is reported to come from China and India.

Claims

The perceived medicinal qualities of ginger have been broadly documented in cultures as diverse as Indian, Chinese, Arabic, Greek, and Roman. It is cited in ancient Ayurvedic, Sanskrit, and Chinese texts as early as the fourth century B.C. for conditions such as stomachache, diarrhea, cholera, toothaches, and nausea. The first-century Roman herbalist Dioscorides included ginger in his herbal text, which became the basis for much of the practice of medicine throughout the Middle Ages.

In addition to its medicinal applications, ginger is also widely used as a spice in foods, beverages, candies, and liqueurs, and is commonly used in many cosmetic products. The Chinese use fresh ginger in many dishes, not only for its spicy flavor and perfume but also as a *yang* ingredient, to balance cooling (or *yin*) dishes. (See Traditional Chinese Medicine, page 279, for an explanation of *yin* and *yang*.) Five-spice powder and many curries contain dried ginger.

Ginger has many reported beneficial pharmacological effects, including antioxidant properties; prevention of abnormal blood clotting; and reduction of prostaglandin levels which cause inflammation. It is also used for loss of appetite and indigestion. Herbalists will also recommend ginger for colic, dyspepsia, gas, rheumatoid arthritis, baldness, snakebites, and rheumatism.

Study Findings

One study (✔✔✔) found ginger provided relief from pain and swelling in osteoarthritis and rheumatoid arthritis. However, most studies (✔✔✔✔) have examined ginger's ability to prevent and treat nausea in a variety of clinical settings, including postanesthetic nausea. Studies (✔✔✔) also were done on vomiting in pregnancy, motion sickness, and seasickness, as well as on (✘✘) chemotherapy-induced nausea.

The way ginger works for the prevention and treatment of nausea is not clear. Studies have shown increased gastric motility, but not increased gastric emptying. Ginger enhances salivary and gastric secretion, and has documented antispasm effects. Unlike most medications that treat nausea, ginger does not affect the central nervous system.

At least four studies of ginger to reduce postoperative nausea and vomiting have been conducted, with conflicting results. All four were with women who had undergone gynecological procedures. The earliest study (✔✔✔) involved sixty women randomized to receive 1 gram of ginger, 10 mg metoclopramide (Reglan®), or placebo. Women receiving both ginger and metoclopramide had significantly fewer episodes of nausea and used less intravenous medications for vomiting after surgery. There was no significant difference between the metoclopramide group and the ginger group, and all three groups had identical side-effect profiles. In 1993, an almost identical study (✔✔✔) was performed, with similar outcomes.

In 1995, yet another study was performed with 108 women randomized to receive placebo, 500 mg ginger, or 1000 mg ginger. This study (✘✘✘) found an increase in incidence of moderate or severe nausea and vomiting in both groups taking ginger compared with placebo. The risk of nausea or vomiting was higher with the higher ginger dose. This was the first negative study published.

The most recent study (✘✘✘) we examined was published in 1998 and randomized 120 patients to placebo, droperidol, 1000 mg of ginger by mouth, or ginger plus droperidol. There were no significant differences in nausea or vomiting between the four treatment groups; in essence, droperidol and ginger showed no improvement over placebo. The side-effect profiles for all four groups also were identical.

Investigators in the only randomized, double-blind, crossover trial (✔✔✔) of ginger for hyperemesis gravidarum (a more serious form of morning sickness in which pregnant women have continuous and uncontrollable vomiting) gave patients 250 mg of ginger or placebo four times a day for four days. Measures of relief were significantly greater with ginger.

Only one study (✘✘) evaluating ginger for nausea associated with chemotherapy has been reported. This study involved a nonrandomized, nonblinded protocol called a "case series." Eleven patients with a history of chemotherapy-induced nausea were undergoing chemotherapy for lymphoma. They were given 1590 mg of ginger thirty minutes prior to chemotherapy, and their symptoms were carefully monitored and recorded. Those given ginger had slightly less nausea, but this difference was not significantly different from the control.

Multiple studies have been performed using ginger to prevent motion sickness. Two randomized, controlled trials (✘✘✘✘) of experimentally induced motion sickness found no effect of ginger on prevention or treatment of motion sickness. A third study (✔✔✔) compared 1 gram of ginger to 100 mg Benadryl® or placebo. Each group was given the test sample one-half hour prior to having motion sickness induced in a revolving chair. The ginger group tolerated being spun around on the revolving chair significantly better than the Benadryl or placebo groups.

The one trial (✔✔✔) of ginger for treatment of seasickness was a double-blind, randomized, placebo-controlled study of eighty naval cadets on rough-sea voyages. Cadets who complained of seasickness were given 1 gram of ginger or placebo every hour for four hours. Ginger significantly reduced seasickness measured by vomiting and cold sweats. Ginger also tended to reduce nausea and vertigo, but these reductions were not significantly different between the two groups.

We should point out that the inconsistency of the results discussed above is also found in studies of conventional medications for nausea and vomiting. This is due, in part, to the difficulty in measuring symptoms such as nausea. In addition, the effect of antinausea medications and herbs is often subtle and difficult to discern unless tested in a homogenous population with a high prevalence of nausea.

Ginger is less effective when given to a patient who is already nauseated. All food forms of ginger can be used, but dried capsules are preferable. Candied ginger is usually not dried well enough to be therapeutic, and the pickled and candied forms have not been tested formally. The liquid sources of ginger (ginger ale or ginger tea) generally have such low concentrations of ginger that large quantities of liquid are required to consume adequate amounts of ginger.

When buying ginger tablets or capsules, look for the amount of ginger in each capsule, and look for a lot number and expiration date. Although some products are standardized, the smell and taste of ginger are better guides to freshness and, therefore, efficacy. A botanical monograph on ginger has recently been approved by the United States Pharmacopoeia for inclusion in the national formulary.

Cautions

The use of ginger in pregnancy for hyperemesis gravidarum is controversial among botanical experts. Ginger's effect on a woman's hormones and blood clotting warrant caution in recommending ginger for pregnant women. The risk of bleeding is slight, but real. However, concerns about ginger increasing bleeding have not been supported by one study done with patients undergoing a laparoscopic gynecological procedure who showed no difference in intra-operative or postoperative bleeding complications.

In the only study of hyperemesis gravidarum, fetal loss rate was not reported, and it is not clear whether investigators even kept track of this. Two authoritative sources categorize ginger as "not to be used during pregnancy." An editor's note in the German Commission E monographs opines that there are no data to support this admonition, but the caution is based upon two Japanese studies in the 1980s showing cancer-causing effects on cells in the lab with certain ginger compounds. This study must be balanced by an earlier study that did not show this effect.

Since there are no conclusive data about ginger in pregnancy, caution must prevail. The Natural Database rates ginger "Likely Safe" in pregnancy and lactation, in the amounts usually contained in foods. However, it is rated "Likely Unsafe" in pregnancy and lactation in medicinal amounts. One case of spontaneous abortion at twelve weeks has been reported with ginger use for morning sickness, and a related plant *(Zingiber cassumunar)* causes uterine contractions in animals.

Ginger also is not recommended for patients with gallstones as ginger increases the flow of bile and may lead to gallbladder obstruction or colic. Finally, large doses of ginger have been known to cause heartburn and may cause central nervous system depression and cardiac arrhythmias. These latter effects have led the Natural Database to rate ginger "Possibly Unsafe" when used in large amounts, but "Possibly Safe" when the dried or fresh root are used orally and appropriately for medicinal use.

Recommendations

Ginger is an ancient spice that has reputed antinausea properties in postanesthesia, pregnancy, hyperemesis gravidarum, chemotherapy, motion sickness, and seasickness. The data are not conclusive in any of these settings, but it seems reasonable to use a trial of ginger for the prevention of postoperative or chemotherapy-associated nausea, motion sickness, and seasickness for two reasons:

1. There is data to support its efficacy and safety.
2. It is relatively inexpensive and readily available.

Despite common food and folk use, experts debate whether ginger should be recommended for nausea during pregnancy. However, this caution becomes a generally agreed upon warning if the pregnant patient has a history of bleeding disorders, gallbladder disease, or miscarriage.

The data on ginger for prevention and treatment of chemotherapy-induced nausea and motion sickness are too poor to draw definitive conclusions. The data on prevention of postoperative nausea is mixed.

Anyone considering taking ginger prior to chemotherapy or surgery should discuss this with his or her physician well in advance. In some cases, patients should not take any form of medication before surgery or other medical procedures.

Dosage

Different doses are recommended for the different uses of ginger. The usual dosage for preventing motion sickness is 1 to 2 grams (tablets or capsules) of dried powdered ginger root taken orally thirty minutes before the journey.

Treatment Categories

Complementary Therapy

Prevention of nausea from seasickness	☺☺
Prevention of nausea from chemotherapy	☺
Prevention of nausea from anesthesia	☺
Prevention of nausea from motion sickness	☺
Prevention or treatment of morning sickness in pregnancy (including hyperemesis)	☹
Pain and increasing motility in rheumatoid arthritis	☺

Scientifically Unproven

Any other medical indication

Further Reading

Ernst, E., and M. H. Pittler, "Efficacy of Ginger for Nausea and Vomiting: A Systematic Review of Randomized Clinical Trials," *British Journal of Anaesthesiology* 84, no. 3 (March 2000): 367–71.

Fetrow, Charles W., and Juan R. Avila, *Professional's Handbook of Complementary and Alternative Medicine* (Springhouse, Penn.: Springhouse, 1999), 274–77.

Jellin, Jeff M., Forrest Batz, and Kathy Hichens, *Pharmacist's Letter/Prescriber's Letter: Natural Medicines Comprehensive Database* (Stockton, Calif.: Therapeutic Research Facility, 1999), 416–18.

GINKGO BILOBA

What It Is

Look into the shopping basket of older health food store shoppers and chances are you will see one or more of three herbal remedies—saw palmetto for prostate and sexual function, St. John's wort for minor depression, and ginkgo biloba for memory. Usually these are not taken because of the suggestion of a physician, though increasingly St. John's wort is being suggested for some patients. Instead, the popular press has helped make these "the big three" for helping an increasingly aging population cope with their fears and anxieties.

The comedians and writers who created the popular cultural image of old people as doddering and forgetful are now in their sixties and seventies themselves. They are active, vibrant, and yet still fear that the myth may be reality. Products such as *Ginkgo Biloba* are symbols of their awareness that mental decline is an unnatural state of aging, not the norm of a person's last two or three decades of life. This may help to explain why, according to *Prevention Magazine*, in 1999 nearly 13 million Americans took ginkgo regularly (the third most common herb after garlic and ginseng).

Ginkgo biloba is a tree native to southeast Asia, where such trees can be hundreds of years old. The leaves, the part used to make the herbal remedy, have a distinctive fan shape. An extract is made from the leaves using alcohol, is dried, and made into capsules. This extract is one of the most popular herbal remedies in Europe, recently approved in Germany for the treatment of dementia. In the United States it has become the main ingredient in a number of "memory boosters."

Claims

The claims for ginkgo center on improvements in mental capacity. It is recommended for general memory-loss related to aging, advancing Alzheimer's disease, and cognitive problems occurring after a stroke or with depression. It has also been used for several types of dementia, including vascular dementia. Ginkgo contains a variety of compounds that prevent oxidation reactions (antioxidants), which are known to play a role in diseases of brain tissue. Herbalists have been known to recommend ginkgo for headache, tinnitus, dizziness, difficulty concentrating, mood disorders, peripheral vascular disease (especially claudication), hearing loss related to vascular disease, PMS, heart disease, high cholesterol, and dysentery. Ginkgo has also been used to reverse sexual dysfunction caused by antidepressants (especially the SSRIs like Prozac®).

Study Findings

A number of animal studies have found that ginkgo does help with learning and memory. Very few studies have been done with humans, and the results have been unclear. The first controlled clinical trial (✔✔✔) in the United States (by Le Bars) found the extract helpful for patients with mild to moderate symptoms related to Alzheimer's disease or multi-infarct (vascular) dementia. After six months to a year of ginkgo, patients' symptoms had remained stable or slightly improved, while those taking the placebo had worsened. However, on one of the three measurements, ginkgo was no better than placebo. A 1998 review of nine randomized, controlled trials (✔✔✔✔) found that ginkgo was more effective than placebo in delaying the onset of dementia.

At the end of 2000, another study (✘✘✘) was published which found that older people with mild to moderate dementia (due to Alzheimer's or other causes) did not benefit from taking ginkgo. This study contradicts the findings of earlier studies, and demonstrates why more studies of ginkgo are needed before firm recommendations can be made.

Ginkgo is believed to work by increasing the flow of blood through arteries and veins in various tissues, including the brain and in arms and legs. In keeping with this, small clinical trials (✔✔) have shown that ginkgo can improve overall functioning in patients with peripheral arterial disease, improve certain aspects of memory in people in their fifties, and even improve some asthmatic symptoms. More than fifteen European trials (✔✔✔✔) have shown improvement in claudication (pain in calf muscles that people with narrowed or blocked arteries get when walking). It has also been shown (✔✔✔) to reduce mountain sickness in climbers.

Ginkgo's antidementia effects are similar to currently available prescription drugs. However, while this effect is statistically significant in clinical studies, it remains uncertain as to whether this is enough to make a noticeable difference in people's lives. So far, while ginkgo has been shown to delay the onset of dementia, it has not been shown to prevent or treat dementia.

Cautions

Ginkgo seeds can cause fatal neurological and allergic reactions and should never be taken. The extract, which comes from the *Ginkgo* leaf, has led to relatively few side effects. In the Le Bars research, though, twice as many patients taking ginkgo reported intestinal problems compared to those taking the placebo. There have been bleeding problems (✘✘) in patients also taking "blood-thinning" drugs (like aspirin or warfarin). Ginkgo is also believed to inhibit an enzyme called "monoamine oxidase" (MAO), meaning it may cause problems with a number of other antidepressant drugs that act the same way. Since people taking both these medications may also be concerned about memory loss, they should consult their physician before taking ginkgo or any other herbal remedy.

Most clinical studies have been conducted with an extract made according to specific German specifications. Because there are no precise standards for the preparation of herbal products sold in the United States, what you buy may not have been made in the same way. Preparation affects what a product contains and how well it works. For example, an independent testing lab, ConsumerLab.com, purchased thirty leading brands of *Ginkgo biloba* during August 1999 and tested them to determine whether they possessed proper amounts of the appropriate plant chemicals. Nearly one-quarter of the thirty brands tested did not have the stated levels of chemical marker compounds.

Those brands that did not pass the testing all bore labels claiming standardization for total flavone glycosides, and most also indicated being standardized for total terpene lactones (specific chemicals thought to be the ones responsible for ginkgo's activity). All the products had less than adequate levels of at least one of the terpene lactones, and three products also lacked adequate levels of at least one flavone glycoside. Some of the labels were correct for total amounts of compounds, but the products did not meet the standards for one or more specific compounds. Products that passed the testing can be viewed by subscribing to the company's Website (*www.consumerlab.com*).

There is no reliable data upon which to determine if ginkgo is safe to use with children or in pregnancy or lactation.

Recommendations

Very few studies have been conducted on ginkgo, with most studies using Kaveri® or Tebonin®. The first product is now available in the U.S., with the second being the main component in GinkoGold®, Ginkgoba®, and Quanterra® ginkgo. While ginkgo looks promising as a means of delaying the memory loss related to a variety of diseases, the most recent study found it had no benefit. The studies which found memory benefits only demonstrated those for about six months, and it has not been shown that these benefits continue for longer.

Ginkgo may prove helpful for retarding age-related memory loss, dementia, asthma, and peripheral arterial disease, and as a mountain sickness preventative. However, the long-term effects of taking an extract with such a large number of active compounds have not been examined.

Dosage

The usual dose is 120 to 240 mg daily, divided into two or three doses.

Treatment Categories

Complementary Therapy

Stabilize or slightly improve cognitive function, at least for the short term, in Alzheimer's disease	☺☺☺
Slightly improve cognitive function in multi-infarct (vascular) dementia	☺☺☺
Improving memory, concentration, and/or learning or retarding age-related memory loss	☺☺☺
Cognitive symptoms of other types of dementia	☺☺

Bronchial spasm in asthma	☺
Increasing walking distance of people with peripheral arterial disease or claudication	☺☺☺
Claudication or peripheral vascular disease	☺☺
Symptoms of dizziness	☺☺
Tinnitus	☺☺
Headache	☺☺
Prevent mountain (altitude) sickness	☺☺
Reverse sexual dysfunction associated with SSRI antidepressants	☺☺

Further Reading

Ernst, E., and M. H. Pittler, "Ginkgo biloba for Dementia: A Systematic Review of Double-Blind, Placebo-Controlled Trials," *Clinical Drug Investigation* 17, no. 4 (1999): 301–8.

Jellin, Jeff M., Forrest Batz, and Kathy Hichens, *Pharmacist's Letter/Prescriber's Letter: Natural Medicines Comprehensive Database* (Stockton, Calif.: Therapeutic Research Facility, 1999), 418–22.

Le Bars, Pierre L., Martin M. Katz, Nancy Berman, Turan M. Itil, Alfred M. Freedman, and Alan F. Schatzberg, "A Placebo-Controlled, Double-Blind, Randomized Trial of an Extract of Ginkgo Biloba for Dementia," *Journal of the American Medical Association* 278, no. 16 (October 1997): 1327–32.

Martien, C. J., M. van Dongen, Erik van Rossum, G. Alphons, H. Kessels, J. Hilde, G. Sielhorst, and Paul G. Knipschild, "The Efficacy of Ginkgo for Elderly People with Dementia and Age-Associated Memory Impairment: New Results of a Randomized Clinical Trial," *Journal of the American Geriatric Society* 48, no. 10 (October 2000): 1183–94.

GINSENG

What It Is

If it can be said that there is a "Fountain of Youth" in an herbal therapy, proponents of ginseng would be first in line to claim the discovery. In China, during the time of Jesus, medical texts identified ginseng as leading to longevity, wisdom, and enlightenment. While few American merchandisers would even consider claiming that you can gain wisdom from a bottle, the connection between ginseng and longevity continues to be made both in the United States and in many parts of the world where the herb is used. In fact, the Chinese still refer to ginseng as the root of immortality. In 1976, a 400-year-old root of Manchurian ginseng was reported to sell for an incredible $10,000 per ounce.

Ginseng preparations are made from five different plants, the most popular being Asian ginseng *(Panax ginseng)* and American ginseng *(Panax quinquefolius)*. Siberian ginseng is made from the botanically unrelated *Eleutherococcus senticosus*, and contains a completely different set of chemicals.

Red ginseng is steam-cured prior to drying, which leaves a reddish color in the product. White ginseng is produced when the roots are bleached and dried quickly.

Claims

According to *Prevention Magazine*, more than 14 million Americans were using ginseng on a regular basis in 1999. Ginseng is the second most popular herb in America (after garlic) and is most widely used as an "adaptogen," an herbal remedy that allegedly restores a wide variety of bodily functions to normal. It has been used to treat nervous disorders, anemia, wakefulness, dyspnea (difficulty breathing), forgetfulness and confusion, prolonged thirst, decreased libido, chronic fatigue, angina, diabetes, and nausea.

In traditional Chinese medicine it is believed to restore deficiencies in a person's *chi*, or life energy. Asian ginseng is said to have more *yin* and to be better suited for women, while American ginseng is said to be better for men because it has more *yang* (see Traditional Chinese Medicine, page 279).

Study Findings

A vast number of studies have been conducted on ginseng, but the results are not consistent. Many studies (✗✗✗✗) found no benefits from ginseng. Others reported some helpful results. One three-month randomized controlled trial (RCT) (✔✔✔) showed a significant increase in subjective "quality of life" scores among 625 ginseng users. Another RCT in college-aged volunteers (✔✔✔) who took 100 mg of ginseng twice a day for twelve weeks experienced a statistically significant improvement in the speed at which they were able to perform math.

Clinical trials (✔✔✔) have suggested that Asian ginseng may be effective in treating type 2 diabetes. One small Canadian trial (✔✔✔) evaluated the effect of American ginseng on blood sugar levels after a feeding of glucose. The researchers found that when nondiabetic subjects took ginseng forty minutes before the glucose challenge, significant reductions were observed in their blood sugar levels. In subjects with type 2 diabetes mellitus, the same was true whether capsules were taken before or together with the glucose challenge. The researchers concluded that for nondiabetic subjects, to prevent unintended hypoglycemia it may be important that the American ginseng be taken with the meal.

European references, including German Commission E reports, cite human studies (✔✔✔) indicating that ginseng improves mental alertness, memory, physical endurance, sleep pattern, and appetite. These reports also say ginseng may be helpful in hyperlipidemia, type 2 diabetes, improving resistance to stress, improving immune response, protecting against some toxins, and in individuals with congestive heart failure. These same sources cite studies (✘✘✘✘) showing that ginseng is ineffective in improving athletic performance in healthy young adults.

Nevertheless, most human studies show no benefit of ginseng. In fact, reviews dealing with the efficacy of ginseng have concluded that while studies with animals show that ginseng, or its active components, may prolong survival under physical or chemical stress, there is a lack of controlled research demonstrating ginseng's ability to improve or prolong performance in either fatigued or nonfatigued humans. The inconsistent results of this research can be explained, at least partially, on the poor methodological design of some of these studies, the lack of adequate controls, and the failure to standardize the ginseng administered. In addition, there is considerable confusion in the literature about the different species of ginseng, with particular indifference to the fact that Siberian ginseng is a completely different genus of plant. Among the few human trials that are of good quality, the results can be considered only suggestive, not conclusive.

Furthermore, plant sources of ginseng contain a large number of closely related compounds called "ginsenosides." These have been shown to have antioxidant properties, which may underlie any beneficial effects. However, in controlled studies, ginseng did not improve exercise or mental performance, although subjects did report feeling less fatigued. In general, none of the other specific health benefits have been verified by research.

Cautions

A number of side effects have been found (✘✘) when people take large doses of ginseng for extended periods of time (in the past this was called the "ginseng abuse syndrome," although experts now discount the existence of such a syndrome). The supposed symptoms include diarrhea, weakness, tremors, palpitations, nervousness, decreased libido, and high blood pressure. Side effects with ginseng are not rare and include insomnia, breast pain, vaginal bleeding, fast heart rate, decreased appetite, diarrhea, headache, vertigo, and skin reactions. Some Russian medical studies (✘✘) have led a number of their practitioners to recommend that their patients not use large doses of ginseng for more than two weeks at a time without a break. However, no specific formula for use and abstinence has been developed.

Ginsenosides are steroid-like, which can cause menstrual problems as well as increase the serum levels of hormones like testosterone. People with diabetes should be very cautious when taking ginseng as it has led to hypoglycemia (very low blood sugar levels). Ginseng also may hinder blood clotting, which is especially problematic in patients taking blood thinners (like aspirin or warfarin).

In addition, ginseng products are notorious for being mislabeled and adulterated, which can cause a whole host of other problems. One study found that one in four ginseng products contained no ginseng. In another study of fifty-four ginseng products, 85 percent were evaluated as being "worthless," containing little or no ginseng. Also, *Eleutherococcus senticosus*, usually labeled as "Siberian ginseng," actually contains no true ginseng. Drinks and chewing gum made from ginseng are now available, but the quantity and quality of the herb they contain is unknown.

In April and May 2000, ConsumerLab.com purchased a total of twenty-two brands of Asian and American ginseng products sold in the United States to determine whether they possessed the claimed amounts and types of ginseng. Only nine products tested met all of the criteria for ginseng quality and purity. Even more problematic, eight products contained unacceptable levels of two pesticides called "quintozene" and "hexachlorobenzene." Two products had pesticide levels more than twenty times the allowed amount. Hexachlorobenzene is believed to cause cancer in humans and has been banned from most food crop use throughout the world. Quintozene is potentially cancer-causing, may also be toxic to various organs, and is generally not allowed in food production in the United States. Two ginseng products also contained lead above the acceptable level.

American consumers are being placed at risk when only nine out of twenty-two products pass the three ConsumerLab.com criteria (i.e., levels of ginsenosides, pesticides, and heavy metals). Five of the products failed two criteria and eight failed a single criterion. All eight of the products that contained lead or pesticides were labeled as containing "Korean" ginseng. In fact, only two of the twelve products containing Korean ginseng passed. The names of the brands that passed the tests can be viewed at the subscription-based ConsumerLab.com Website (*www.consumerlab.com*).

There is insufficient reliable data to conclude that ginseng is safe in childhood, pregnancy, or lactation—and therefore ginseng should be avoided by these individuals.

Recommendations

When taken in moderate amounts, quality ginseng products appear to be relatively harmless to most people, except for those with the conditions mentioned above. It may have some benefits in helping type 2 diabetics and may help some people feel better and more energetic, although none of the "well-being" benefits have been conclusively verified in research. Therefore, people who take ginseng risk paying a high price without proven benefit, as preparations cost up to $20 per ounce and vary tremendously in quality. If you are going to purchase ginseng, make sure you use a reputable brand that can demonstrate that it contains the correct amount of the appropriate plant and is free of cancer-causing compounds.

Dosage

For most indications, 0.25 to 0.5 grams of the root are taken twice a day. Large quantities, up to about 3 grams two or three times daily, have been recommended, including for diabetes.

Treatment Categories

Complementary Therapy

Feel better or improve energy	☺
Type 2 diabetes	☺☺
Mental alertness	☺
Memory	☺
Physical endurance	☺
Sleep pattern	☺
Appetite	☺
High cholesterol levels	☹
Improving resistance to stress	☺
Improving immune response	☺
Protecting against some toxins	☺
Congestive heart failure	☺

Scientifically Unproven

Improving athletic performance in healthy young adults	☹☹
Any other medical indication	

Further Reading

Bahrke, M. S., and W. R. Morgan, "Evaluation of the Ergogenic Properties of Ginseng: An Update," *Sports Medicine* 29, no. 2 (February 2000): 113–33.

Jellin, Jeff M., Forrest Batz, and Kathy Hichens, *Pharmacist's Letter/Prescriber's Letter: Natural Medicines Comprehensive Database* (Stockton, Calif.: Therapeutic Research Facility, 1999), 422–28.

Schiedermayer, David, "Ginseng for the Improvement of Constitutional Symptoms," *Alternative Medicine Alert* 1, no. 4 (April 1998): 37–40.

GLUCOSAMINE

What It Is

Glucosamine is an important component of proteoglycans and other compounds used to make connective tissue. Proteoglycans are important lubricants within joints and integral to the makeup of healthy cartilage. Glucosamine is available on its own or in a number of salt forms, including glucosamine sulfate and glucosamine hydrochloride. All are converted into glucosamine in the stomach and are therefore believed to be equivalent.

Claims

Glucosamine sulfate came to widespread public attention as part of the "medical miracle" promoted in the book *The Arthritis Cure* (New York: St. Martin's Press, 1997). The subtitle of the book claimed that a combination of glucosamine and chondroitin sulfate "can halt, reverse, and may even cure osteoarthritis." Since then, glucosamine has become available in many formulations as a way to treat and cure arthritis. According to a *Consumer Reports* survey done in 2000, nearly 36 percent of the people surveyed who had arthritis were using glucosamine regularly, with 42 percent using over-the-counter medications and 64 percent using prescription medications.

Study Findings

At least twelve randomized controlled trials have been conducted using glucosamine sulfate for osteoarthritis. We are aware of only two clinical studies with glucosamine hydrochloride—one using glucosamine hydrochloride compared to placebo and the other using a combined product (glucosamine, chondroitin, and manganese) called Cosamine DS® compared to placebo.

While some of these (✔✔✔) have involved relatively small numbers of subjects and had some methodological problems, they have produced consistent results. Higher quality studies have found positive results, though not to the degree of the smaller studies. Either way, the studies have shown that there are benefits from this treatment. Glucosamine was always more effective in relieving pain and promoting joint mobility than placebo, and was of comparable effectiveness to ibuprofen. A 2001 study (✔✔✔) showed with X-rays the preservation of cartilage in the knees of patients with osteoarthritis.

Most of these studies were conducted with a patented glucosamine sulfate product produced in Italy and not yet available in the U.S. In some of the studies, injectable preparations were used, and these also are not available in the U.S.

In America, glucosamine is sold in many forms, including glucosamine sulfate, glucosamine hydrochloride, and N-acetylglucosamine. According to ConsumerLab.com, "there appears to be no conclusive evidence that one form is better than another." However, two relatively large studies (✘✘✘) published in 1999 and 2000 found that glucosamine hydrochloride was no better than placebo in relieving osteoarthritis pain. In the trial using the combination product Cosamine DS (✔✔✔), the combination was more effective than placebo in reducing the pain of arthritis. However, the effect could theoretically have been from the chondroitin portion of the combination. Glucosamine hydrochloride is less expensive than glucosamine sulfate, which was used in all the trials finding it to be effective. The 1999 trial was also important because it was the first one conducted in the United States and lasted longer (eight weeks) than most others. Since osteoarthritis lasts for many years, people will take medications for it for prolonged periods, and long-term assessment of remedies is essential.

A potential problem with glucosamine products obtained in the United States is poor product quality. If this is true, then Americans may not be able to obtain the same results seen in studies in other countries. In December 1999 and January 2000, ConsumerLab.com purchased a total of twenty-five brands of glucosamine and combined glucosamine/chondroitin products. These products were then tested to determine whether they possessed the labeled amounts of the glucosamine and/or chondroitin ingredients. Overall, nearly one-third of the products did not pass testing. Among glucosamine/chondroitin combination products, however, almost half (six out of thirteen) did not pass—all due to low chondroitin levels. In contrast, all ten of the glucosamine-only products passed testing. The brand names of the products which passed the test are available at *www.consumerlab.com,* which is subscription based. One possible explanation for the low pass rate for chondroitin-containing products is economic—chondroitin costs manufacturers approximately four times as much as glucosamine.

The failure of many American manufacturers to meet certain quality standards may explain one large United States survey that revealed a high degree of consumer dissatisfaction with glucosamine for arthritis. In May 2000, *Consumer Reports* surveyed nearly 47,000 Americans. Of those taking glucosamine for back pain, only 18 percent said it helped "much" and 51 percent said it helped "little or none." Of those taking glucosamine regularly for arthritis, only 24 percent reported it helped "much" (about what one would expect with a placebo) and a surprising 48 percent said it helped "little or none."

Cautions

Adverse reactions to glucosamine have been mild and infrequent, with gastrointestinal problems being most frequently reported. However, glucosamine is involved in a number of metabolic processes, warranting close monitoring of patients taking it for long periods. For example, animal studies and at least one human study (✗✗) have found that glucosamine can play a role in worsening insulin resistance, which underlies some cases of diabetes. People with osteoarthritis tend to gain weight, which also makes them susceptible to type 2 diabetes mellitus.

Therefore, people with diabetes, or at risk for developing it, should be cautious when using glucosamine and at the very least inform their physician they are taking glucosamine. Blood sugar problems have not been reported in the other clinical trials of glucosamine, although this problem would only be expected after prolonged use.

Furthermore, there is a theoretical concern that glucosamine derived from marine exoskeletons may cause allergic reactions in people allergic to shellfish. However, no such reactions have been reported. Unfortunately, most producers of glucosamine do not list the source of the product on the label.

An unexpected concern was raised when, in January 2001, the Institute of Medicine issued a new Tolerable Upper Intake Level (UL) for manganese, which is contained in the Cosamine DS product mentioned above. The manufacturer quickly adjusted its formulation to bring it into compliance with the new UL. But adults taking Cosamine DS manufactured before that adjustment was made would exceed the new manganese UL of 11 mg per day. This points to the importance of examining the list of all ingredients in a remedy, and checking the date of manufacture. Older batches of Cosamine DS have too much manganese. Vegetarians should be particularly cautious as their diet likely includes more manganese, present mostly in nuts, legumes, tea, and whole grains.

There is insufficient reliable information about the use of glucosamine in childhood, pregnancy, and lactation, and it therefore should not be used by these individuals.

Recommendations

Overall, there is some evidence to suggest that glucosamine sulfate may provide relief from the symptoms of osteoarthritis. McAlindon's 2000 review concluded that although the positive effects of glucosamine are "exaggerated," "some degree of efficacy appears possible." There is no evidence to suggest that it cures arthritis, as has been suggested in popular literature.

Use of glucosamine in combination with chondroitin sulfate is recommended, but has not been well studied to date. Glucosamine alone appears to produce a smaller benefit than chondroitin alone. However, chondroitin products in America are often substandard. Only reputable brands, certified by independent labs, should be used. There is no information on the safety and effectiveness of taking glucosamine for prolonged periods of time.

Dosage

The most frequently recommended dosage of glucosamine alone is 500 mg three times daily. The dose depends on the person's weight, and is usually in combination with chondroitin. An average daily dose would be 1200 mg chondroitin and 1500 mg glucosamine. This is usually divided into two to four doses, taken with food.

Treatment Categories

Complementary Therapy

Osteoarthritis, when glucosamine hydrochloride
  is used in combination with chondroitin and manganese ☺☺☺

Osteoarthritis, when combined with chondroitin ☺☺☺

Osteoarthritis, when used alone ☺☺☺

Rheumatoid arthritis, when glucosamine
  sulfate is used in combination with chondroitin ☺

Scientifically Unproven

Use of glucosamine hydrochloride or N-acetylglucosamine alone for osteoarthritis

Topical use for arthritis, orally for any other medical indication

Further Reading

Delafuente, Jeffrey C., "Glucosamine in the Treatment of Osteoarthritis," *Rheumatic Disease Clinics of North America* 26, no. 1 (February 2000): 1–11.

Jellin, Jeff M., Forrest Batz, and Kathy Hichens, *Pharmacist's Letter/Prescriber's Letter: Natural Medicines Comprehensive Database* (Stockton, Calif.: Therapeutic Research Facility, 1999), 430–32.

McAlindon, Timothy E., Michael P. LaValley, Juan P. Gulin, and David T. Felson, "Glucosamine and Chondroitin for Treatment of Osteoarthritis: A Systematic Quality Assessment and Meta-analysis," *Journal of the American Medical Association* 283, no. 11 (March 2000): 1469–75.

GOLDENSEAL

What It Is

Goldenseal is one of the most popular herbal remedies in the United States, being native to the woodland areas of the eastern and midwestern states. It was standard antiseptic medicine for both Native Americans and the pioneer families who settled the west, learning the indigenous ways as they traveled. The Cherokees also used goldenseal for stomach ailments, an idea that the settlers adopted much later in a patent medicine for intestinal upsets.

Goldenseal *(Hydrastis canadensis),* part of the buttercup family, is a small herb with a bright yellow underground stem, from which it gets its name. Other names for it include golden root, eye root, and ground raspberry (because it has a small red fruit).

Claims

Native-American tribes commonly used goldenseal as a diuretic and stimulant, eyewash, mouthwash, for stomach ulcers, and as a dye. It was included among official lists of medicinal herbs until 1955.

Today, goldenseal is regarded as a natural antibiotic, antiseptic, and antidiarrheal. Its most popular use is for colds, especially combined with echinacea. Some Internet promoters market it as a panacea, for example: "Goldenseal is a cure-all type of herb that strengthens the immune system, acts as an antibiotic, has anti-inflammatory and antibacterial properties, potentiates insulin, and cleanses vital organs. It promotes the functioning capacity of the heart, the lymphatic and respiratory system, the liver, the spleen, the pancreas, and the colon." Herbalists use goldenseal as an eyewash for conjunctivitis, and as a diuretic and laxative. It is also recommended for tinnitus, nasal congestion, sore gums, hemorrhoids, gastritis, anorexia, peptic ulcer, colitis, painful menses, urinary tract infections, flatulence, fever, pneumonia, and cancer. Topically it has been used for eczema, itching, acne, dandruff, ringworm, fever blisters, and wounds. Goldenseal has also received a boost in popularity from the faulty but prevalent belief that it can mask illicit drugs in urine drug screens.

Study Findings

No clinical studies have been conducted on goldenseal. However, it contains a drug called "berberine," which has been shown to have broad antimicrobial activity. Berberine is found in many herbs with antimicrobial reputations, including barberry, Oregon grape root, goldenthread, and a number of Chinese herbs. In one randomized controlled trial, a single dose of berberine (400 mg) significantly reduced stool volume and duration of diarrhea among patients with bacterial dysentery. In another trial, berberine was more effective than placebo and as effective as a standard prescription antibiotic in treating children with the parasite *Giardia*.

However, the studies of berberine used quantities far greater than the amount found in goldenseal and its products. It has been estimated it would take twenty-five or more commercially available goldenseal capsules to obtain the same amount of berberine used in these studies. There is also the problem that the studies did not examine berberine's effects within the body, and there is evidence it is very poorly absorbed from the digestive tract. More importantly, there are no reports of berberine being active against viruses, which cause the colds and flu goldenseal is said to prevent and cure.

Cautions

The popularity of goldenseal has led to its overcollection. It is difficult to cultivate and is becoming increasingly rare in its natural habitats. This has driven prices up to $100 per pound and has led some producers to use other, less expensive berberine-containing herbs in their goldenseal products. Some of these herbs are more toxic than goldenseal.

Large amounts of goldenseal cause nausea, vomiting, numbness, high blood pressure, and breathing problems. A few fatalities have been reported, and goldenseal has also been used to cause abortions. It should therefore be completely avoided during pregnancy or when a woman might become pregnant. Nor should goldenseal be given to babies or nursing mothers.

Berberine increases bilirubin levels in the blood, and bilirubin causes jaundice. While there is little or no indication that goldenseal can cause jaundice, the fact that one of the active ingredients increases bilirubin means that goldenseal is likely to cause someone who has jaundice to worsen.

Recommendations

Goldenseal may have some use as an antibiotic when applied externally to the body or as an antidiarrheal. There is no evidence that its ingredients are absorbed into the bloodstream when taken internally, or that it works against viral infections. The long list of adverse effects and potential toxicity, as well as the plant's endangered species status, make its popular use for diarrhea, colds, and flu unwarranted.

The use of goldenseal for colds should be discouraged for other reasons. As a nation, we already use so many antibiotics for minor, short-lasting ailments that we now have antibiotic-resistant organisms. Resorting to natural products just extends the concerns. If you have a cold, take plenty of liquids and rest, letting the minor ailment run its course. Then, when you truly need medication, there is a greater chance that it will work with the minimum dose possible.

Dosage

Orally, a wide variety of doses are recommended, with 0.5 to 1 gram three times a day being most common.

Treatment Categories

Complementary Therapy
Colds	☹☹☹
Flu	☹☹☹

Scientifically Unproven
Other indications

Further Reading

Bergner, Paul, *The Healing Power of Echinacea, Goldenseal, and Other Immune System Herbs* (Rocklin, Calif.: Prima, 1997).

Jellin, Jeff M., Forrest Batz, and Kathy Hichens, *Pharmacist's Letter/Prescriber's Letter: Natural Medicines Comprehensive Database* (Stockton, Calif.: Therapeutic Research Facility, 1999), 440–41.

O'Mathúna, Dónal P., "Goldenseal for Upper Respiratory Infections," *Alternative Medicine Alert* 3, no. 5 (May 2000): 56–58.

GRAPE SEED EXTRACT

What It Is

A relative newcomer to the top ten best-selling herbal remedies is grape seed extract. Interest in this product arises from what has been called the "French Paradox." Studies in the 1970s showed that when a country's citizens enjoyed a diet that contained relatively high proportions of fat, they also suffered a higher than average incidence of, and deaths from, heart disease. The one extreme exception to all this was France and, to a lesser degree, other Mediterranean countries. They had relatively high amounts of fat in their diet, but a relatively low incidence of heart disease. When researchers looked to see how the French high-fat meals differed from similar high-fat meals in countries plagued with heart disease, the one consistent difference was not on the plate, but in the glass. French men, women, and children tended to drink one or more glasses of wine with their meals, something citizens of other countries did not.

However, recommending a daily glass of wine raised concerns about negative effects and the potential for abuse. Certainly the myth of the safety of wine consumption was shattered when it was found that the French have a relatively high incidence of alcoholism. In fact, the higher alcohol-related death rate in France completely eliminates any benefit due to the lower death rate from heart disease. Others are now questioning whether the "French Paradox" is actually just a statistical anomaly due to the way the original surveys were conducted. In spite of this, interest in grape products remains high, with grape seed extracts identified as the most likely candidate to have potentially beneficial effects.

Pycnogenol is another name used for some grape seed extract products, although the name is also used for pine bark extracts that contain compounds similar to those in grape seed extracts. Interestingly, the French are again credited with discovering this possible remedy. In 1534, Jacques Cartier, a famous French explorer, was trapped by ice on the Saint Lawrence River. He and his men had plenty of stores of biscuits and salted meat to survive the harsh winter. Although they were able to eat their fill, they developed scurvy, a disease caused by a deficiency of vitamin C. Some of Cartier's men died. Those who survived recovered when they met Native Americans who advised them to drink a tea made from the bark and needles of pine trees.

No one knew why this helped, but four centuries later, Professor Jacques Masquelier of the University of Bordeaux in France determined that the pine bark and needles contained vitamin C. He then found bioflavonoids and other components he termed pycnogenols. Grape seed extract contains these same types of components.

Claims

Proponents claim the grape seed extracts improve circulation, protect against heart disease, treat arthritis, allergic reactions, and varicose veins, and fight cancer. All of these effects are said to result from the extract's antioxidant activity. These effects have been traced to a group of compounds called "flavonoids." The particular ones found in grape seed extracts are also called "procyanidins" or "OPCs." These are present in much greater amounts in red wine compared to white wine or grape juice. These are believed to work via the same general antioxidant effect as discussed under "Antioxidants" (see page 298).

Study Findings

Grape seed extracts contain antioxidants, and these have been shown to have beneficial effects on the hearts of animals fed high-fat diets. However, very few studies have been conducted on humans. The only double-blind studies (✔✔✔) date from the 1980s and showed improvements in blood flow. A recent study (✔✔✔) showed that the concentration of antioxidants in the blood was increased after five days of taking the supplements. However, the longest of these studies lasted just one month. No studies have examined whether taking grape seed extracts leads to lower incidence of heart disease or any of the other diseases for which the extracts are recommended.

Cautions

No adverse effects or drug interactions have been reported from grape seed extracts. Rats and mice fed very large quantities suffered no ill effects. One theoretical concern is that the use of grape seed extract may increase the blood-thinning effect of warfarin (Coumadin) due to the presence of vitamin E in the extract. These issues have not been investigated. Caution should be exercised since beta-carotene is another antioxidant of natural origin that was promoted widely until large-scale studies showed it could have harmful effects when taken by long-term smokers.

As with all dietary supplements, quality is a concern. One study examined the quality of six grape seed and pine bark products. The total flavonoid content of these products ranged from 2 to 804 mg per gram of extract. When the researchers tested the ability of these products to prevent oxidation, they ranged from 16 to 8392 (in technical units of μmol TE/g [micromole trolox equivalents per gram]), a remarkable 525-fold difference in strength!

Grape seed extract should be avoided in amounts greater than found in food sources in childhood, pregnancy, and lactation, as insufficient reliable information is available.

Recommendations

Antioxidants appear to play an important role in preventing heart disease and other illnesses. The Bible recognizes the value of a little wine for stomach problems (1 Timothy 5:23). Grape seed extract is a potentially useful product of this type and appears to be very safe. However, there is little evidence that taking antioxidants from one particular source has the same benefit as eating a diet rich in a variety of antioxidants. Until properly designed clinical trials show that grape seed extract prevents the incidence or severity of heart disease, it should only be taken as part of a balanced diet rich in fruits and vegetables.

Dosage

Doses vary considerably, with 25 to 300 mg daily being suggested for up to three weeks. After this, 40 to 80 mg daily is recommended.

Treatment Categories

Complementary Therapy
Dietary source for essential fatty acids and tocopherols ☺☺☺
Cardiovascular disease treatment or prevention ☺

Scientifically Unproven
Other indications

Further Reading

Fetrow, Charles W., and Juan R. Avila, *Professional's Handbook of Complementary and Alternative Medicine* (Springhouse, Penn.: Springhouse, 1999), 310–12.

Jellin, Jeff M., Forrest Batz, and Kathy Hichens, *Pharmacist's Letter/Prescriber's Letter: Natural Medicines Comprehensive Database* (Stockton, Calif.: Therapeutic Research Facility, 1999), 447–49.

Law, Malcolm, and Nicholas Wald, "Why Heart Disease Mortality Is Low in France: The Time Lag Explanation," *BMJ* 318 (May 1999): 1471–80.

O'Mathúna, Dónal P., "Grape Seed Extract for the Prevention of Cardiac Disease," *Alternative Medicine Alert* 2, no. 8 (August 1999): 91–94.

Prior, Ronald L., and Guohua Cao, "Variability in Dietary Antioxidant Related Natural Product Supplements: The Need for Methods of Standardization," *Journal of the American Nutraceutical Association* 2, no. 2 (Summer 1999): 46–56.

HAWTHORN

What It Is

Hawthorn might be called a "living fence." The name is a corruption of the translation from the German where it was called the Hedgethorn. This spiny shrub grows to a height of thirty feet if not regularly trimmed, and was used in Germany to mark off plots of land. The bush provided beauty and, because of its spiny nature, security from trespassers.

By either name, hawthorn is the name used for a number of *Crataegus* species. The most popular one used for medicinal purposes is *Crataegus laevigata;* however, many of the *Crataegus* species are interchanged in remedies. The leaves, flowers, and fruit of most species contain a number of biological substances that may dilate blood vessels and lower blood pressure. Antioxidant flavonoids are found in the highest concentrations in the young buds and leaves. Hawthorn is best known in many parts of the world as a heart or cardiac tonic.

Claims

Hawthorn has been used to treat various heart diseases, particularly angina. It has been said to relax smooth muscle in coronary vessels and thus may help avoid angina. Hawthorn berries have been used for centuries in Europe and the Orient for their beneficial effects on the cardiovascular system. It has been used by European physicians for hypertension, heart failure, cardiomyopathy, and angina.

Study Findings

Laboratory studies in animals have shown that *Crataegus* extracts contain antioxidants and are able to prevent abnormal blood clotting. The extracts have also been shown in animals to improve abnormal cholesterol levels and atherosclerosis via a variety of mechanisms. In several animal studies, highly concentrated extracts have been shown to have a protective effect on the heart without increasing cardiac blood flow.

Animal studies have also shown that hawthorn dilates blood vessels and inhibits angiotensin-converting enzyme (thereby making it an ACE inhibitor, similar to prescription ACE inhibitors). It has also been shown to have a mild diuretic effect.

In humans, case studies (✔✔✔) have shown that hawthorn increases the strength of the contraction of the heart and increases coronary blood flow while decreasing the heart rate and the consumption of oxygen. A recent randomized, placebo-controlled, double-blind study (✔✔✔) in patients with heart failure showed a clear improvement in cardiac function in patients taking an extract of *Crataegus*. However, hawthorn appears to be most effective for milder cases of heart failure and may be inappropriate for more advanced stages. Physicians use a system called the New York Heart Association (NYHA) stages to describe the severity of heart disease. In Stage I, heart disease patients only have symptoms with strenuous activity, and in Stage II the symptoms occur with less strenuous activity. More advanced heart disease leads to symptoms with moderate activity (Stage III) or any activity (Stage IV). The symptoms experienced include palpitations, trouble breathing, fatigue, or chest pain.

Cautions

Hawthorn has been shown to be tolerated, relatively free of adverse effects and, in fact, when compared with other drugs that increase heart function, may have benefits for the heart. However, using (✘✘) hawthorn along with digitalis can markedly increase the activity of the latter and should never be tried unless under medical supervision.

Recommendations

Further studies of hawthorn in humans with heart disease are now ongoing at a number of medical centers. European studies supporting hawthorn used two products, Crategult® (sold as HeartCare®) and Faros® (not available in the U.S.). Because of its apparent favorable side-effect profile, hawthorn is probably safe to be used with NYHA Stage I or II heart failure; however, it should only be taken under a physician's supervision and probably should not be used with NYHA Stage III or IV heart failure.

The Natural Database rates hawthorn as "Likely Unsafe" during pregnancy as it may increase uterine contractions. It is recommended that it not be used in children or during lactation as there is insufficient information available to establish that it is safe in these individuals.

Dosage

A powder containing 300 to 1000 mg of dried extract is usually taken orally three times a day or used to make a tea.

Treatment Categories

Complementary Therapy
    Coronary artery disease   ☺☺
    Improve ejection fraction, exercise
        tolerance, and to reduce subjective
        symptoms in NYHA Stages I and II heart failure   ☺☺☺

Scientifically Unproven
    Other indications, including NYHA Stages III or IV heart failure

Further Reading

Jellin, Jeff M., Forrest Batz, and Kathy Hichens, *Pharmacist's Letter/Prescriber's Letter: Natural Medicines Comprehensive Database* (Stockton, Calif.: Therapeutic Research Facility, 1999), 475–80.

Loew, D., "Phytotherapy in Heart Failure," *Phytomedicine*, 4, no. 3 (1997): 267–71.

Mashour, Nick H., George I. Lin, and William H. Frishman, "Herbal Medicine for the Treatment of Cardiovascular Disease," *Archives of Internal Medicine* 158 (1998): 2225–34.

HONEYBEE VENOM

What It Is

Bee venom differs from bee pollen, which is commonly available in health food stores as a nutritional supplement. Honeybee venom therapy (BVT) has reportedly been known since the time of Aristotle. In fact, illnesses of Charles the Great and Ivan the Terrible are said to have been cured by bee stings.

Claims

The actual number of users of BVT in the United States is unknown. BVT is said to be common in Romania as well as in China and the former Soviet Union. The American Apitherapy Society has been established "for advancing the investigation of apitherapy" as well as monitoring adverse reactions to BVT.

Many proponents point to the benefits of BVT, claiming it possesses an anti-inflammatory effect. They claim success in treatment of a wide variety of illnesses such as arthritis, multiple sclerosis, Bell's palsy, and irritable bowel syndrome. Others use it for rheumatoid arthritis, cervicobrachial neuralgia, fibromyositis and fibromyalgia syndrome, abnormal hardening of the muscles (myogeloses), tendinitis, tenosynovitis, and for desensitization to bee stings. However, critics point to potentially harmful side effects and warn of its potential to be a form of quackery.

Anecdotal reports of BVT on symptoms of multiple sclerosis (✔) have led many patients to seek therapy by repeatedly subjecting themselves to bee stings, reportedly as many as twenty-five to thirty stings per session, a practice that has been common in many Eastern countries for centuries; although most practitioners use subcutaneous, intra-dermal, or intra-articular (into the joint) injections of a purified, sterile bee toxin called "apitoxin." In China, bee venom is administered through the skin using electrophoresis, ultrasonophoresis, or acupuncture.

Study Findings

Bee venom is composed of several substances that have been proposed to reduce inflammation. Animal studies suggest that bee venom may work by stimulating the adre-nal glands to release natural steroids. Case reports (✔) cite improvement in patients with rheumatoid arthritis, multiple sclerosis, cervicobrachial neuralgia, fibromyositis or fibromyalgia syndrome, myogeloses, and tendinopathies. Therefore, one respected source, the Natural Database, formerly rated honeybee venom as "possibly effective" for rheumatoid arthritis, cervicobrachial neuralgia, fibromyositis, myogeloses, tendinitis, and tenosynovitis. It has since changed this to "possibly ineffective" as new studies have been released. We know of no controlled clinical trials looking at the effectiveness of BVT on arthritis in humans. There also is no reliable information that would indicate that orally administered BVT (tablets, capsules, or drops) is safe or has any effect at all.

Two nonprofit organizations, the Multiple Sclerosis Association of America and the National Multiple Sclerosis Society, are funding new research into the possible use of injectable bee venom in the treatment of multiple sclerosis.

Although controlled clinical trials on humans have not been performed, numerous studies have assessed the effect of BVT on adjuvant-induced arthritis (AID) in rodents, which is thought to be a close experimental model for human rheumatoid arthritis. These studies suggest that BVT may exert a beneficial impact on AID. Purified bee venom (as opposed to whole bee venom) may not be as effective as whole bee venom in suppressing adjuvant-induced arthritis.

Cautions

Administration of bee venom obviously carries the risk of an allergic reaction and should not be given without the immediate availability of injectable epinephrine and oral antihistamines. BVT injections have caused inflammation at the shot site, swelling, pain, itching, fatigue, congestion, headache, nausea, vomiting, fainting, low blood pressure, fever, and chills. It can also cause anaphylaxis, which can be deadly. The cumulative stings of many honeybees may also provoke any of these reactions. The American Apitherapy Society monitors adverse reactions and requests that reports of such reactions be sent to them.

There is no information concerning the administration of honeybee venom to children or women who are pregnant or lactating. Therefore, BVT should be avoided in these individuals.

Recommendations

Many anecdotal reports exist about the benefits of using BVT for arthritis and multiple sclerosis, diseases that affect many Americans and cause considerable disability and health care expenditures. Laboratory studies provide evidence that BVT may have a beneficial impact on arthritis, at least in animals.

No human studies have been conducted and much remains to be learned about BVT, including its effectiveness and appropriate dose. Users should understand the possibility of severe allergic reactions to bee stings as well as how to recognize and deal with them. Furthermore, BVT users should have an allergy kit (e.g., EPI-PEN) readily available, and they should be instructed in its use. All allergic reactions to BVT should be reported to the American Apitherapy Society. Individuals with particular chronic medical conditions (e.g., hypertension and heart disease) should be cautious about initiating BVT without discussing the risks with their physician.

Dosage

There is little information available on the appropriate dose of honeybee venom. People vary in how they respond to the venom, which is usually injected, making it advisable to only receive doses from physicians who are well trained in the therapy.

Treatment Categories

Complementary Therapy
Rheumatoid arthritis
Cervicobrachial neuralgia

Fibromyositis or fibromyalgia syndrome ☺
Myogeloses ☺
Tendinopathies ☺

Scientifically Unproven
Multiple sclerosis ☹
Any other medical indication

Possible Fraud or Quackery
In the hands of some practitioners

Further Reading

Jellin, Jeff M., Forrest Batz, and Kathy Hichens, *Pharmacist's Letter/Prescriber's Letter: Natural Medicines Comprehensive Database* (Stockton, Calif.: Therapeutic Research Facility, 1999), 497.

Somerfield, Stanley D., "Bee Venom and Arthritis," *Journal of Rheumatology* 13 (1986): 477.

Yoirish, N., *Curative Properties of Honey and Bee Venom* (San Francisco: New Glide Publications, 1977).

KAVA

What It Is

The history of kava is a blend of myth, magic, marketing, and reality. What is certain is that it was the ceremonial drink of choice in the Pacific Islands from sometime before their written history through the eighteenth century when Europeans first made contact with the people. Kava is said to have been first reported by Captain James Cook, who called it "intoxicating pepper." Kava drinking was the equivalent of happy hour, the liquid used in the manner of friends taking their first, slow sips of their favorite alcoholic beverages at the end of a day of hard work. Kava caused the natives to relax and become more social, and because of its effect, there were many stories about its origins.

One story claims that kava grew from the grave of the corpse of a Tonga king's servant. She had been killed and used for a royal feast that the king had respectfully declined. Instead, after her burial, the plant that rose from the grave was supposed to be used to make a ceremonial drink.

Less ... well ... disgusting is another legend in which a Samoan woman witnessed a rat radically changing his behavior after nibbling on the plant. She brought it back to her people and they discovered the stimulating benefit of the plant.

The actual preparation of the ceremonial drink, at least by the eighteenth century, was not a pleasant one. The root of a species of pepper tree was cut into small pieces and passed among the islanders preparing the drink. They chewed the pieces to gain the juice and a rather pulpy mass, all of which was spit into a bowl. None of the juice was consumed by the "cooks." Coconut milk was then poured over all this, after which it was strained through coconut fibers. The pulpy pieces were squeezed to get as much of the juice mixed in with the milk as possible, then set aside. Finally the coconut milk and kava juice mix was poured into a second bowl and quickly consumed. Fortunately, contemporary kava preparation is far more sanitary.

Kava, or kava-kava, or "intoxicating pepper," is an up-and-coming herbal remedy made from the shrub that grows primarily in the South Pacific islands. The underground parts (roots and rhizome) of *Piper methysticum* are used to make the extract.

Claims

Herbal manufacturers claim kava is "nature's stress buster" and a natural way to relieve anxiety (as an alternative to such drugs as Valium®). It is also used to promote sleep. One promoter claims it is the herbal equivalent of having a soak in a hot tub and a massage. Others recommend kava for promoting wound healing, treating headaches (including migraines), colds, rheumatism, tuberculosis, chronic cystitis, menstrual problems, and as an aphrodisiac.

Study Findings

More than a dozen compounds isolated from the plant have been shown to cause muscle relaxation and pain relief. No clinical trials have been conducted in the United States. A systematic review published in 2000 found seven randomized, controlled studies on patients with a variety of disorders associated with anxiety: agoraphobia, specific phobia, generalized anxiety disorder, and adjustment disorder with anxiety. These studies were limited because they used relatively small numbers of patients, but they all showed that kava was somewhat effective at relieving generalized anxiety. One study (✔✔✔) found kava was as effective as oxazepam, a Valium-like drug. Another (✔✔✔) showed that kava reduced the "psychosomatic dysfunctions" associated with menopausal symptoms. However, the clinical studies that have shown kava to be effective have all used formulations which contain 30 to 55 percent of kava lactones. Extracts containing 70 percent kavapyrones may be even more effective.

Cautions

Side effects are relatively mild, with the most common being intestinal disturbances, muscle weakness, and allergic reactions. Other less common side effects include headache, dizziness, enlarged pupils, dysequilibrium, and (rarely) allergic skin reactions. Drowsiness can be a problem, especially when taken along with alcohol or other depressants, although one randomized controlled trial showed no side effects from combining kava and alcohol. Nevertheless, those driving or operating machinery while taking kava should be cautious and alert to any possible changes it may induce. As with any medication affecting the brain, an abuse syndrome can develop. As with all herbal remedies, there can be great variability in the strengths of different kava preparations.

Chronic abuse of kava leads to a syndrome called "kawaism," which is characterized by reddened eyes, dry and scaly skin, and a yellowish discoloration of the skin, eyes, and nails. If kava use is stopped, the signs of the syndrome slowly are resolved. A case report (✘) of liver disease after consuming kava for two months has recently been published.

The Natural Database rates kava as "Possibly Unsafe" when used orally for more than three months, and as "Possibly Unsafe" during pregnancy or lactation.

Recommendations

Kava holds out some promise as a mild way to treat anxiety. However, very little clinical research has been conducted on it, and no studies have examined its long-term effects. Generalized anxiety is a common disorder, but can have many causes. Using herbs or drugs exclusively may result in relief of symptoms without addressing the underlying emotional and spiritual causes. Use of kava usually results from self-diagnosis, which may not be reliable or accurate. Anxiety is also one of the conditions for which placebos are most effective, which also may contribute to kava's overall effectiveness.

Dosage

Most studies have used a dose of about 100 mg kava extract three times a day. However, products vary widely in the concentration of kava lactones they contain.

Treatment Categories

Complementary Therapy
Mild anxiety	☺☺☺
Stress	☺☺
Restlessness	☺☺

Scientifically Unproven
Other indications

Further Reading

Escher, Monica, Jules Desmeules, Emile Giostra, and Gilles Mentha, "Hepatitis Associated with Kava, A Herbal Remedy for Anxiety," *BMJ* 322 (January 2001): 139.

Jellin, Jeff M., Forrest Batz, and Kathy Hichens, *Pharmacist's Letter/Prescriber's Letter: Natural Medicines Comprehensive Database* (Stockton, Calif.: Therapeutic Research Facility, 1999), 549–50.

Pittler, Max H., and Edzard Ernst, "Efficacy of Kava Extract for Treating Anxiety: Systematic Review and Meta-Analysis," *Journal of Clinical Psychopharmacology* 20, no. 1 (February 2000): 84–89.

LICORICE

What It Is

Most of us think of ropelike red and black candy when we think of licorice. However, the candy is not licorice, but anise-flavored "sticks." European licorice is more likely to be the "real thing." In America, the most common use for licorice is as an ingredient in tobacco products in order to counteract the bitter flavor and add some sweetness.

Commercial licorice is extracted primarily from the roots and rhizomes of what is called Italian or Spanish licorice *(Glycyrrhiza glabra typica)*, along with a number of other closely related species—including Persian or Turkish licorice *(Glycyrrhiza glabra violacea)*, Russian licorice *(Glycyrrhiza glabra glandulifera)*, and Chinese licorice *(Glycyrrhiza uralensis)*. The plant grows in subtropical areas, with most commercial licorice coming from eastern Mediterranean countries.

Claims

Licorice has been used for centuries in China, Egypt, Greece, and Rome as an expectorant and carminative (antiflatulence agent). It has also been used to mask bitter flavors (it is still added to pharmaceutical cough and cold preparations). The primary medicinal use was as a natural treatment for peptic ulcers. Others recommend licorice for bronchitis, gastritis, colic, arthritis, lupus, tuberculosis, hepatitis, and in formulations to increase fertility in women with polycystic ovarian syndrome. In has been used intravenously to treat hepatitis B and C and topically as a shampoo for a number of scalp disorders.

Study Findings

Licorice root contains between 5 and 9 percent glycyrrhizin, a compound fifty times sweeter than glucose (a form of sugar). Glycyrrhizin can be broken down (chemically or during digestion) to glycyrrhetic acid, which is not sweet. Both of these compounds have mild anti-inflammatory effects and stimulate the secretion of mucous in the stomach. A number of randomized controlled trials (✘✘✘✘) looked at the effect of deglycyrrhizinized licorice in treating gastric and peptic ulcers. In general it was no more effective than placebo—although it had significantly fewer side effects than glycyrrhizin. Glycyrrhizin's potential for treating ulcers led to much research and even the development, in the 1960s, of a semisynthetic derivative called "carbenoxolone." While clinical studies (✔✔✔✔) showed that the licorice derivatives were effective, they were less effective than standard drugs like cimetidine. Glycyrrhizin also had much more serious side effects (✘✘✘✘), including edema, high blood pressure, and causing excessive secretion of potassium.

There are at least two randomized controlled trials (✔✔✔✔) of intravenous glycyrrhizin in hepatitis C patients. In both studies, glycyrrhizin lowered serum liver enzyme elevations (a sign that it might be relieving some of the liver damage that hepatitis C can cause). Clinical trials (✔✔✔) have also shown benefit in patients with hepatitis B. However, during treatment there were no changes in the levels of the hepatitis virus in the blood. In these trials the drug appeared to be safe and well tolerated.

Cautions

Other side effects than those mentioned above have been found when people ingest large quantities of licorice for extended periods. Headache, lethargy, water retention, electrolyte imbalances, high blood pressure, and heart failure have been noted (✘✘) in people consuming about 1 gram of glycyrrhizin daily. These symptoms have occurred in people eating a quarter-pound of some European licorice candy daily, or swallowing their saliva while continuously chewing tobacco.

Licorice, taken chronically, can theoretically interact with a number of prescription and over-the-counter drugs (such as aspirin, NSAIDS, steroids, female hormones, diuretics, heart drugs, insulin, and MAO inhibitors). Individuals taking prescription drugs should not take licorice without first discussing this with their physician.

More recently (✘✘), seven young men given 0.5 gram of glycyrrhizin daily had reduced testosterone levels and other changes in their steroid levels. These could have far-reaching health effects.

Licorice has been rated "Contraindicated" in pregnancy by the Natural Database, as it can have abortifacient, estrogenic, and steroid effects in humans and has been shown to stimulate the uterus in animal studies. Licorice, in amounts greater than in foods, is not recommended in lactation, as there is no information on the safety of taking it while breast-feeding.

Recommendations

Licorice candy in the United States will provide a lot more sugar than licorice. If you enjoy licorice, it may actually be the anise flavor you like. Products that contain real licorice extract should not be used for extended periods of time. The extract may have some expectorant and antiulcer effects, but other products are readily available which do not carry the same risks. The use of glycyrrhizin for hepatitis B or C should be coordinated with a hepatologist (expert in liver disease).

Dosage

A typical dose of licorice is whatever gives a person 200 to 600 mg glycyrrhizin. A tea made from 1 to 4 grams of powdered root gives roughly this amount of glycyrrhizin.

Treatment Categories

Complementary Therapy
Upper respiratory mucous membrane inflammation

Some forms of cough	☺☺
Peptic ulcer disease	☺
Gastric ulcers	☺
Duodenal ulcers	☺
Indigestion	☺
Hepatitis B or C	☺

Scientifically Unproven
    All other uses

Further Reading

Fetrow, Charles W., and Juan R. Avila, *Professional's Handbook of Complementary and Alternative Medicine* (Springhouse, Penn.: Springhouse, 1999), 393–96.

Foster, Steven, and Varro E. Tyler, *Tyler's Honest Herbal: A Sensible Guide to the Use of Herbs and Related Remedies*, 4th ed. (New York: Haworth Herbal Press, 1999), 241–43.

Jellin, Jeff M., Forrest Batz, and Kathy Hichens, *Pharmacist's Letter/Prescriber's Letter: Natural Medicines Comprehensive Database* (Stockton, Calif.: Therapeutic Research Facility, 1999), 580–82.

MARIGOLD

What It Is

While marigold has been used medicinally for centuries, not all types of marigolds are considered effective. The common marigold found in gardens throughout America consists of a number of related species (the *Tagets* species). But it is the marigold plant with orange and yellow flowers, a variety sometimes called pot marigold and known by the scientific name *Calendula officinalis,* that is most commonly used for healing.

The part of the flower used is the ligulate floret, which is often mistakenly called the flower petal. This part of the flower is used to make tinctures and extracts, or sometimes is dried and used as a seasoning like saffron.

Claims

The oldest and most common use of marigold tinctures is for treating a variety of skin conditions, to promote healing, and to reduce inflammation. It is also said to prevent infections in open wounds. When taken internally, it has been used to relieve fever and spasm, control dysmenorrhea (painful menstrual periods), and to treat cancer. It has also been recommended for treating fever, initiating menstrual periods, stomach ulcers, nosebleeds, varicose veins, hemorrhoids, and conjunctivitis.

Study Findings

A number of studies in animals have shown that calendula extracts have an anti-inflammatory effect. The particular compounds causing this effect have not been identified. In fact, little is known about what the active ingredients in calendula could be, even though much research has been conducted in this area. However, few studies have examined the tinctures and extracts on humans, and those studies that have been published have been small and limited. These studies (✔✔✔) show that calendula ointment does promote healing of burns, including sunburn, and can positively affect other types of wounds. Studies (✔✔✔) on sunburn also showed the ointment promotes healing.

Cautions

Only one report (✘) of a serious adverse effect with calendula exists. This was a case of anaphylactic shock after an extract was gargled. Marigolds belong to the aster and daisy families (like ragweed, echinacea, and feverfew) to which some people are allergic. Anyone allergic to any of these should apply calendula products cautiously at first. Theoretically, concomitant use of marigold with herbs or prescriptions that cause sedation might enhance adverse effects.

The Natural Database rates marigold as "Likely Unsafe" for oral use in pregnancy due to possible abortifacient effects. There is insufficient reliable information for use orally by children or lactating women or for use topically by pregnant women; therefore, it should not be used by these individuals.

Recommendations

Before the development of antibiotics, extracts of calendula were widely used to prevent infections and promote healing of wounds. Even with its widespread use, there is little evidence of it being harmful. Although there is little clinical evidence to support its effectiveness, its long history and its few studies do support calendula's wound-healing properties.

Dosage

The most common products are teas, tinctures, and ointments, leading to a variety of dosage recommendations.

Treatment Categories

Complementary Therapy
    Topical application for superficial skin wounds   ☺☺☺
    Bug bites   ☺☺☺

Orally for inflammation of the oral mucosa ☺☺
Topical for poorly healing wounds ☺☺
Leg ulcers ☺☺

Scientifically Unproven
Other indications—such as colitis, duodenal and gastric ulcers, and dysmenorrhea

Further Reading

DerMarderosian, Ara, ed., "Calendula," in *The Review of Natural Products* (St. Louis, Mo.: Facts and Comparisons, January 1995).

Dietz, Vance, "Calendula Preparations to Treat Cutaneous Infections," *Alternative Medicine Alert* 1, no. 11 (November 1998): 140–42.

Jellin, Jeff M., Forrest Batz, and Kathy Hichens, *Pharmacist's Letter/Prescriber's Letter: Natural Medicines Comprehensive Database* (Stockton, Calif.: Therapeutic Research Facility, 1999), 186–87.

MARIJUANA

What It Is

Marijuana hardly needs any introduction. Whether it's called pot, grass, weed, Indian hemp, or any number of other names, the plant in question is *Cannabis sativa* (sometimes called *Cannabis indica*). In some ways it could be viewed as the most popular herbal remedy of them all even though it is illegal to grow marijuana, illegal to have it in your possession, illegal to use it, and illegal to sell. We have great concern about *any* use of marijuana because, as we've just emphasized, marijuana is an illegal substance. Anyone using it or prescribing it is breaking the law. Only under the tightest restrictions are a small number of people legally allowed to use marijuana in research. We have included marijuana here to explore the medical claims being made and to provide a scientific evaluation of its active ingredients.

Marijuana's illegal use in the United States peaked in the 1960s, but it remains popular. About half of all people living in the United States are believed to have tried marijuana (most illegally) at some time in their lives. The 1992 National Household Survey on Drug Abuse found that approximately 5 million Americans illegally use marijuana on a weekly basis. Nearly 70 percent of high school students reported using it illegally in the previous month. Use drops off dramatically as people enter their thirties.

Marijuana differs from all of the other herbal remedies we discuss because of its illegal status. Marijuana has been very difficult to obtain medically since passage of the Marijuana Tax Act of 1937. It is currently regulated in the United States as a Schedule I drug, which means it is viewed as having a high potential for abuse, to lack an accepted medical use, and to be unsafe for use under medical supervision. This means marijuana is unavailable even for physicians to prescribe.

Starting as far back as the 1970s, efforts were made to reclassify marijuana as a Schedule II drug, which would allow doctors to prescribe it for certain conditions. These efforts were quashed by the Drug Enforcement Agency in 1992, which led to proponents going directly to voters to change the laws. In 1996, voters in California and Arizona passed ballot initiatives permitting the use of marijuana as a medicine. Arizona's referendum was invalidated, but in 1998 another initiative passed there, along with similar initiatives in Alaska, Nevada, Oregon, Washington, and Colorado. The Colorado vote has since been dismissed as it was determined that not enough valid signatures were collected to put the initiative on the ballot.

However, all these initiatives received a setback in August 2000 from the U.S. Supreme Court. In a 7-to-1 ruling, the Supreme Court determined that the potential benefits of legalizing distribution of marijuana by physicians did not warrant the violation of federal law that prohibits distribution of marijuana. This ruling came in response to an emergency appeal from the Clinton administration to uphold the federal law.

Marijuana has a very long history of medicinal use, being mentioned in ancient records from China and India. Both its illegal and medicinal uses involve smoking or eating the unpurified leaves and flower tops. As with all herbs, there is great variability in the strength and quality of samples. However, it is generally acknowledged that the potency of marijuana available today is much higher than what was available on the street a couple decades ago.

The active ingredients in marijuana are a group of about thirty compounds called "cannabinoids." The most abundant and active of these is Δ^9-THC (delta-9-tetrahydrocannabinol, or delta-9-THC). A manufactured form of Δ^9-THC has been available since 1985 as a Schedule II drug called Marinol®, or dronabinol. Marinol is FDA-approved for the treatment of chemotherapy-induced nausea and vomiting, and AIDS-induced weight loss. In 1999, this product was reassigned to Schedule III, meaning it is viewed as having less potential for abuse and dependence. (Schedule II drugs include narcotics, amphetamines, and barbiturates, which are viewed as highly susceptible to abuse with severe dependence.) Some of the marijuana research has been conducted on pure Δ^9-THC and other cannabinoids, and must be distinguished from that done on whole marijuana itself. Unless otherwise stated, "marijuana" in this entry refers to smoking or eating marijuana plant material.

Claims

During the nineteenth century, medical journals and pharmacopoeias recommended marijuana as an appetite stimulant, muscle relaxant, pain reliever, hypnotic agent, and anticonvulsant. Most of marijuana's current use centers around its ability to induce euphoria, relaxation, sexual arousal, and give a general "high." Although some would like to see marijuana legalized as a recreational drug, we will address only the controversy about its medical use.

On the one side are those who claim marijuana should be available under medical supervision for nausea and vomiting associated with chemotherapy, to lower intraocular pressure in glaucoma, to stimulate appetite in AIDS patients who have difficulty maintaining their weight, as an anticonvulsant and muscle relaxant with certain spastic disorders, and to relieve chronic pain.

On the other side of this issue are those who might agree that marijuana has some of these effects, but would argue that it should still not be legalized for three reasons.

- There are more effective treatments available for all these conditions.
- Marijuana, especially smoking marijuana, can have negative effects, not the least of which is dependence. For this reason, they would prefer that purified substances like Marinol be used, not marijuana joints.
- Marijuana is believed to be a "gateway" drug. Those who use other illicit drugs have usually tried marijuana earlier. The claim is that marijuana acts as a "gateway" to these other drugs, and that making it available medically would lead to patients and others trying other illicit drugs.

The debate over whether marijuana has a legitimate medical use is very similar to that over other herbal remedies. Some people give compelling anecdotal reports of people with cancer or AIDS being helped by smoking marijuana, who then have to face the anxiety and embarrassment of obtaining marijuana from drug dealers. Even if its medical use were legalized, the familiar questions arise concerning quality and consistency. But this herbal debate is complicated by claims that marijuana is addictive and harmful.

Equally compelling stories exist of people's lives being ruined by marijuana. Some of these people started using marijuana out of curiosity or due to peer pressure. There are great fears that legitimizing the herb in any way will lead to more people getting hooked on it. However the legal and political situation gets resolves, the first step is to resolve the medical debate, and that centers around the results of research on marijuana and its cannabinoids.

Study Findings

After California voters legalized medical marijuana in 1996, the White House Office of National Drug Control Policy asked the Institute of Medicine (IOM) to review the scientific evidence concerning marijuana. The IOM is the same organization that issues the

Recommended Dietary Allowances for vitamins and nutrients (see page 301). It is a private, nonprofit organization that advises the federal government on medical issues, especially those involving controversy over the scientific evidence.

In March 1999, the IOM released a report, *Marijuana and Medicine: Assessing the Science Base*, that has become the focus of much of this controversy. The report concluded, "Until a non-smoked, rapid-onset cannabinoid drug delivery system becomes available, we acknowledge that there is no clear alternative for people suffering from chronic conditions that might be relieved by smoking marijuana, such as pain or AIDS wasting. One possible approach is to treat patients as 'n-of-1' clinical trials, in which patients are fully informed of their status as experimental subjects using a harmful drug delivery system, and in which their conditions are monitored and documented under medical supervision, thereby increasing the knowledge base of the risks and benefits of marijuana use under such conditions."

As will become clear, we have serious reservations about much of the recommendation of the IOM. Without doubt, a lot of progress was made during the 1980s and 1990s on understanding how marijuana might work. Researchers discovered that Δ^9-THC interacts with very specific proteins in the brain called "receptors." Other receptors interact with compounds called "endorphins," which our bodies produce as natural painkillers and which also cause euphoria (they are believed to play a big role in the so-called "runners' high"). Researchers have discovered that Δ^9-THC works in the brain on what is now called a "cannabinoid receptor." We naturally make at least one compound that interacts with this receptor, called "anandamide" (the name comes from *ananda*, which means "bliss" in Sanskrit).

This very new area of research is showing that the human brain has a cannabinoid system that is naturally involved in controlling pain, movement, and memory. The excitement in this area of research is similar to when steroids were discovered. We can see that the traditional uses of marijuana are based on real interactions between cannabinoids and this system in people's brains. There's a good chance this research may lead to new treatments. However, much remains unknown in this area. The fact that our brains have a cannabinoid system means that marijuana may influence us in many different ways that we currently are not aware of or don't understand.

The second area of research has been with pure cannabinoid drugs, like Δ^9-THC, or Marinol, which is FDA-approved for two indications. Anorexic AIDS patients who took Marinol in randomized controlled trials recovered their appetite significantly more compared to those taking placebo. They also had less nausea, improved mood, and regained some of their lost weight. Marinol was not as effective as another pharmaceutical drug used to stimulate the appetite (megestrol acetate, or Megase®).

Other studies with chemotherapy patients also showed significant improvements in reducing nausea and vomiting. However, when researchers compared Δ^9-THC to another antiemetic drug (metoclopramide, or Reglan®), three times as many patients receiving metoclopramide reported effective relief. So, while Marinol works, it is not as effective as other available drugs. In addition, the researchers noticed that different people responded very differently to the same dose of Marinol. A lot of people also reported unpleasant feelings while taking Marinol. Recreational users of marijuana report these same unpleasant effects. This drug therefore has to be closely monitored until individualized doses are determined.

The use of Δ^9-THC for pain relief has very little controlled research. The IOM reviewers could find only one study conducted since 1981 using Δ^9-THC, and none with marijuana. The studies conducted prior to then were poorly designed. The results of studies with acute pain were contradictory, and in some cases those taking Δ^9-THC reported feeling increased pain. Studies of Δ^9-THC for chronic pain were more encouraging, though still limited. Three small double-blind studies reported significantly more pain relief for cancer patients.

Controlled studies of smoking marijuana have been conducted with cancer patients as a way of controlling nausea and vomiting. One study found smoking marijuana to be similar in effectiveness to taking Δ^9-THC capsules. Other studies comparing marijuana to antiemetic drugs have found marijuana effective in about one-quarter of the patients, and much less effective than pharmaceutical drugs. During the 1970s, when interest in medical marijuana increased, acute nausea and vomiting occurred in almost 100 percent of chemotherapy patients. Since then, and especially in the 1990s, much more effective drugs have been developed which control these side effects in 70 to 80 percent of chemotherapy patients. However, some patients remain unresponsive to these newer drugs.

Medical marijuana use is probably more popularly reported to counteract the wasting syndrome experienced by AIDS patients. However, this area has received very little controlled research, with most of the claims being based on anecdotal reports. The only controlled evidence is that for Marinol. Overall, there is little evidence to support the claim that marijuana is medically useful. However, a small proportion of patients do not respond well to pharmaceutical agents. The euphoric effect of marijuana might help some people feel better in addition to any other direct effect. These factors will be taken into consideration in our conclusion.

Cautions

Advocates of medical marijuana use point out that no one has ever reported a lethal overdose from marijuana. Estimates based on animals have put the amount needed to kill someone at about 20,000 times the amount normally used medically. This compares with some drugs whose lethal dose is only a few times the amount commonly prescribed. While this may be the case, it would be analogous to claiming that since few people die from alcohol poisoning (from an overdose) there are no serious problems with the use of alcohol below its toxic levels.

Marijuana use can lead to problems after both acute and chronic use. The high for which marijuana is used recreationally has many similarities to intoxication. People are sedated and less coordinated, making it unwise to drive or operate equipment while under its influence. Coordination problems may last up to 24 hours, long after the person no longer feels intoxicated. Many people report euphoria and positive feelings from the high, but 40 to 60 percent of people also report unpleasant experiences. This has been the case with marijuana smoked for medical reasons and with Marinol.

Chronic use of marijuana can lead to dependence, although relatively few users develop this. When people stop using marijuana after chronic use, they can have withdrawal effects. Compared to other abused drugs, these can be mild and short-lived, with symptoms like restlessness, insomnia, nausea, and cramping. The IOM report concluded that there was no conclusive evidence that marijuana is a "gateway" drug. The frequent finding that users of illicit hard drugs report having earlier used marijuana can be explained by marijuana being so commonly used. Underage tobacco smoking and alcohol drinking act as "gateway" drugs just as much as marijuana. At the same time, there is no evidence that allowing the medical use of marijuana might not lead to undesirable changes in its illicit use.

Other physical effects of smoking marijuana are also of significant concern. The dangers of smoking tobacco are widely acknowledged, and all-out efforts are under way to reduce its use. Marijuana smoke does not contain nicotine, but it has a significantly higher tar content that is usually not filtered, except when water bongs are used. The smoke contains carcinogens and has been associated with a number of types of cancer.

The first study to document that marijuana smoking puts people at higher risk for cancer was published in December 1999. This epidemiological study compared the rate of marijuana use among adults with head and neck cancer to similar people without cancer. Only those younger than fifty-five years of age were studied because this group includes those who were teenagers when marijuana was most popular (the 1960s). The researchers found that after they made allowances for other risk factors like smoking cigarettes and alcohol, those who had used marijuana at any time had 2.6 times the risk of these cancers compared to those who never used marijuana. The risk increased with frequency of use, with those who smoked marijuana more than once a day having 4.9 times the risk of these cancers compared to those who abstained. Current smokers of marijuana and cigarettes had thirty-six times the risk of head and neck cancer. Those who had cancers of the larynx or tongue had the highest prevalence of marijuana use. These tissues had previously been suspected to be at highest risk for cancer because the rapid and deep inhalation characteristic of marijuana smoking deposits four times as much tar on the larynx and tongue as cigarette smoking.

Other negative effects have been reported. Children have ten times the risk of leukemia if their mothers smoked marijuana shortly before or during pregnancy. Students regularly using marijuana have lower grades, more traffic accidents, higher use of alcohol and sex as coping mechanisms, and more psychiatric problems than nonusers. These conclusions come from epidemiological studies that do not establish cause and effect, but have been cited as evidence of what is called "amotivation syndrome." More seriously, there is growing evidence of a connection between marijuana use and psychosis. The relationship is complicated, with uncertainty over whether marijuana causes psychoses, or whether people with psychosis tend to experiment with marijuana.

A number of concerns have been expressed that marijuana negatively impacts the immune system, leading to higher risks of infections. This would be particularly problematic since the people for whom medical marijuana is most frequently recommended (AIDS and chemotherapy patients) are already at very high risk for infections. Research is not as yet clear about this connection.

According to the Natural Database, marijuana is rated as "Unsafe" in pregnancy due to the fact that it can cause a reduction in the growth rate of the preborn child and is associated with childhood leukemia. It is "Likely Unsafe" for use by lactating women as Δ^9-THC is concentrated and excreted in the breast milk.

Recommendations

Obey the law. That is first and foremost. Marijuana is illegal—to grow, possess, use, or sell. Our recommendations in no way ignore this most important aspect of any discussion on marijuana.

Recommendations about marijuana use must be carefully subdivided. First, there is clear evidence that marijuana contains powerful drugs with much potential for relieving nausea, vomiting, chronic pain, and loss of appetite, along with bringing mood elevation and other beneficial effects. However, very few preparations are currently available to safely deliver these components. The one FDA-approved drug (Marinol) is effective for some of these conditions, but other—much more effective—pharmaceuticals are already available. Patients in whom these more effective pharmaceuticals do not work, or who do not tolerate them well, might benefit from Marinol.

Our second recommendation concerns patients for whom these pharmaceuticals do not work well. For example, patients who already have nausea might not be able to tolerate any oral medicine. Should doctors be able to prescribe marijuana smoking for patients in these situations? The evidence does not indicate that large numbers of people would benefit from smoking marijuana, although a few might. The serious adverse effects from smoking marijuana must also be taken into account. The most reasonable compromise seems to us to allow seriously ill patients who do not respond to conventional drugs to try marijuana as part of a short-term clinical trial.

However, as Christians we should obey the laws of our governments unless they conflict seriously with our faith. Paul stated it succinctly: "Everyone must submit himself to the governing authorities, for there is no authority except that which God has established. The authorities that exist have been established by God. Consequently, he who rebels against the authority is rebelling against what God has instituted, and those who do so will bring judgment on themselves" (Romans 13:1–2; see also Matthew 22:21). Considering the availability of other medical approaches in most cases, we see no need for anyone to break the law to provide marijuana for medical reasons, and we strongly urge that the law be honored.

This general approach to highly restricted availability of marijuana for medical use was allowed in thirty-six states between 1978 and 1992 under an FDA program called the Compassionate Investigational New Drug (IND) application. This is also the final recommendation of the IOM review, which added that these patients should be fully informed that they are in an experimental study and being given a harmful drug-delivery system. Meanwhile, research is urgently needed to develop new products that deliver the active ingredients in marijuana in effective, standardized, fast-acting systems that are legal.

Our third recommendation is that marijuana not be licensed as a medical drug. We reiterate the conclusion of the IOM review: "If there is any future for marijuana as a medicine, it lies in its isolated components, the cannabinoids and their synthetic derivatives. Isolated cannabinoids will provide more reliable effects than crude plant mixtures. Therefore, the purpose of clinical trials of smoked marijuana would not be to develop marijuana as a licensed drug but rather to serve as a first step toward the development of non-smoked rapid-onset cannabinoid delivery systems." In this way, the issue of medical marijuana would quickly become a thing of the past.

Our fourth recommendation is that a consistent effort should be maintained to discourage all use of marijuana even if at some future time its illegal status is changed. The risks of using marijuana are great. Every year, about 100,000 people seek help in kicking the marijuana habit. The church could play a significant role here as only Jesus Christ can fill the void that marijuana abusers experience.

Dosage

Marinol is usually prescribed by physicians in doses of 5 to 15 mg every two to four hours for nausea and vomiting due to chemotherapy, or 2.5 to 10 mg twice a day for appetite stimulation in people with AIDS.

Treatment Categories

Conventional Therapy
> Orally as pure cannabinoid (Marinol, not the marijuana plant) for moderately effective relief of nausea and vomiting with chemotherapy and AIDS-related weight loss

Complementary Therapy
> When inhaled in rare, very specific instances for chronic disease-caused nausea and vomiting or appetite loss associated with weight loss, *provided marijuana is legal in that jurisdiction* and the patient fully understands the physical and mental risks, and that possible benefits exceed the risks

When inhaled to produce a euphoric effect, in rare, specific instances of terminal or severe chronic disease *provided marijuana is legal in that jurisdiction* and the patient fully understands the physical and mental risks, and that possible benefits exceed the risks

When inhaled for anorexia and appetite loss associated with AIDS wasting, *provided marijuana is legal in that jurisdiction* and the patient fully understands the physical and mental risks, and that possible benefits exceed risks

Scientifically Unproven
Other indications

Further Reading

Grinspoon, Lester, and James B. Bakalar, "Marihuana as Medicine: A Plea for Reconsideration," *Journal of the American Medical Association* 273, no. 23 (June 1997): 1875–76.

Hubbard, John R., Sharone E. Franco, and Emmanuel S. Onaivi, "Marijuana: Medical Implications," *American Family Physician* 60, no. 9 (December 1999): 2583–93.

Jellin, Jeff M., Forrest Batz, and Kathy Hichens, *Pharmacist's Letter/Prescriber's Letter: Natural Medicines Comprehensive Database* (Stockton, Calif.: Therapeutic Research Facility, 1999), 619–20.

Joy, Janet E., Stanley J. Watson, and John A. Benson, *Marijuana and Medicine: Assessing the Science Base* (Washington, D.C.: National Academy Press, 1999).

Physicians' Desk Reference, "Marinol®," (Montvale, N.J.: Medical Economics, 2000), 2709–11.

Zhang, Zuo-Feng, Hal Morgenstern, Margaret R. Spitz, Donald P. Tashkin, Guo-Pei Yu, James R. Marshall, T. C. Hsu, and Stimson P. Schantz, "Marijuana Use and Increased Risk of Squamous Cell Carcinoma of the Head and Neck," *Cancer Epidemiology, Biomarkers & Prevention* 8, no. 12 (December 1999): 1071–78.

MEGAVITAMIN THERAPY

What It Is

Megavitamin therapy, also called "orthomolecular therapy," involves taking large doses of vitamins, minerals, and amino acids to treat a variety of physical and psychological illnesses. The therapy is based on the belief that when a group is given the identical diet, rich in nutrients and everything needed to sustain good health, some individuals in the group will actually absorb fewer nutrients than others. This inability to absorb adequate nutrients from proper diet alone is believed to lead to the development of different illnesses.

Some of the proponents of megavitamin therapy maintain that vitamins and minerals can cure illnesses in the same manner as drugs. Instead of thinking of them as nutrients required for normal metabolism, the practitioners prescribe vitamins and minerals tailored to believed medical needs. The doses recommended are vastly higher than the Recommended Dietary Allowance (RDA). The RDAs for vitamins were originally in large part an arbitrary measurement. If you compare the original RDAs for various vitamins with the same figure today, you will see differences in some cases. Our knowledge about vitamin supplements, our bodies' nutritional needs, and the long-term impact of various quantities of nutrients has increased over the years. There may be solid evidence that what was once considered safe is actually causing problems for some. And other substances, like chromium, are being added to the list of required nutrients. Megavitamin therapy goes far beyond the RDA recommendations.

For example, in the 1960s, Nobel Prize winner Dr. Linus Pauling, a biochemist, promoted his belief that the use of megadoses of vitamin C could do everything from cure the common cold to treat some forms of cancer. At that time he was taking at least 10 grams (10,000 mg) of vitamin C per day. Studies later indicated many benefits from vitamin C, but did not validate his anecdotal comments or such high doses. In fact, the megadoses Pauling was consuming are believed to cause an increased risk of kidney stones for some people.

The RDA has gone from an often arbitrary number to one that is more scientifically refined. Though not yet perfect, doses dramatically higher than the RDA put users at risk for potentially serious problems. Proponents of megavitamin therapy, when discussing why they feel it should be ignored, stress the early nature of the RDA as an "educated guess" and not the present reality.

Claims

The earliest uses of megavitamin therapy were in the treatment of schizophrenia, for which vitamin B_3 (niacin) was recommended. Soon after this, Dr. Linus Pauling made his recommendations about vitamin C.

Megavitamin therapy became popular in the 1970s for developmentally challenged children, especially those with attention deficit hyperactivity disorder (ADHD). The therapy appears to come and go in popularity, claiming effectiveness in a wide range of conditions from acne and mild depression to arthritis and Down's syndrome.

Study Findings

Some diseases are caused by drastically reduced abilities to absorb or use vitamins. However, these are not very common and are well known to physicians. The vast majority of illnesses for which megavitamin therapy is recommended have not been linked to vitamin deficiencies at all. Even if the vitamins were acting by some unknown mechanism, studies have not found megavitamin therapy to be effective.

A number of controlled studies (✗✗✗✗) in the 1980s examined megavitamin therapy in ADHD children, and consistently found little evidence for any improvements. Some children had poorer behavior when on the therapy. The evidence is just as unconvincing in other areas.

A *Consumer Reports* survey (✗✗) in May 2000 of nearly 47,000 Americans looked at megavitamin therapy. For problems in which megavitamins were reported to "help much," allergic disorders were helped only 32 percent of the time, whereas prescription drugs helped "much" 51 percent of the time and "somewhat" 32 percent of the time. Respiratory infections were helped "much" only 25 percent of the time, whereas prescription drugs helped "much" 60 percent and "somewhat" 23 percent of the time. For arthritis, the megavitamins helped "much" only 27 percent of the time. The responses to megavitamins are about what we would expect with a placebo effect.

One of the explanations for this poor response may be poor product quality. Concerns about the quality and purity of multivitamins sold in the United States are being addressed. ConsumerLab.com is an independent testing company that permits promoters to use its flask-shaped seal of approval on products that pass its criteria—usually meeting generally accepted standards concerning the quantity of active ingredients in the preparation. It released the results of tests of multivitamin products in 2001, which can be viewed on the company's subscription based Website. Twenty-seven multivitamin products were tested, of which nine failed to contain the amounts of vitamins listed on the label. Another four had amounts of some vitamins that exceeded the Tolerable Upper Intake Level (UL), although the products were made before some new ULs were set. Nonetheless, half of the products did not meet accepted standards. Those taking megadoses of vitamins must be aware of this lack of quality.

Cautions

The Dietary Reference Intake recommendations issued in 2000 for antioxidant vitamins included a UL. This is the highest level likely to pose no risk of adverse health effects for almost everyone. Intakes exceeding the UL have increased risks of adverse effects. The UL for vitamin C was set at 2000 mg per day based on the risk of serious diarrhea and the possibility of pro-oxidant effects. The UL for vitamin E is 1000 mg per day based on the increased risk of hemorrhage due to its anticoagulant properties.

A number of other vitamins are known to have toxic effects in high doses. Vitamin D in large quantities can lead to muscle weakness, bone pain, and high blood pressure. Chronic overdosing of vitamin A can result in joint pain, cracked skin, bone abnormalities, and anemia. A single overdose can lead to nausea, vomiting, headache, blurred vision, and lack of muscle coordination. Large doses of vitamin A can lead to visual problems in children, and are suspected of causing deformities in unborn babies. In January 2001, the UL for vitamin A was set at 3 mg per day.

A number of vitamins, especially the B group, can interfere with one another's absorption. High doses of one can lead to deficiencies of others. The same is true of certain minerals. Use of megavitamin therapy in children is particularly popular, yet unwarranted. The February 2000 issue of *Pediatrics* reported (✘) the death of a two-year-old due to excessive magnesium from megavitamin therapy recommended by a dietitian, but without the child's physician being informed.

Recommendations

Vitamins (derived from the combination of the terms "vital" and "amines") are an essential part of our diet, but adequate amounts are usually available from a healthy, balanced diet. A general multivitamin preparation is more than adequate to make up for any shortages most people in developed countries might have. Megavitamin therapy has been tested as a treatment for numerous conditions, ranging from ADHD and mental retardation in children to the flu and cancer in adults, and found to have little or no benefit. The risks of overdosing on some of the vitamins are significant, warranting avoidance of this therapy. This is especially the case with children.

Some of the conditions for which megavitamin therapy is recommended are chronic and difficult to endure. Patients are willing to try anything, especially something "natural" that seems safe. These products are no more natural than pharmaceuticals and are not regulated to ensure their quality. Unfortunately the treatments are ineffective and will not provide relief. Anyone who does try this approach should inform his or her physician so that any related developments can be monitored.

Treatment Categories

Scientifically Unproven
For any indication ☹☹

Scientifically Questionable

Quackery
As promoted by some proponents

Further Reading

Institute of Medicine, *Dietary Reference Intakes for Vitamin C, Vitamin E, Selenium, and Carotenoids* (Washington, D.C.: National Academy Press, 2000).

Nutrition Committee, Canadian Paediatric Society, "Megavitamin and Megamineral Therapy in Childhood," *Canadian Medical Association Journal* 143, no. 10 (November 1990): 1009–13.

MILK THISTLE

What It Is

Milk thistle has long been a staple of folk medicine throughout Europe, and it still is a top-selling herbal supplement (more than $18 million in annual sales in Germany alone, which is roughly six times the rising U.S. sales). For many years it was considered valuable for lactating women who needed a boost in their milk production, though studies have now proven that it is ineffective for this purpose. Still common is its use as a liver tonic and digestive aid.

Milk thistle of the variety called *Silybum marianum* (previously called *Carduus marianus*) is found widely in Europe, Eastern Africa, and North America. A member of the aster family, milk thistle grows to a height of up to ten feet. It bears a bright purple brushlike flower, and, in summer, it produces black seeds from which the drug is derived.

Milk thistle has been known by a number of other common names, including holy thistle, St. Mary thistle, marian thistle, lady's thistle, and royal thistle. Its spiritual names stem from the belief that the white veins on the plant's leaves carried the milk of the Virgin Mary. Its chivalrous names come from the fact that in England it was found growing near Dumbarton Castle.

Claims

For 2000 years, the milk thistle has been used as a medicinal herb. The Latin name, *Silybum*, was derived by Dioscorides, an herbalist in ancient Greece who used the term *silybon* to describe thistle-like plants. Pliny the Elder, a Roman writer (A.D. 23–79), recorded that the plant's juice was excellent for "carrying off bile." Culpepper (1787), an English herbalist, described its use in removing obstructions to the liver and spleen and as a remedy for jaundice. The Eclectics, a late nineteenth-century school of medical herbalists, used milk thistle for congestion in the liver, spleen, kidney, varicose veins, and in menstrual disorders. Milk thistle is widely used in Europe, where it has been commercially available for almost thirty years for such problems as dyspepsia, hepatitis, liver protection, loss of appetite, and diseases of the spleen. It has been used intravenously to treat people poisoned by the *Amanita phalloides* mushroom (also called Death Cap).

Study Findings

In searching for ways to use milk thistle medicinally, a number of properties and biochemical actions have been considered. These include antioxidation, liver cell regeneration through protein synthesis, and membrane stabilization. Many of these studies have used a compound isolated from milk thistle called "silymarin," which is not the same as using the plant material itself. One study (✔✔✔) of acute viral hepatitis treated with silymarin suggested improved outcomes. However, more recent studies (✘✘✘✘) of people with acute hepatitis B infections and people with alcoholism did not confirm these results.

The results of studies of silymarin and chronic liver disease are likewise mixed. One study (✔✔) in alcoholics with cirrhosis showed improvement of liver function with silymarin (140 mg three times a day). However, a larger and randomized controlled trial (✘✘✘) in alcoholics showed that both silymarin and placebo gave similar improvements in laboratory and liver biopsy. In one case series (✔✔) in which milk thistle was used in patients with hepatitis C, it was purported to help, while in another series (✘✘) it was of no help.

Two studies are frequently quoted to support the use of milk thistle, but both have been criticized for having weaknesses. One recently published study (✘✘✘) was unable to confirm an improved life expectancy benefit with silymarin for cirrhosis, but suggested an improved life expectancy for hepatitis C patients (no deaths in thirteen patients receiving silymarin, versus four deaths in sixteen receiving placebo), although this difference was not statistically significant.

Another recent study (✔✔✔) looked at silymarin to see if it reduced the side effects of a drug called "tacrine" when it is used in patients with Alzheimer's disease. Although silymarin was not shown to prevent tacrine-induced liver inflammation, it did reduce the rate of gastrointestinal and other side effects (like dry mouth, drowsiness, and dizziness) without any impact on the mental status of these Alzheimer's patients. These authors concluded that silymarin (at a dose of 420 mg per day) could be coadministered with tacrine to improve tolerability in the initial phases of treating Alzheimer's disease.

The German Commission E, an expert committee responsible for evaluating the safety and efficacy of herbal medicines, has recommended milk thistle as supportive treatment for chronic inflammatory liver conditions.

Cautions

No serious adverse effects have been seen with milk thistle. Animals subjected to high doses of milk thistle have shown no toxic effects. Some patients report loose stools. In the largest clinical trial, joint aches, headaches, and hives were rarely reported. There are no reported drug interactions. There is no reliable information showing that it is safe for children or women who are pregnant or lactating.

Recommendations

Milk thistle has become a popular herbal supplement for hepatitis and cirrhosis. There is extensive laboratory and animal data suggesting a liver protective benefit with silymarin. However, the clinical studies in humans are mixed. Most European studies used Legalon®, available in the U.S. as Thisylin®. The positive studies in alcoholic hepatitis and cirrhosis showing improved liver function tests and longer life must be viewed alongside studies that are equally well done and that show milk thistle to be no better than placebo.

There are no published controlled trials of milk thistle for hepatitis C, although investigators at Cedars-Sinai in Los Angeles have recently initiated one. For patients with hepatitis or cirrhosis, milk thistle appears to be safe and inexpensive. For patients with alcoholic liver disease, abstinence from alcohol remains the cornerstone of therapy, and, for patients at risk for hepatitis A and B, vaccines are available. For patients with chronic hepatitis C, milk thistle remains unproven. For patients with acute viral hepatitis, alcoholic hepatitis, and cirrhosis, a modest benefit may exist, but the evidence remains inconclusive.

Patients may wish to try milk thistle for chronic hepatitis but should know the evidence only suggests a benefit in early cirrhosis and chronic hepatitis.

Dosage

A typical dose is 200 to 400 mg of extract per day, although up to 800 mg daily has been evaluated in studies. German Commission E recommends a formulation standardized to at least 70 percent silymarin. Unfortunately, there is no guarantee in the United States that products so labeled actually contain this much silymarin. Therefore, buy only reputable brands. No one makes recommendations for duration of therapy.

Treatment Categories

Complementary Therapy (based on silymarin content)

Acute viral hepatitis	☺☺☺
Alcoholic hepatitis	☺☺
Cirrhosis	☺☺
Dyspeptic complaints	☺☺
Treating toxic liver damage	☺☺
Supportive treatment for chronic inflammatory liver disease and chronic hepatitis	☺☺
Hepatitis C	☺
Reducing side effects of tacrine in patients with Alzheimer's disease	☺☺

Scientifically Unproven
Other indications

Further Reading

DerMarderosian, Ara, ed., "Milk Thistle," in *The Review of Natural Products* (St. Louis, Mo.: Facts and Comparisons, January 1997).

Jellin, Jeff M., Forrest Batz, and Kathy Hichens, *Pharmacist's Letter/Prescriber's Letter: Natural Medicines Comprehensive Database* (Stockton, Calif.: Therapeutic Research Facility, 1999), 641–43.

Schulz, Volker, Rudolf Hänsel, and Varro Tyler, *Rational Phytotherapy: A Physician's Guide to Herbal Medicine*, 3d ed. (Berlin, Germany: Springer-Verlag, 1998), 214–16.

PENNYROYAL

What It Is

People who grow their own mint for use as a salad garnish or for tea occasionally become all too familiar with the herb pennyroyal. Both mint and pennyroyal are from the variety of plants scientifically known as the *Mentha* genus. However, while mint is quite harmless, pennyroyal, known officially as either *Hedeoma pulegioides* or *Mentha pulegium*, can cause poisonings when consumed (as sometimes occurs when it is mistaken for mint tea).

Claims

Pennyroyal is commonly available as an herbal remedy for skin diseases in children and to control fleas in pets. It has been used in the past for colic, gas, bowel stimulation, stomach pain, colds, digestive disorders, respiratory ailments, and as a diuretic. Most problematically, however, pennyroyal has been recommended since Roman times as a way to induce abortions despite its potentially lethal effects on the liver.

Study Findings

No studies support any use of pennyroyal. Its oil contains a number of compounds called "monoterpenes." One called "pulegone" is present in larger quantities in pennyroyal than in any other mint oil. Pulegone is highly toxic to the liver, lungs, and nervous system. Pennyroyal has been reported to cause abdominal pain and cramping, fever, nausea and vomiting, confusion, delirium, seizures, loss of consciousness, hallucinations, elevations in blood pressure and heart rate, lung congestion, liver failure, kidney failure, bleeding, respiratory failure, and death.

Cautions

Pennyroyal poisonings (✗✗) are regularly encountered at poison centers around the United States. People have died from taking pennyroyal, including many women who have tried to self-induce an abortion. When larger amounts are taken, people experience severe liver damage, which can lead to multiple organ failure. Poisonings also occur with smaller amounts when people mistakenly use pennyroyal to make mint tea. Symptoms are less severe for adults in these cases, although in young children even small amounts of pennyroyal tea have been fatal.

Recommendations

Pennyroyal is highly toxic and should *not* be used under any circumstances. The consequences of using the wrong plant material should lead people to be very careful in selecting their mint and be cautious about giving any form of mint tea to children.

Dosage

Avoid completely. Poisonous.

Treatment Categories

Scientifically Unproven
WARNING: DEADLY ☹☹☹☹

Further Reading

Anderson, Ilene B., W. H. Mullen, J. E. Meeker, S. C. Khojasteh-Bakht, S. Oishi, S. D. Nelson, and P. D. Blanc, "Pennyroyal Toxicity: Measurement of Toxic Metabolite Levels in Two Cases and Review of the Literature," *Annals of Internal Medicine* 124 (1996): 726–34.

Jellin, Jeff M., Forrest Batz, and Kathy Hichens, *Pharmacist's Letter/Prescriber's Letter: Natural Medicines Comprehensive Database* (Stockton, Calif.: Therapeutic Research Facility, 1999), 716–18.

PYRUVATE

What It Is

Most American herbal remedy buyers who are not experiencing a short-term or chronic illness are usually seeking to influence one of three factors in their lives—weight, sex, and longevity. A best-selling book could be created around the title *How to Live Forever Loving Your Way to a Slimmer You*. This is why anytime someone can promote a compound that influences one of these three areas, you will see a rush to buy it in health food stores. Websites will tout the positive history for the alleged therapy. And newspapers and magazines will have full-page advertisements for one brand or another.

Such is the case with pyruvate (also called "pyruvic acid"), one of the compounds normally formed when your body breaks down glucose to obtain energy from your diet. In the 1970s it was noticed that animals gained less weight and stored less body fat when their diets were supplemented with pyruvate along with a similar compound called "dihydroxyacetone" (DHA). Interest in pyruvate exploded in late 1997 after the previous "big thing" in weight loss, an inappropriate mix of drugs popularly called Fen-Phen, was taken off the market. Fen-Phen was supposed to increase weight loss and seemed to achieve that end for many people. It also caused heart valve damage in some patients and was suspected of causing the death of one twenty-nine-year-old woman. Although each drug alone had been shown to be relatively safe, using the two drugs in combination had neither been tested nor approved.

Pyruvate rapidly began to replace Fen-Phen as the Holy Grail of dieters.

Claims

Internet sites abound with claims that pyruvate is a powerful "fat burner." It's said to boost overall weight loss by 37 percent and increase fat loss by 48 percent. These numbers are quoted straight from one of the research studies, adding much supposed credibility to the advertisements. Pyruvate is also supposed to lower cholesterol levels, improve the health of the heart, and increase exercise endurance by 20 percent (making it popular among athletes). One Website promotes pyruvate to "inhibit tumor growth."

Study Findings

The Internet sites we have seen state that their claims are based on twenty-five years of scientific research, published in respectable journals. This is true. What is not noted is that most of the research was done on animals, which is only one of the earliest steps in the evaluation process. Such positive results lead to hopeful conclusions and then to testing on humans, but unfortunately with pyruvate, the human tests are neither extensive nor conclusive.

For example, seven human studies were published before 1999, and all were coordinated by the same researcher. Two studies (✔✔✔) found some improved athletic endurance with pyruvate, but they used few subjects and they were all untrained males. The effects in trained athletes could be very different, and they are usually the ones taking the supplement for this purpose. For example, a study (✘✘✘) published on the effect of pyruvate on American football players concluded that it was ineffective for anaerobic performance and body composition.

Pyruvate's effect on weight loss has received the most attention, leading to four published studies (✔✔✔). However, these were conducted under conditions very different from everyday life. For example, three of the studies involved women weighing more than 220 pounds (on average), who were on severely restricted liquid diets while confined to bed in a special research unit in a hospital. Control groups in similar conditions were included. Those given the supplement received between 15 and 44 grams of pyruvate daily, along with similar amounts of DHA. This is many times the 1 to 5 grams of pyruvate daily recommended by the promoters of the supplement, and most commercial pyruvate products contain no DHA. Therefore, the commercial products are completely different from what was tested in research.

Moreover, the research results were unimpressive. The women taking the supplements lost between 1.3 and 3.5 pounds more than the control group. The percent values quoted by promoters only arise because of how *little* weight all the participants lost. This inappropriate use of percentages may be seen better in an everyday example.

Suppose you are told you will be given $1 to spend the next hour cleaning a neighbor's garage. You are outraged. The garage is filthy and stacked with junk that needs to be hauled to the street-side for the trash collectors coming the next morning. The money is far from even the minimum wage.

"Okay," says the person seeking to have the work done. "I'll give you a 50 percent raise."

You are still outraged. The percentage sounds wonderful, but 50 percent more than a dollar is only $1.50, still far less than minimum wage for a difficult job.

On the other hand, suppose the offer is $1,000. When you are offered a 50 percent raise, you will be paid $500 more, a substantial increase.

The statistics used by the promoters of pyruvate for weight loss are quoting the equivalent of the $1 example. The patients in both groups only lost a few pounds, so losing 37 percent more with pyruvate makes little practical difference, especially since these women all wanted to lose much more weight. This is a good example of a study showing statistical significance, but *not* clinical (or real-world) significance. Promoters don't make this clear in their advertisements. Beware advertisements with percents that don't also include the actual numbers measured!

Very small clinical trials (✔✔✔✔) report that dietary supplementation with dihydroxyacetone and pyruvate increased arm and leg exercise endurance. Animal studies suggest that a liquid diet supplemented with pyruvate might inhibit breast tumor growth. One other study (✔✔✔) found that pyruvate reduced cholesterol levels, but other studies (✘✘✘✘) found no effect on cholesterol levels.

Cautions

Between one-half and two-thirds of the research subjects (✘✘) receiving pyruvate had diarrhea or other intestinal disturbances. While not too harmful, these could become more serious if they continued for very long. Other side effects include gas and bloating. Weight-loss supplements are often taken for extended periods, and no studies have been done on pyruvate's long-term safety, or effectiveness. Pyruvate should not be taken during pregnancy or lactation as there is insufficient information available to establish its safety. Pyruvate should not be given to children as there is no data to establish its safety. In addition, there has been one reported death in a child given pyruvate intravenously.

Recommendations

Anyone who struggles with weight knows how complicated and difficult it can be to lose weight. While drugs and supplements may have a place in dieting regimens for some people, long-term success requires significant lifestyle changes, including diet and exercise, as well as psychological and spiritual considerations (see Diets and Dieting, page 181). Quick-fix pills are not realistic answers. You should be very cautious using any "diet pill" without proper medical supervision.

Dosage

Studies have used 22 to 44 grams a day along with DHA, although proponents often recommend much lower doses.

Treatment Categories

Complementary Therapy
High cholesterol	☹
Promoting weight loss	☹☹
Improving athletic performance	☹
Increasing arm or leg endurance	☺

Scientifically Unproven
Other medical indications

Possible Quackery or Fraud
Weight loss
Athletic performance enhancement

Further Reading

Jellin, Jeff M., Forrest Batz, and Kathy Hichens, *Pharmacist's Letter/Prescriber's Letter: Natural Medicines Comprehensive Database* (Stockton, Calif.: Therapeutic Research Facility, 1999), 772–73.

O'Mathúna, Dónal P., "Pyruvate for Weight Loss," *Alternative Medicine Alert* 2, no. 3 (March 1999): 31–34.

Sukala, William R., "Pyruvate: Beyond The Marketing Hype," *International Journal of Sport Nutrition* 8 (1998): 241–49.

RED YEAST RICE

What It Is

Lovers of Chinese food have long been familiar with red yeast rice, though they usually do not realize that fact. A number of Chinese fish and meat dishes have a red color that comes from red yeast. Red yeast rice is the product of rice fermented with the *Monascus purpureus* yeast. It is used as a food preservative and flavor enhancer and for making red rice wine.

In the United States, a proprietary dietary supplement containing red yeast is called Cholestin™ and is sold as capsules filled with the red-orange-colored red yeast rice. Use of this natural medicine is mentioned in a traditional Chinese medicine book called the *Ben Cao Gang Mu*, written during the Ming Dynasty (1368–1644). The medical text states that red yeast rice is helpful in improving blood circulation and reducing blood clotting.

The red yeast rice is used as either a dried powder called "Zhitai," or extracted with alcohol to remove the rice gluten and called "Xuezhikang." Cholestin most closely resembles Zhitai.

Claims

Red yeast rice is sold as a dietary supplement, which means that it is not subject to the testing required by the FDA of all drugs. That designation also means the manufacturer cannot claim it cures or treats any disease. However, a claim that it improves the functioning of the body is acceptable. The FDA has contested in court the validity of the manufacturer's claim that Cholestin, one particular brand of red yeast rice, is a dietary supplement, but lost the case. The FDA claimed that Cholestin is actually a drug and should be regulated like pharmaceutical agents. The judge disagreed, ruling that Cholestin, as defined under the Dietary Supplement Health and Education Act of 1994, is a dietary supplement.

Red yeast rice is said to promote healthy blood cholesterol levels. Some say that it both controls high cholesterol levels in patients with elevated levels and maintains desirable levels of cholesterol in those with normal levels. This is important because high cholesterol levels are known to promote the buildup of plaque in arteries (atherosclerosis). This restricts the flow of blood through the vessels, which can lead to increased blood pressure and a higher chance of heart attacks or strokes.

Study Findings

Cholesterol is actually present in the blood in a number of different forms, including low-density lipoproteins (LDL) and high-density lipoproteins (HDL). Blood tests are reported in terms of total cholesterol, LDL cholesterol, and HDL cholesterol. Studies

(✔✔✔) have found that having low values for the first two measures (total cholesterol and LDL) and a high value for the third (HDL) is most desirable. A number of studies in China (✔✔✔) have shown that both Zhitai and Xuezhikang reduce total cholesterol and LDL cholesterol levels, while simultaneously increasing the HDL cholesterol level.

The first clinical trial of Cholestin (✔✔✔), the United States product, was published in February 1999, and reported that it reduced total cholesterol by 16 percent and LDL cholesterol by 22 percent, but left HDL cholesterol levels unchanged.

These are very encouraging results, but not unexpected. Conventional medicine has been using a group of drugs called "statins" since 1987 to reduce cholesterol levels. The first of these was isolated from yeast of the same genus as that used in red yeast rice. That compound was called "lovastatin," and is commercially available as a drug called Mevacor®. Analysis of Cholestin reveals that it also contains lovastatin, along with several other statinlike compounds. Taking the daily recommended dose gives a person the equivalent of about 10 mg of statins. Patients (✔✔✔✔) given 10 mg of Mevacor had a 17 percent reduction in LDL cholesterol, almost the same as that obtained from Cholestin. Therefore, taking Cholestin may be practically the same as taking low-dose Mevacor. The FDA sought to have Cholestin regulated like Mevacor, in the belief that its active ingredients are basically the same, but lost their case in court.

While evidence supports the medical use of statins by people with high cholesterol levels, we are not aware of any evidence demonstrating that healthy people with normal cholesterol levels will benefit from taking any red yeast rice product.

Cautions

Studies of Cholestin and its Chinese equivalents reported no adverse effects other than stomach disturbance in a small number of patients. However, Mevacor has been found to cause liver damage, muscle pain, and kidney damage in a small number of patients. For these reasons, patients taking Mevacor are cautioned to have their livers checked regularly.

Because developing fetuses require cholesterol in unique ways, these drugs may harm the unborn. Animal studies have found abnormalities in developing bones. Hence, these products are not recommended for women who might become, or already are, pregnant. The FDA rating for lovastatin is an X rating, meaning that it should never be taken in pregnancy. We can find no studies showing the products are safe in lactating women, and therefore they would best be avoided while breast-feeding.

Given that red yeast rice contains the same type of drugs as contained in the pharmaceutical statins, the same cautions and concerns should exist with it. While the presence of other constituents in the preparation may act to prevent some of these side effects, this has not been demonstrated in long-term studies. One of the reasons why some drugs are available only on prescription is to ensure adequate monitoring by physicians. Since red yeast rice is available as an unregulated dietary supplement, people will use it to self-medicate without having the blood tests necessary to monitor for any liver damage. While this will not be a problem for the majority of people, it may be for others—and we have no way of predicting whose liver might be damaged by any of the statins. Furthermore, without monitoring of blood cholesterol levels, some people may take it without needing to, and others with very high cholesterol levels may not reduce their cholesterol enough.

Last, but not least, taking red yeast rice within 24 hours of ingesting grapefruit products may dramatically increase the levels of red yeast rice in the bloodstream and increase the risk of adverse effects. If you choose to take red yeast rice, avoid grapefruit products.

Recommendations

Cholestin appears to be a natural remedy that does what it claims to do—at least for those with elevated cholesterol levels; however, there is no evidence that it helps those with normal levels of cholesterol or triglycerides (a general term for all blood lipids). People with mildly elevated cholesterol levels may benefit from it. It is less expensive than the pharmaceutical products, but then it also comes unmonitored. While Cholestin is manufactured under high-quality conditions and is of standardized strength, nothing prevents the sale of low-quality products by less scrupulous companies. For those taking red yeast rice, we recommend they ask their personal physician about regular blood tests. Also, as its producers state, cholesterol levels are best kept in check by a combined strategy of diet, exercise, stress reduction, and, in some cases, drug therapy.

Dosage

The usual dose is 1200 mg twice a day, taken with food.

Treatment Categories

Complementary Therapy
Lowering elevated cholesterol or triglyceride levels ☺☺☺☺

Scientifically Unproven
Controlling normal cholesterol or triglyceride levels
Any other indication

Further Reading

Heber, David, *Natural Remedies for a Healthy Heart* (Garden City Park, N.Y.: Avery, 1998).

Jellin, Jeff, M. Forrest Batz, and Kathy Hichens, *Pharmacist's Letter/Prescriber's Letter: Natural Medicines Comprehensive Database* (Stockton, Calif.: Therapeutic Research Facility, 1999), 786–87.

SAW PALMETTO

What It Is

Saw palmetto might be called the "great berry hope" of the aging male population. Rumored to at least maintain and possibly improve a man's sex life (some herbalists consider it to be an aphrodisiac), it has a history of use for genital and urinary tract problems. This was especially true with the Native Americans who also used the berries to create a tonic that was believed to improve nutritional health. In the first half of the twentieth century, saw palmetto tea was included in *The United States Pharmacopoeia* and *The National Formulary.*

Saw palmetto is a small palm tree found along the southeastern coasts of the United States and in the West Indies. It is also called the American dwarf palm tree, the palmetto shrub, or the Cabbage Palm. Its most common scientific name is *Serenoa repens;* however, scientific synonyms include *Sabal serrulata* and *Serenoa serrulata.* It produces blue-black berries early in the winter, and the herbal remedy is extracted from these.

Claims

Saw palmetto extract has been used traditionally as an aphrodisiac, a tonic for the male reproductive system, and a remedy for respiratory complaints, urinary conditions, migraine headaches, genital problems, and cancer. It has also been promoted to restore hair growth and to increase breast size. It is currently used most commonly for problems related to enlargement of the prostate gland. Benign prostatic hyperplasia (BPH) is the most common nonmalignant tumor in men (which means it does not spread, and thus is usually less serious than metastatic cancers).

Most men over sixty years of age have BPH resulting in numerous urinary problems, which are irritating, frustrating, and embarrassing. While conventional pharmaceuticals are available, most commonly drugs called "finasteride" (Proscar®) or "alpha blockers" (Hytrin®, Cardura®, Flomax®), these have the potential for serious side effects such as impotence and dizziness. Recently the alpha blockers have been associated with increased death rates in patients with hypertension or heart disease. A natural, safe treatment available without a prescription is a very attractive option for many patients.

Study Findings

Most of the studies on saw palmetto extract have been done in Europe with a standardized preparation called Prostagult®. Many of these used small numbers of patients, but recent studies have been larger and better controlled. A review of this research found eighteen controlled trials, nine of which were evaluated as well controlled. Overall, these studies (✔✔✔) found saw palmetto extract almost twice as effective as placebo for improving urinary flow and relieving the symptoms of BPH.

When studies (✔✔✔) compared the extract to finasteride, they were equally effective, but people taking the berry preparation reported fewer problems with impotence. However, these studies used numerous types of saw palmetto preparations, and were for relatively short duration (almost all for less than six months).

Some experts feel that saw palmetto may be most useful in stages I and II (early stage) BPH. Stage I is characterized by increased frequency of urination during the day and night, delayed onset of urination, and a weak stream. Stage II is characterized by the symptoms of stage I accompanied by failure to completely empty the bladder.

How saw palmetto might affect BPH is not precisely known. The extract contains a number of steroids that act somewhat like estrogen, the female sex hormone. The most active one of these, beta-sitosterol, was found (✔✔✔) to be as effective as pharmaceutical drugs used for BPH. It is felt to inhibit dihydrotestosterone (DHT). Increased levels of DHT in the prostate gland are believed to be one cause of BPH. Theoretically, decreasing DHT could reduce the symptoms of BPH. In addition, saw palmetto may inhibit an enzyme (5-alpha-reductase) in the prostate gland that breaks down testosterone to DHT.

There is no convincing evidence that saw palmetto is effective in the treatment or prevention of prostate cancer.

Cautions

Side effects reported in clinical trials have been relatively mild, including headache, nausea, and dizziness. The compounds in saw palmetto that are most likely to be beneficial for BPH are water insoluble—not water soluble—so teas made from the plant material are not likely to have any benefit. Concerns that saw palmetto might falsely raise the PSA (prostate specific antigen) level in men have not proven to be true.

Almost all the clinical research was done on standardized European extracts, which may differ from products available in the U.S. Therefore, caution is needed in choosing reliable products. For example, one independent group, ConsumerLab.com, purchased twenty-seven leading brands of saw palmetto in November and December 1999 in order to determine whether they possessed the minimum amounts of specific fatty acids and sterols commonly found in saw palmetto products used in published clinical trials. These compounds should make up at least 85 percent of the weight of the plant material used in a product. Six of the twenty-seven saw palmetto products were not tested because their labels claimed they had been standardized to levels of fatty acids below this 85 percent minimum—some claiming to have only 20 to 25 percent fatty acids. These products admitted they were below the recognized standard. Of the twenty-one remaining products tested, four did not contain the minimum amount used in published clinical trials.

Among the seventeen products that passed, most contained additional oils that were generally identified as being part of a "prostate formula." These combinations may or may not have additional benefit, as they have generally not been clinically tested. Only two products that passed appeared to contain only saw palmetto extract similar to that used in most clinical trials. The brand names of these products can be viewed at the subscription-based ConsumerLab.com Website (*www.consumerlab.com*).

This apparent poor product quality may explain the high rate of American dissatisfaction with saw palmetto. In May 2000, *Consumer Reports* published a survey (✗✗) of nearly 47,000 Americans. Nearly 37 percent of those with prostate problems reported using saw palmetto. Of these, 46 percent reported that it helped "little to none" and only 21 percent reported it helped "much."

The Natural Database rates saw palmetto as "Likely Unsafe" in pregnancy and contraindicated lactation because of its steroids.

Recommendations

Saw palmetto appears to be beneficial for relief of an enlarged prostate gland in many men. However, the evidence for this is based on a Prostagult (German). This is now available in the U.S. as ProstActive® and a Quanterra® product. BPH is a condition for which treatment may be needed for many years. No studies have been done on people taking saw palmetto for extended periods of time. Caution is therefore needed, along with monitoring of vital functions. Before using saw palmetto, check with a health care professional for a proper diagnosis as symptoms of BPH may signal other more serious conditions that require treatment. Given its lower cost and few side effects, saw palmetto extract may be a helpful alternative for people with mild to moderate BPH.

Dosage

An extract is recommended at a dose of 160 mg twice a day or 320 mg once daily.

Treatment Categories

Complementary Therapy
   Benign prostatic hyperplasia (BPH)   ☺☺☺☺
Scientifically Unproven
   Prostate cancer
   Other indications

Further Reading

Barrette, E. P., "Use of Saw Palmetto Extract for Benign Prostatic Hyperplasia," *Alternative Medicine Alert* 1, no. 1 (January 1998): 1–4.

Jellin, Jeff M., Forrest Batz, and Kathy Hichens, *Pharmacist's Letter/Prescriber's Letter: Natural Medicines Comprehensive Database* (Stockton, Calif.: Therapeutic Research Facility, 1999), 820–22.

Wilt, Timothy, Areet Ishani, Gerold Stark, Roderick MacDonald, Joseph Lau, and Cynthia Mulrow, "Saw Palmetto Extracts for Treatment of Benign Prostatic Hyperplasia: A Systematic Review," *Journal of the American Medical Association* 280, no. 18 (November 1998): 1604–9.

SELENIUM

What It Is

Selenium is a naturally occurring mineral. The most abundant sources of what is known as organic selenium (chemically bonded to amino acids) are seafood, cereal grains, liver, and Brazil nuts. The last one is the richest source. Amino acids are the chemical building blocks of all proteins. Selenium also occurs in inorganic forms (as salts) and is thus, in many ways, similar to sulfur. It is required in the diet, with a number of diseases linked to its deficiency. Selenium plays a role in the body's antioxidant system, which may be how it impacts health. It attaches itself to certain enzymes (which are proteins) that are involved in the body's natural antioxidant system.

Claims

The main claim regarding selenium is that it helps prevent cancer. This has made it one of the best-selling dietary supplements. It is also reported to protect against heart disease, infertility, muscular dystrophy, rheumatoid arthritis, depression, and aging. Some alternative practitioners recommend selenium to treat AIDS and to prevent heart disease, atherosclerosis, macular degeneration of the eye, and premature graying of hair. Selenium is also said to protect the skin from the damaging effects of ultraviolet light.

Study Findings

For a long time, people have believed that selenium protects against cancer, heart ailments, and other diseases. But studies report conflicting conclusions. Animal studies have clearly demonstrated that selenium reduces the risk of cancer. Uncontrolled studies (✔✔) have found that those who have lower blood levels of selenium have higher incidences of cancer. However, in controlled studies, the results have been less positive, although some lowering of cancer rates has been found compared to placebo.

For example, a 1996 study using selenium came out of the University of Arizona and caused quite a stir. The Arizona Cancer Center started a randomized trial to study the ability of selenium supplements to protect against basal-cell and squamous-cell skin cancers. The researchers recruited 1,312 patients from the eastern United States, where selenium levels in the soil and crops are low and skin cancer rates are high. All the patients had a history of skin cancer. Half the group received a placebo pill every day for an average of 4.5 years, and the other half took pills with 200 micrograms of selenium each day.

The study (✗✗✗), published in the *Journal of the American Medical Association*, found that the selenium supplements had no effect on skin cancers; however, halfway through the study (✔✔✔), the researchers decided to look at other types of cancers and cancer mortality. They found some surprising results. The people who had taken selenium had 63 percent fewer prostate cancers, 58 percent fewer colorectal cancers, and 46 percent fewer lung cancers than the placebo treated group.

Overall, there were 39 percent fewer new cancers among those taking selenium and half as many died from their cancer. Since the selenium seemed to be so beneficial, the researchers stopped the placebo phase of the trial early so that everyone could benefit.

One clinical trial (✔✔✔) evaluated a combination of vitamin E with selenium and found it relieved joint pain and morning stiffness in arthritis patients when compared to placebo. However, it is not clear whether the effect was from one or both compounds.

There were many weaknesses in the Arizona study we just mentioned. For example, few women were included. Furthermore, the results are not consistent with those of other studies—even though those studies used lower doses of selenium. Therefore, the researchers and other cancer specialists are calling for further trials before any national recommendations are made about selenium supplementation to prevent cancer.

Cautions

A condition called selenosis occurs (✗✗) when people take more than 1 mg (1000 micrograms) of selenium daily. The effects range from a garliclike odor on the breath to loss of hair and nails, diarrhea, skin lesions, nausea, vomiting, fatigue, irritability, muscle tenderness, tremor, light-headedness, facial flushing, liver and kidney dysfunction, and, in the extreme—death. Those with thyroid problems are particularly prone to these side effects.

Selenium interacts with many drugs and other vitamins, such as vitamins E and C. Most dietary selenium occurs in its organic form, but commercial supplements often use inorganic selenium. The two do not act in the same way, with organic selenium being preferable.

The Natural Database rates selenium as "Likely Unsafe" when used in doses exceeding 400 micrograms per day. However, for practitioners recommending up to 1000 micrograms per day, blood levels can be followed to assess the risk of toxicity prior to the onset of symptoms. Selenium is rated "Likely Safe" in doses up to 400 micrograms per day. For women who are pregnant or lactating, doses above the RDA (65 micrograms for pregnancy, 75 micrograms for lactation) should not be exceeded. In the case of pregnancy, higher doses may cause birth defects or miscarriage.

Recommendations

It seems to us that there is sufficient evidence to warrant supplemental selenium in the diet. If you prefer to get your supplements in food, then you can get 120 micrograms of selenium in just one Brazil nut. However, remember to buy the shelled kind as they are grown in the region of Brazil that has soil rich in selenium. Other good sources are tuna, seafood, wheat germ, and bran.

Although more studies are needed, especially into the long-term effects of supplementation, selenium does appear to protect people against some types of cancers. However, caution should be exercised as this is one mineral producing toxicity at a relatively low level. If you take selenium and notice any changes in the strength or appearance of your fingernails, especially your thumbnails, you should immediately stop taking the selenium and discuss the matter with your primary health care provider.

Dosage

The Institute of Medicine report in early 2000 on antioxidants set the daily recommended intake level for selenium at 55 micrograms per day (65 micrograms for pregnancy and 75 micrograms for lactation). The old level was 70 micrograms for men and 55 micrograms for women. Food sources include seafood, liver, meat, and grains. The report also set the upper intake level for selenium at 400 micrograms per day. This maximum level is based on nutrients from all sources. More than this amount could, according to the report, cause selenosis, the toxic reaction described under cautions.

Treatment Categories

Conventional Therapy
    In doses up to 75 micrograms
        per day as an antioxidant   ☺☺☺☺

Complementary Therapy
    In doses up to 200 micrograms per day to
        prevent cancer mortality, total cancer incidence,
        and the incidence of lung, colon, rectal, and
        prostate cancers   ☺☺☺
    In doses up to 200 micrograms per day
        for arthritis pain and stiffness   ☺

Scientifically Unproven
    Other indications

Further Reading

Cirigliano, Michael D., and Philippe O. Szapary, "Selenium Supplementation for Cancer Prevention," *Alternative Medicine Alert* 2, no. 1 (January 1999): 3–7.

Clark, L. C., B. Dalkin, A. Krongrad, G. F. Combs Jr., B. W. Turnbull, E. H. Slate, R. Witherington, J. H. Herlong, E. Janosko, D. Carpenter, C. Borosso, S. Falk, and J. Rounder, "Decreased Incidence of Prostate Cancer with Selenium Supplementation: Results of a Double-Blind Cancer Prevention Trial," *British Journal of Urology* 81, no. 5 (May 1998): 730–34.

Clark, Larry C., Gerald F. Combs Jr., Bruce W. Turnbull, Elizabeth H. Slate, Dan K. Chalker, James Chow, Loretta S. Davis, Renee A. Glover, Gloria F. Graham, Earl G. Gross, Arnon Krongrad, Jack L. Lesher Jr., H. Kim Park, Beverly B. Sanders Jr., Cameron L. Smith, and J. Richard Taylor, "Effects of Selenium Supplementation for Cancer Prevention in Patients with Carcinoma of the Skin: A Randomized Controlled Trial," *Journal of the American Medical Association* 276, no. 24 (December 1996): 1957–63.

Jellin, Jeff M., Forrest Batz, and Kathy Hichens, *Pharmacist's Letter/Prescriber's Letter: Natural Medicines Comprehensive Database* (Stockton, Calif.: Therapeutic Research Facility, 1999), 833–34.

SENNA

What It Is

The senna shrub, known technically as *Cassia senna* (scientific synonyms include *Senna alexandrina* and *Cassia acutifolia*), has long been a part of medicine in the Middle East and northern Africa. The plant grew along the Nile River in the Sudan and Egypt where the leaves and berries were found to be a gentle laxative. Another form of senna, *Cassia angustifolia,* is found in India where its properties are said to be similar.

The Arab nations introduced senna throughout Europe around the ninth or tenth centuries. Since then it has remained a popular natural laxative and is available in many over-the-counter pharmaceutical products.

Claims

Senna has long been used to treat constipation and remains a popular laxative. In addition, senna has traditionally been used as a cathartic to clear toxins from the bowels. Native Americans used a senna species *(Cassia marilandica)* indigenous to eastern North America to reduce fevers. In a few cultures senna also has been used to kill intestinal worms, alleviate indigestion, and treat ringworm and hemorrhoids. Traditional healers in northern Africa used it to heal various types of stomach pain. An unlikely traditional use, given that senna tastes awful, was to use it as a mouthwash to freshen the breath.

Today, senna is used almost exclusively to treat constipation and constipation-related disorders like hemorrhoids and anal fissures. Senna is considered more potent than another widely used stimulant laxative, cascara sagrada bark (from the bush *Rhamnus purshiana*). Senna is sometimes combined with herbs such as ginger or coriander to avoid intestinal cramps. Senna is included for its laxative properties in some diet teas; however, the value of a laxative in promoting weight loss is considered questionable by most practitioners.

Study Findings

Compounds in senna called "anthracenes" stimulate the colon to contract more frequently, moving material through the intestines faster. These compounds also cause secretion of electrolytes and water into the intestines to facilitate movement. A small number of randomized controlled trials (✔✔✔) support the use of senna as an effective, relatively safe laxative when used occasionally.

Two recent studies have compared senna to other laxatives for treating the constipation suffered by patients with advanced cancer who are taking opioid drugs. In one study (✔✔✔), Spanish researchers determined that senna had similar efficacy and adverse effects when compared to the prescription laxative drug lactulose, but recommended senna due to its lower cost. In another study (✘✘✘), researchers in India found similar efficacy with senna and a liquid Ayurvedic herbal preparation, but recommended the latter due to its better taste and fewer side effects.

Researchers in France compared senna with polyethylene glycol to clear the bowels prior to surgery of the colon or rectum. In the randomized controlled trial (✔✔✔), the colons of the patients who took senna were cleaner and those patients reported it was easier to take than those taking the polyethylene glycol. Scientists in Egypt tested (✔✔✔) a species of senna *(Cassia italica)* found in Africa and parts of Europe for its potential effects on the central nervous system. They found that extracts had mild pain-relieving and sedative effects.

Cautions

Potential side effects (✘✘) from senna include diarrhea, nausea, and abdominal cramps or pains. Because of these side effects, most practitioners recommend trying milder laxatives before resorting to senna.

Pregnant or lactating women should avoid senna, as should anyone with acute or chronic intestinal diseases and persons taking diuretics, steroids, or licorice because senna interferes with their intestinal absorption. The Natural Database rates senna "Possibly Unsafe" in pregnancy and lactation. Senna should be used with caution by children under the age of twelve and not at all by children under six; however, it is rated

"Likely Safe" when the standardized nonprescription products are used orally and short-term following the directions on the label. Most practitioners recommend that senna not be taken for more than seven days at a time because after this people may lose their ability to have bowel movements without the help of a stimulant laxative.

Extended use can also lead to more serious adverse side effects from dehydration, potassium loss, and electrolyte imbalance, including muscle and heart ailments. In fact in 1996, California became the first state to require warning labels for products containing senna and other stimulant laxatives. Chronic use is also suspected of increasing the chances of getting colon cancer.

Recommendations

Senna is a readily available and inexpensive laxative. However, its effects may not occur for a number of hours and can then be rather dramatic! Less drastic products are commonly available. Senna teas contain varying amounts of active ingredients, while results with standardized laxative preparations are much more predictable and reliable. As with any laxative, senna should not be used for more than a week and is not a safe way to lose weight.

Dosage

Tablets usually contain 187 mg extract, with adults recommended to take two tablets at bedtime.

Treatment Categories

Conventional Therapy
Short-term treatment of constipation and constipation-
related disorders such as hemorrhoids and anal fissures ☺☺☺☺

Complementary Therapy
Evacuation of the bowel for medical indications and procedures ☺☺☺☺
Mild pain ☺
Sedative effects ☺

Scientifically Unproven
Other indications

Further Reading

Agra, Y., A. Sacristan, M. Gonzalez, M. Ferrari, A. Portugues, and M. J. Calvo, "Efficacy of Senna Versus Lactulose in Terminal Cancer Patients Treated with Opioids," *Journal of Pain Symptom Management* 15, no. 1 (January 1998): 1–7.
Foster, Steven, and Varro E. Tyler, *Tyler's Honest Herbal: A Sensible Guide to the Use of Herbs and Related Remedies*, 4th ed. (New York: Haworth Herbal Press, 1999), 355–57.

Jellin, Jeff M., Forrest Batz, and Kathy Hichens, *Pharmacist's Letter/Prescriber's Letter: Natural Medicines Comprehensive Database* (Stockton, Calif.: Therapeutic Research Facility, 1999), 836–37.

Valverde, Alain, Jean Marie Hay, Abe Fingerhut, Marie Jeanne Boudet, Roberta Petroni, Xavier Pouliquen, Simon Msika, and Yves Flamant, "Senna vs Polyethylene Glycol for Mechanical Preparation the Evening Before Elective Colonic or Rectal Resection: A Multicenter Controlled Trial," *Archives of Surgery* 134, no. 5 (May 1999): 514–19.

SHARK CARTILAGE

What It Is

Shark cartilage is a cancer therapy made popular by Dr. William Lane in his books *Sharks Don't Get Cancer* (1992) and *Sharks Still Don't Get Cancer* (1996). Lane believed that sharks do not get cancer, and noted that their skeletons don't contain bones. Instead, they are made of cartilage that contains no blood vessels. Other research has shown that cancers require extensive blood supplies to grow. This occurs through a process called "angiogenesis." If cartilage contains something that prevents the growth of blood vessels, this might be able to stop cancers from growing by cutting off their blood supply.

Claims

Shark cartilage is sold in the United States as a dietary supplement and therefore does not have to be tested or regulated by the FDA. For this reason, it is advertised as beneficial for the health of bones and joints. However, its most popular reputation is as a treatment for cancer, especially breast, colon, intracranial, and spinal cancers. It is estimated that about 50,000 Americans use it every year for this purpose. It is also used for psoriasis, intestinal inflammation, retina problems of the eye related to diabetes, and wound healing.

Study Findings

Although Dr. Lane claims to have research support for his claims about shark cartilage, the results of these studies are not very convincing. Research on animals has shown that cartilage from a variety of animals does slow the growth of blood vessels. Lane extracted shark cartilage and tested the product on humans in cancer clinics in Cuba and Mexico. This research led to three publications used to support shark cartilage's effectiveness against cancer. One study (✔✔) contained only eight patients and no control group. The second reported only differences in microscope slides made of tumors in treated and untreated animals. The third (✔✔) reported interviews with twenty-one cancer patients who contacted Lane to express their appreciation for his product. Taken together, these constitute extremely weak evidence for effectiveness.

A small number of other studies supporting shark cartilage's efficacy have been published, but they have been uncontrolled or had significant design problems. A 1998 study published by Miller (✗✗✗) tested the safety and efficacy of shark cartilage in sixty patients with advanced forms of cancer. They found that shark cartilage was inactive with all forms of cancer studied, primarily breast, colon, and lung cancer. A small proportion of patients became stable during the study, but this was about the same percent as respond to placebos in other studies. The Natural Medicines Comprehensive Database, an independent publication that evaluates the safety and effectiveness of natural treatments, rates shark cartilage as "Likely Ineffective."

However, the search for effective antiangiogenic agents continues, and promising agents appear to be on the horizon. One of these has been isolated from an extract of shark cartilage and is being tested for anticancer activity. This approach, however, is very different from the current way that shark cartilage is used as a dietary supplement. People are said to need 60 to 90 grams of shark cartilage per day. The experimental extract is being tested at a dose of less than 0.1 gram per day of the purified antiangiogenic compounds.

Cautions

No serious adverse effects have been reported in the trials conducted on shark cartilage. The recommended amounts of shark cartilage needed to treat cancer are very large, and it is not very palatable. Hence, the most common side effects are nausea, vomiting, a bad taste in the mouth, dyspepsia, dizziness, elevated blood sugar and calcium levels, decreased strength and performance, weakness and fatigue, altered consciousness, and constipation. Almost half the patients in Miller's study (✗✗) reported problems of this type. The biggest danger with shark cartilage, and other alternative cancer therapies, is that people may avoid effective treatments while taking these ineffective ones.

Recommendations

Shark cartilage costs about $700 a month. This is a high price to pay for a therapy that shows little evidence of effectiveness. While cancer remains a devastating disease, conventional medicine has developed reliable and effective treatments for some types of cancer. If the cancer progresses to the point where no treatments remain, Miller's study suggests that supportive care is as effective as shark cartilage. This approach to the end of one's life is more likely to produce spiritual and relational blessings than the continued pursuit of elusive "cures."

Dosage

The most common doses recommended to prevent cancer range from 0.5 to 4.5 grams daily, divided into a number of small doses taken with meals. To treat cancer, proponents recommend taking much higher doses.

Treatment Categories

Complementary Therapy
    Cancer   ☹☹☹☹

Scientifically Unproven
    For any indications   ☹☹☹☹

Quackery and Fraud
    In certain instances   ☹☹☹☹

Further Reading

Jellin, Jeff M., Forrest Batz, and Kathy Hichens, *Pharmacist's Letter/Prescriber's Letter: Natural Medicines Comprehensive Database* (Stockton, Calif.: Therapeutic Research Facility, 1999), 837–38.

McCutcheon, Lynn, "Taking a Bite out of Shark Cartilage," *Skeptical Inquirer* 21, no. 5 (September/October 1997): 44–48.

Miller, Denis R., et al., "Phase I/II Trial of the Safety and Efficacy of Shark Cartilage in the Treatment of Advanced Cancer," *Journal of Clinical Oncology* 16, no. 11 (November 1998): 3649–55.

SLIPPERY ELM

What It Is

The slippery elm tree *(Ulmus rubra* and *Ulmus fulva)* has long been considered one of the most versatile available in nature. It is native to eastern North America and is found most commonly in the Appalachian mountains. Over the centuries, both Native Americans and early settlers used the trees (including the red elm, or Indian elm, as well as white elm, *Ulmus americana*) for construction and medicinal purposes. The latter included turning it into a burn salve, a cure for chapped skin, poultices, and drinks.

Claims

Slippery elm became extremely popular in the 1700s and 1800s in colonial America as a cough and cold remedy. Some early Americans also mixed the ground bark with water or milk to make a nutritious, oatmeal-like food. Early American folk healers said this gruel was especially helpful to eat while recovering from illness because it was easily digested.

Slippery elm was also used as a digestive tonic and said to be a common treatment for dysentery and acid indigestion. It was less commonly sold as a remedy for baldness, broken bones, constipation, syphilis, hemorrhoids, stomach ulcers, and typhoid fever.

The "slippery" in the name is a clue to its major medicinal use. A mucilage material from the slippery elm swells on contact with water and forms a slimy coating over surfaces. This was used to coat irritated tissues, either externally on wounds or internally for sore throats or ulcers. It was believed to be soothing to all types of inflamed tissues and to draw toxins, splinters, and other irritants from tissues.

Study Findings

The mucilage made from slippery elm bark contains a number of carbohydrates that are believed to be the source of the soothing effects. Controlled clinical trials have not been conducted to give us evidence about how well these products might work. However, slippery elm products once held official status in *The United States Pharmacopoeia* and *The National Formulary*. Slippery elm has been consumed as a food for a long time and seems to be nontoxic. The FDA considers it a safe and effective over-the-counter demulcent, a soothing agent for the more sensitive membranes in the mouth, nose, and eyes.

Cautions

Slippery elm products have generally proven to be safe, although some people have had allergic reactions. Of more serious concern is the tradition of using the whole bark of slippery elm to induce abortions. Although its effectiveness is not known, women of childbearing age would do well to avoid these products. Pregnant and nursing women should be hesitant to take any herbal remedy, as little is known about how they affect pregnancy and early development. The Natural Database rates slippery elm bark products as "Likely Unsafe" in pregnancy. It is rated as "Possibly Safe" if the inner bark is used as a food.

Dutch elm disease has ravaged slippery elms in recent years, making the product more expensive to produce and somewhat more difficult to obtain. Because of this, it is usually easier to find less expensive options than slippery elm.

Recommendations

Slippery elm products have a long history of relieving skin and gastrointestinal irritation, and soothing sores and wounds. They may provide adequate relief for milder cases of irritation and inflammation. Other than those cases mentioned above, the products appear to be safe and well tolerated.

Dosage

No reliable recommendations can be made about dosage.

Treatment Categories

Complementary Therapy
    Superficial external skin irritations or wounds   ☺
    Mild sore throat   ☺
    Gastrointestinal irritation   ☺

Scientifically Unproven
    Other indications

Further Reading

DerMarderosian, Ara, ed., "Slippery Elm," in *The Review of Natural Products* (St. Louis, Mo.: Facts and Comparisons, February 1999).

Fetrow, Charles W., and Juan R. Avila, *Professional's Handbook of Complementary and Alternative Medicine* (Springhouse, Penn.: Springhouse, 1999), 605–6.

Jellin, Jeff M., Forrest Batz, and Kathy Hichens, *Pharmacist's Letter/Prescriber's Letter: Natural Medicines Comprehensive Database* (Stockton, Calif.: Therapeutic Research Facility, 1999), 846–47.

ST. JOHN'S WORT

What It Is

For centuries anyone who felt plagued by emotions that led them to despair turned to St. John's wort *(Hypericum perforatum)* for relief. At first this meant using St. John's wort to fight demons and evil spirits blamed for the problem. The word "hypericum" is derived from the Greek words *hyper* and *eikon,* which translate to "above" and "icon," an allusion to the herb's ancient use for protection against evil spirits. "St. John's" derives from the fact that the flower of the plant blooms around St. John's Day (June 24). Also, when the buds and flowers are squeezed, they exude a red pigment that was associated with the blood of John the Baptist.

More recently and for the same reasons, some call the herb "St. Joan's wort" for Joan of Arc's martyrdom.

Today, with our more sophisticated knowledge of biochemistry, many people consider that consuming St. John's wort is the perfect answer to reversing mild depression. The remedy, made from an extract of the flowers of *Hypericum perforatum,* is the most widely prescribed antidepressant in Germany, being used even more than Prozac®. In the United States it is quickly becoming one of the best-selling herbal remedies. In 1999, according to *Prevention Magazine,* it was the fourth most commonly used herb in America (after the "3 G's": garlic, ginseng, and ginkgo).

Claims

St. John's wort is used primarily for mild to moderate forms of depression and anxiety. It is also recommended for people with insomnia and generalized chronic fatigue. The medicinal benefits have been cited by herbalists for at least 400 years. In the United States, the earliest recorded mention of St. John's wort may have been by Griffith (1847), who stated that the herb can be taken as an oil or ointment for ulcers, tumors, and as a diuretic. Over the centuries, St. John's wort has been used for ailments such as nervous disorders, depression, neuralgia, kidney problems, wounds, and burns.

More recently, St. John's wort has been postulated as a treatment for viruses. Testing is in the very earliest stages to see if it—in particular, one of its active ingredients, hypericin—will have an impact against HIV infections. However, pending the outcome of the research that is just beginning, this remains conjecture.

Study Findings

Numerous clinical studies (✔✔✔) have been conducted in Germany, and the randomized ones were reviewed in Linde's article listed below. At the time of Linde's writing, four additional large-scale clinical trials were under way in the United States. Linde found much variation in the quality of the trials examined and the types of depression studied. However, he concluded that St. John's wort is better than placebo, although it could not be determined if it works better for one type of depression over another. However, experts warn that Prozac (or similar SSRI antidepressants or MAO inhibitors) should never be used in conjunction with St. John's wort.

A number of new, larger studies have been published since Linde's review. Four of these had more than 150 subjects, making their conclusions more reliable. In all of these studies (✔✔✔), St. John's wort was effective in relieving mild to moderate depression and anxiety. Furthermore, one study found St. John's wort to be as effective as Prozac, another found it as effective as a closely related drug, sertraline, and two studies found it as effective as imipramine, an older tricyclic antidepressant. In these last two studies, subjects reported significantly fewer side effects with St. John's wort. The authors of the more recent *BMJ* study concluded that St. John's wort "should be considered for first-line treatment in mild to moderate depression, especially in the primary care setting."

In spite of increasing evidence that St. John's wort works, how it works is not certain. One advantage with this remedy over many other herbal products is that it is available in a standardized form. This means that each batch contains a specified amount of one chemical, usually hypericin. However, no one knows if hypericin is the actual active ingredient in the remedy. This is one of the questions that researchers hope to determine in future studies.

Some manufacturers of St. John's wort standardize their products against a second compound, hyperflorin. In addition to hypericin and hyperflorin, there are a number of other compounds in St. John's wort with biological activity, including flavonoids, essential oil components, and carotenoids. The question becomes whether the hypericin, the hyperflorin, the other components, or a combination of all these, are the active ingredients in the plant. Until this is discovered, evaluation and standardization of products will be difficult.

Furthermore, because of the lack of regulation of dietary supplements in the United States, there is significant variation in products available in this country. One study, commissioned by the *Los Angeles Times,* found dramatic variation in the percentage of active ingredients in a number of different brand names of St. John's wort. This variation might explain why Americans seem to have less favorable responses to the herb than their European neighbors. A large survey (✗✗) of more than 46,000 Americans was reported by *Consumer Reports* in May 2000. Among those who responded and reported they had depression 30 percent said they had tried St. John's wort. Of these, only 17 percent said it helped "much," while 55 percent said it helped "little to none." ConsumerLab.com, an independent testing company that permits promoters to use its flask-shaped seal of approval on products that pass its criteria—usually meeting German testing standards concerning the quantity of active ingredients in the preparation—is planning to test St. John's wort products in 2001. Results, when available, can be viewed by subscribing to their Website (*www.consumerlab.com*).

Cautions

Side effects from St. John's wort are infrequent and relatively mild. However, studies have generally only lasted eight weeks, so long-term effects are not known. The most common symptoms are intestinal discomfort, fatigue, dry mouth, dizziness, skin rash, and (with very high doses) hypersensitivity to sunlight. Although how St. John's wort combats depression is not known, it probably has an effect similar to pharmaceutical antidepressants, which means it will probably affect how they work. Therefore, patients on prescription antidepressants should alert their physicians before starting St. John's wort or any other herbal remedy.

The FDA warned doctors in early 2000 of a study conducted by the National Institutes of Health that showed a significant drug interaction between St John's wort and indinavir, a protease inhibitor used to treat HIV infection. In this study, patients taking St. John's wort along with indinavir had substantially decreased levels of indinavir in their blood. This was probably due to induction of the cytochrome P450 metabolic pathway. Now, before you turn the page (after all, who cares about a P450 pathway?), let us explain how important this finding might be.

Many prescription drugs used to treat conditions such as heart disease, depression, seizures, and certain cancers, or to prevent conditions such as transplant rejection or pregnancy (oral contraceptives), are metabolized via this P450 pathway. The pathway is one of the body's important ways to eliminate foreign compounds from the body. If it is induced (a form of stimulation suspected to occur with St. John's wort), it will cause many other drugs to be broken down more quickly than usual, possibly even before they can have their proper effect. A significant and potentially dangerous drug interaction could occur between St. John's wort and many prescription medications. The following table lists the drug interactions that have already been reported due to P450 induction. Many other drugs are likely to be affected. To prevent loss of therapeutic effect of any drug metabolized via the cytochrome P450 pathway, patients on these drugs should not take St. John's wort. Likewise, patients on St. John's wort should not take any of these prescriptions.

Drug Whose Blood Levels Were Lowered	Most Common Use for This Drug
Indinavir	Treatment of HIV
Cyclosporin	Prevention of organ transplant rejection
Ethinylestradiol	Contraceptive pill
Theophylline	Bronchodilator in asthma and lung diseases
Warfarin	Prevention of blood clots
Phenprocoumon	Prevention of blood clots
Digoxin	Treatment for congestive heart failure

Another potential side effect of St. John's wort is that it may cause phototoxicity in fair-skinned people. In Europe, prescribers of the herb suggest that it may be prudent for these people not to expose themselves to strong sunlight when taking the herb. The Natural Database, for example, rates St. John's wort as "Possibly Unsafe" at doses larger than 1800 mg per day "because of the risk of photosensitive reactions." However, there has been only one reported case of phototoxicity in a human despite its wide use. In fact, in one study of 3,250 people using St. John's wort, only 2.4 percent experienced side effects of any kind. To date, no studies have examined the long-term effects of using the herb. It is rated "Possibly Unsafe" in pregnancy and lactation.

Recommendations

St. John's wort appears to be a mild and relatively safe treatment for mild forms of depression, anxiety, or insomnia. Certain types of depression may respond better than others. However, no information is available on the long-term effects of taking this herb, so it should only be used as a short-term option. Given the complicated nature of depression and anxiety, taking St. John's wort, or any other pill, alone should not be viewed as an adequate way to deal with these conditions. The psychological, relational, and spiritual issues should also be addressed.

Furthermore, St. John's wort should never be taken with any prescription medication without a doctor or pharmacist first checking to be sure there is no possible interaction. When deciding on a product, remember that most studies have been conducted with German formulations. These are available in the U.S. under the brand names Kira®, Perika®, Movana®, and Quanterra® St. John's Wort.

Dosage

Most studies have used 300 mg of extract three times daily. These extracts have been standardized to contain 0.3 percent hypericin.

Treatment Categories

Complementary Therapy

Mild depression	☺☺☺☺
Anxiety	☺☺
Indigestion	☺
Topically for bruises, abrasions, mild burns, and muscle aches	☺

Scientifically Unproven

AIDS	☹☹☹
Any other indication	

Further Reading

Ernst, E., "Second Thoughts About Safety of St John's Wort," *Lancet* 354 (December 1999): 2014–16.

Jellin, Jeff M., Forrest Batz, and Kathy Hichens, *Pharmacist's Letter/Prescriber's Letter: Natural Medicines Comprehensive Database* (Stockton, Calif.: Therapeutic Research Facility, 1999), 864–66.

Linde, Klaus, Gilbert Ramirez, Cynthia D. Mulrow, Andrej Pauls, Wolfgang Weidenhammer, and Dieter Melchart, "St. John's Wort for Depression—An Overview and Meta-Analysis of Randomised Clinical Trials," *BMJ* 313 (August 1996): 253–58.

Schrader, E., "Equivalent of St. John's Wort Extract (Ze 117) and Fluoxetine: A Randomized, Controlled Study in Mild-Moderate Depression," *International Clinical Psychopharmacology* 15, no. 2 (March 2000): 61–68.

Woelk, Helmut, "Comparison of St. John's Wort and Imipramine for Treating Depression: Randomised Controlled Trial," *BMJ* 321 (September 2000): 536–39.

TEA TREE OIL

What It Is

The tea tree is native to Australia and got its name from the first British sailors under Captain James Cook, the first to report its use (and kava) to Westerners. Cook and his crew used it to make a hot tea. Later, wanting a stronger drink, Captain Cook and his men made a beer from spruce leaves, which they found "too astringent," according to the captain's account. To correct this, they mixed tea tree leaves with the spruce leaves. The beer made from the mix was still not very good, though they found it drinkable, something that could not be said for the spruce brew alone.

Captain Cook did not realize that the native tribes had used the tea tree for its antiseptic properties. In fact, it would not be until 1930 that the tree's medicinal potential was noted in an Australian medical journal.

The tea tree has the official name *Melaleuca alternifolia,* and the oil is obtained from its leaves. The oil is sometimes sold as Melaleuca Oil, a substance that should not be purchased without a careful check. There are several species of tea trees, and the oils from species other than *Melaleuca alternifolia* contain high concentrations of skin irritants.

Tea tree oil has a faint lemon color and a nutmeglike odor. The oil is a complex mixture of almost 100 compounds called "terpenes."

Claims

Tea tree oil is used as a general antimicrobial agent. It became known outside of Australia during World War I because of its widespread use by Australian troops for burns, wounds, and infections. Based on this history, tea tree oil remains popular as a natural antiseptic and is added to many "natural" cosmetics, toothpaste, and hair products.

Tea tree oil is believed to be effective against a wide range of bacterial, viral, and fungal conditions, including athlete's foot, ringworm, respiratory infections, and vaginitis. As a first-aid remedy it readily penetrates the skin and is believed useful for treating burns, scrapes, bites, stings, and various skin irritations. Some people feel it is an effective insect repellent.

Tea tree is among the most popular essential oils used in aromatherapy, whether by inhalation or in various body care products. Tea tree also has been used in dental care. Diluted in water it is used as a mouthwash and gargle, and in more concentrated forms it is used to relieve canker sores, cold sores, and gum disease.

Tea tree oil is used to help prevent or treat acne, colds and the flu, yeast infections, warts, nasal congestion, and sore throats.

Study Findings

Tea tree oil has been shown in laboratory tests to kill a variety of microorganisms. A number of studies (✔✔✔✔) have found that tea tree oil can help to eradicate fungal infections of the nails, which are relatively difficult to control even with conventional prescription drugs. For example, 10 percent tea tree oil has been shown in one study (✔✔✔) to be as effective as 1 percent tolnaftate cream for reducing the symptoms of athlete's foot (tinea pedis). In yet another study (✔✔✔), 100 percent tea tree oil was as effective as 1 percent clotrimazole in improving nail appearance and symptoms. However, both treatments are known to have high rates of recurrence. Furthermore, there is at least one study (✘✘✘) showing that tea tree oil was no better than placebo against fungal foot infections. Clinical studies (✔✔✔) have also shown it to be somewhat effective against acne. In one study (✘✘✘), comparing 5 percent tea tree oil to benzoyl peroxide lotion, the tea tree oil was better tolerated, but was less effective and had a slower onset of action. Case reports (✔) of tea tree oil pessaries relieving vaginal yeast infections have been reported. There are no demonstrated benefits (✘✘) from adding tea tree oil to toothpaste.

Cautions

Tea tree oil should never be taken internally, and should always be diluted when applied to broken skin. Research on how it kills microbes has revealed that it also kills certain types of human cells. This may result in slower healing and increased scarring when used for burns. All of these findings should caution against its use in toothpaste, mouthwashes, and lozenges, all of which can easily be ingested. A relatively small number of allergic reactions have been reported, and long-term use can lead to dermatitis.

Since tea tree oil may irritate the skin, test it first with a tiny amount on a small patch of skin. Tea tree oil can safely be applied full strength in drops to fingernails or toenails (for treating fungal infections, for example). It should not be applied to broken skin or near the eyes.

The Natural Database rates tea tree oil as "Likely Unsafe" for oral use in children and in women who are pregnant or lactating. It is rated as "Possibly Safe" when used topically, except in pregnancy and lactation, for which there is insufficient reliable information.

Recommendations

This natural oil is effective against a number of microorganisms and may be a helpful agent for minor skin infections. However, it should be used cautiously, if at all, with open wounds, more serious infections, and burns. Tea tree oil should never be ingested.

Dosage

The oil should be applied to the affected areas twice a day. It should not be taken internally.

Treatment Categories

Complementary Therapy
　　Topically for fungal nail or skin infections　　☺☺
　　Mild acne　　　　　　　　　　　　　　　　☺
　　Infections within the mouth　　　　　　　　☹
　　Ingested for any reason　　　　　　　　　☹☹☹

Scientifically Unproven
　　Other indications

Further Reading

Foster, Steven, and Varro E. Tyler, *Tyler's Honest Herbal: A Sensible Guide to the Use of Herbs and Related Remedies*, 4th ed. (New York: Haworth Herbal Press, 1999), 369–70.

Jellin, Jeff M., Forrest Batz, and Kathy Hichens, *Pharmacist's Letter/Prescriber's Letter: Natural Medicines Comprehensive Database* (Stockton, Calif.: Therapeutic Research Facility, 1999), 901–2.

Schiedermayer, David, "Tea Tree Oil as a Topical Antimicrobial Agent," *Alternative Medicine Alert* 1, no. 5 (May 1998): 52–56.

VALERIAN

What It Is

Both cats and their humans have long delighted in the use of valerian. The roots and rhizomes of Common Valerian *(Valeriana officinalis)* form the number one over-the-counter sedative in Germany, with a chemical similar to catnip. Other forms of valerian are harvested, including Indian Valerian *(Valeriana jatamansii,* synonym *Valeriana wallichii),* Mexican Valerian *(Valeriana edulis),* and Pacific Valerian *(Valeriana sitchensis).* Humans use valerian for a gentle sleep. Some Native American tribes also used it to treat cuts and wounds, while ancient Greeks used it for urinary tract and digestive disorders. The cats simply like to "get high."

The pink-flowered perennial valerian grows wild in temperate areas of the Americas and Eurasia. The root, which is politely described as "pungent" or "malodorous," smells terrible—unless you're a cat.

Claims

Valerian has been used as a sedative and to treat anxiety. It is said to act as a central nervous system depressant, binding to benzodiazepine receptors. Benzodiazepine is the active ingredient in the prescription drug Valium®, once the most commonly prescribed tranquilizer in the United States. However, unlike Valium-like prescription drugs, valerian is said to be nontoxic and does not interact with alcohol.

Hippocrates and other early Greek physicians apparently used valerian for a variety of ailments. Some of these ancient uses (particularly as a remedy to soothe digestive ailments) have survived into modern times, while others (as treatments for urinary tract disorders and epilepsy) have not. Valerian was not well recognized as a sedative and muscle relaxant until relatively recently. In the eighteenth and nineteenth centuries, valerian was indispensable as a treatment for various types of nervous conditions, not only insomnia but also anxiety, nervous headache, exhaustion, and hysteria. Doctors often recommended it to women who suffered from emotionally induced exhaustion of the nervous system. The association between women, nervous conditions, and valerian was so strong that valerian has been called the "Valium of the nineteenth century."

Valerian is now the most prominent herbal remedy for insomnia as well as nervous conditions related to anxiety, tension, and stress. It is believed to work well as a nerve tonic for people who suffer from nervous exhaustion, panic attacks, and emotional disturbances. It is used as a pain-relieving agent for conditions such as tension-related headache, nerve pain, and menstrual cramps. Valerian is felt by some to soothe the digestive system and relieve indigestion, constipation, irritable bowel, and stomach cramps, especially those that may be due to excess nervousness.

Valerian is used by some herbalists to prevent or treat high blood pressure, cough (often in combination with other herbs such as licorice), attention deficit disorder (ADD and ADHD), and altitude sickness.

The most unpleasant aspect of valerian may be its odor. It is said to smell like well-worn, though long-unwashed socks or a sharp cheese even starving mice might avoid. It may be used as a tea, tincture (alcohol-based solution), or extract in capsules.

Study Findings

The active ingredient in valerian is thought to be isovalerenic acid, but this has not been established completely. Valerian has been studied in several small, double-blind clinical trials (✔✔✔) that showed improvement of sleep quality. A review of this research found nine controlled studies of valerian alone used to assist sleep. Three of these (✔✔✔) examined the effects of taking valerian over a number of weeks by those who had difficulty sleeping. All showed better sleep patterns after about two weeks, compared to those taking placebo. The six other studies gave a single dose of valerian to people who did not have sleep problems. Three of them (✔✔✔) found valerian improved their sleep, but three (✘✘✘) found it was no different than placebo. A rigorous study published after the above review measured sleep patterns objectively in people with insomnia after giving them valerian. After a single dose (✘✘✘), no differences were noted, but after two weeks (✔✔✔), sleep was significantly improved.

A number of other studies (✔✔✔) have examined valerian used in combination with regular brewing hops (*Humulus lupulus*) and St. John's wort. In one controlled clinical trial, an herbal formula containing hops and valerian was just as effective as a benzodiazepine (the class of tranquilizers that includes Valium and Xanax®) for patients suffering from nonchronic and nonpsychiatric sleep disorders. The valerian preparation and the benzodiazepine got the same ratings from patients for sleep quality and quality of life, while withdrawal symptoms were evident only with the benzodiazepine.

In laboratory experiments, compounds extracted from valerian interact with a substance called gamma-aminobutyric acid (GABA). GABA is a neurotransmitter that plays an important role in mood, relaxation, and sleep. The ability to affect GABA levels is one of the ways benzodiazepines work. Valerian compounds act in similar ways, though with weaker effects.

German health officials have approved valerian for use as a mild sedative and sleep aid, based on several European clinical trials (✔✔✔) that demonstrate these effects. In contrast, the U.S. Pharmacopoeia in 1998 decided there was too much conflicting data to recommend the use of valerian as a short-term treatment for insomnia.

Cautions

In the United States, valerian is approved for use in flavoring foods and beverages such as root beer. No serious side effects have been reported. However, in medicinal doses (✘✘) unusual side effects include morning sleepiness, headache, cardiac disturbances, and trouble walking. One of the consistent findings in clinical trials (✔✔✔) is that people report fewer side effects with valerian than pharmaceuticals, with less residual sedation in the morning. For unknown reasons, a small minority of people may find valerian stimulating instead of calming, causing insomnia, restlessness, or uneasiness. These people become restless and get palpitations, particularly with long-term use. Addiction has not been reported, but rare cases of liver toxicity and withdrawal symptoms have been reported.

Whether valerian interacts with alcohol or not is disputed. Most experts recommend not taking valerian and alcohol together. Valerian has been reported to slow the metabolism of barbiturates and should not be used with these medications. A few people experience stomach complaints from taking valerian.

Some components display cancer-causing activity in the laboratory; however, these effects have not been reproduced in laboratory animals, even at extremely high doses. Nevertheless, most experts warn that valerian probably should not be used by pregnant women. Nor should valerian be given to children under the age of twelve.

Recommendations

Valerian has very few reported side effects and may be an effective over-the-counter treatment for sleep problems or anxiety, as it appears to have mild sedating and tranquilizing effects. It appears to take a week or two before most people notice its effect, so it will not work as well for those with occasional sleep problems as it does for those with chronic insomnia. No studies have examined the side effects of taking valerian long-term. Valerian should not be taken with other sedatives or before driving or in other situations when alertness is required.

Dosage

The studies have used a variety of doses, ranging from 60 mg to over 1200 mg (which is a problem in assessing overall effect). A 400 to 450 mg dose of valerian one to two hours before bedtime is most commonly used.

Treatment Categories

Complementary Therapy

Accelerating onset of sleep and improving quality of sleep after being taken for at least a week	☺☺☺
Accelerating onset of sleep and improving quality of sleep taken on single occasion	☹☹☹
Restlessness and sleep disorders caused by nervous conditions or behavioral disorders	☺☺
Insomnia associated with anxiety	☺☺
Anxiety or mood disorders	☺

Scientifically Unproven

Other indications

Further Reading

Donath, F., S. Quispe, K. Diefenbach, A. Maurer, I. Fietze, and I. Roots, "Critical Evaluation of the Effect of Valerian Extract on Sleep Structure and Sleep Quality," *Pharmacopsychiatry* 33, no. 2 (March 2000): 47–53.

Foster, Steven, and Varro E. Tyler, *Tyler's Honest Herbal: A Sensible Guide to the Use of Herbs and Related Remedies*, 4th ed. (New York: Haworth Herbal Press, 1999), 377–79.

Jellin, Jeff M., Forrest Batz, and Kathy Hichens, *Pharmacist's Letter/Prescriber's Letter: Natural Medicines Comprehensive Database* (Stockton, Calif.: Therapeutic Research Facility, 1999), 926–28.

Stevinson, Clare, and Edzard Ernst, "Valerian for Insomnia: A Systematic Review of Randomized Clinical Trials," *Sleep Medicine* 1 (2000): 91–99.

VITAMIN C

What It Is

Vitamin C, also called "ascorbic acid," is most commonly found in citrus fruits, but large quantities also exist in strawberries, kiwi fruit, and tomatoes. As a vitamin, a certain amount is required in everyone's diet to maintain health. A lack of vitamin C in the diet leads to scurvy, as James Lind demonstrated in one of the first controlled trials in the eighteenth century (see page 117). Vitamin C is required for many functions in the body, including tissue repair, metabolism of carbohydrates, and synthesis of proteins.

Claims

The importance of vitamin C in the diet is well understood and scientifically proven. The only controversy is the amount we need, both from day to day and when our bodies are exposed to unusual stress. Some people claim high daily doses prevent colds.

Linus Pauling, a dual Nobel Prize winner for chemistry and for peace, was the most outspoken proponent of this view, recommending that everyone take 1 gram of vitamin C daily, and increasing this to 2 grams a day as soon as someone felt a cold coming on. Pauling himself took far greater quantities, often appearing on television talk shows with a pocketful of the vitamin, one or more of which he would take during an interview. Pauling claimed that by the end of his life he was taking 18 grams of vitamin C daily, which he increased to 40 grams when he felt a cold start. He also claimed vitamin C could treat everything from cancer to schizophrenia. Although his brilliance was in fields other than medicine, his stature in the field of science led to many independent studies of his theories. In addition to its use with colds, some advocates believe that large amounts of vitamin C improve athletic performance, mood, and cardiovascular health. Vitamin C is believed by some to prevent cancer, increase longevity, prevent cataracts, and enhance brain function.

In the past, the recommended vitamin C intake was 60 mg a day, the equivalent of a glass of orange juice. Recently, this recommended daily allowance was increased somewhat by the Institute of Medicine (IOM). The institute, a private nonprofit organization that advises federal health officials, is part of the National Academy of Sciences, which has set the nation's Recommended Dietary Allowances, or RDAs, for nutrients since 1941. The Food and Drug Administration (FDA) uses these recommendations to set "daily values" that appear on food labels. The IOM recommended that women should consume 75 mg per day, and men 90 mg. Because smokers are more likely to suffer from biological processes that damage cells and deplete vitamin C, they need an additional

35 mg per day. The researchers said these levels can easily be met without taking supplements, and people can get vitamin C by eating citrus fruits, potatoes, strawberries, broccoli, and leafy green vegetables. An 8 oz. glass of orange juice provides about 100 mg of vitamin C. Any amount of the vitamin above the RDA is likely to be excreted by the body unused.

The report also set the upper intake level for vitamin C, from both food and supplements, at 2000 mg per day for adults. Intakes above this amount may cause a number of medical problems.

Study Findings

In 1992, researchers at the University of California, Los Angeles (UCLA), reported that among 11,000 participants surveyed over a ten-year period (✔✔), those getting the most vitamin C (300 mg per day) had the lowest rates of heart disease and cancer and lived the longest. These findings took differences in exercise, diet, and lifestyle into account.

Although vitamin C appears to have only a small effect in preventing the common cold, taken at the onset it can reduce the duration and severity of a cold. Linus Pauling made his original claims about vitamin C and the common cold in a book published in 1970. He based his conclusion on four studies (✔✔✔). (See page 128 for a detailed discussion of the problems in his review.)

Since then, dozens of other high-quality clinical studies have been conducted on vitamin C. There are three consistent findings from these studies.

- 1 gram vitamin C daily does not lower someone's chances of getting a cold (✘✘✘).
- Taking 1 to 2 grams daily as soon as someone gets a cold may shorten the length of time a person has the cold and reduce the severity of the symptoms (✔✔✔). However, the benefit is still not huge, working out on average to reduce the length of the cold by about half a day.
- Megadoses of vitamin C (more than 2 grams daily) do not have any beneficial effects (✘✘✘).

Optimal levels of vitamin C have been suggested in a number of studies (✔✔) to benefit a wide range of health conditions, including cataracts, diabetes, eczema, periodontal disease, glaucoma, gout, high cholesterol, menopause, heavy menstruation, minor injuries, morning sickness, recurrent ear infections, and (✔✔✔) urinary tract infection. Vitamin C also helps recycle the antioxidant vitamin E and promotes the absorption of other nutrients (such as iron).

Confirming earlier population studies, a study of 247 older women (✔✔) determined that vitamin C supplementation use over a ten- to twelve-year period was associated with a dramatically reduced prevalence of age-related cataracts. Another human study (✔✔)

confirmed earlier animal research in finding that eight days of combined vitamins C (2000 mg per day) and E (1000 IU per day) protect the skin from sunburn. Another recent study (✔✔) conducted in a retirement community in Australia found that consumption of vitamin C supplements was associated with a lower percentage of severe cognitive impairment, although not with any effects on tests of verbal fluency.

Vitamin C comes in a wide variety of forms, including tablets, capsules, powders, liquids, and chewable wafers. Buffered vitamin C provides added calcium and magnesium, which helps to reduce irritation from increased stomach acids, and buffered chewable tablets protect teeth from ascorbic acid—an especially important feature for children and anyone with soft enamel. "Corn-free" vitamin C is designed for those who are sensitive to corn (unlike most vitamin C, it's derived from sago palm rather than corn).

Vitamin C can be extracted from natural sources (rose hips, acerola), but no research has proved any nutritional difference between synthetic and "natural" forms of vitamin C. Vitamin C is often combined with plant bioflavonoids (e.g., rutin, hesperdin, quercetin) to enhance absorption or activity, but this claimed biological effect has not been proven. There is no proof that sublingual vitamin C sprays or tablets (which are much more expensive) have any additional benefit.

The body's cells routinely transform dietary vitamin C into other forms called "metabolites." Some research indicates supplements that combine vitamin C with its metabolites may permit it to be absorbed better and faster into the blood and immune cells, and last longer in body tissues. A patented supplement called Ester-C® is composed of esters of vitamin C and its metabolites (an ester is a slightly modified form of any acid group, one of which is in vitamin C, or ascorbic acid). However, we are aware of no proven clinical benefit of this more expensive form of vitamin C.

Furthermore, there can be great variability in different products. For example, in March 2000, ConsumerLab.com tested a total of twenty-six brands of vitamin C. Seven of these products claimed USP quality on their labels. The twenty-six products were tested to determine whether they possessed 100 percent of the labeled amounts of vitamin C and disintegrated sufficiently in solution. Four of the products did not pass this testing. One did not break down quickly enough to release its vitamin C, and three had insufficient vitamin C in the pills. Among these three, one indicated that it was of USP quality but it appeared to contain only 88 percent of its claimed amount of vitamin C. Fifteen percent of the products did not pass testing. Surprisingly, this rate was about the same for USP and non-USP labeled products. Furthermore, USP-labeled products that passed testing tended to have amounts slightly less than 100 percent of the claimed amount and non-USP labeled products that passed tended to have somewhat more than 100 percent of their labeled amounts of vitamin C. The brand names of these products can be viewed at the ConsumerLab.com subscription based Website (*www.consumberlab.com*).

A number of studies in humans (✘✘) have demonstrated that it is very unlikely that high doses of vitamin C could benefit people. A dose of up to 200 mg is absorbed well from the digestive tract. At higher doses, some of the vitamin C is not absorbed. For example, only about half of the vitamin C from a 1000 mg dose will be absorbed into the body, and the rest is excreted. Taking 1000 mg per day leads to the maximum possible amount dissolved in the blood plasma. All the rest is excreted in the urine. Overall, this means that taking any more than 500 mg vitamin C per day will result in hardly any of the additional vitamin C making it to your cells. All the rest will get flushed down the drain.

Cautions

Vitamin C does not cause serious adverse effects, even when taken in very high doses. However, some people report (✗) nausea, heartburn, diarrhea, and other intestinal problems. People who are prone to get kidney stones should be cautious about how much vitamin C they take as high doses (2000 mg per day or more) may cause kidney stones and may be associated with deep vein blood clots (thromboses). Some researchers feel that amounts of vitamin C exceeding 1000 mg per day may actually induce a pro-oxidant effect, instead of an antioxidant effect. For example, at least one study (✗✗) has shown an increase in atherosclerosis in people taking only 500 mg a day of vitamin C.

Vitamin C at the RDA of 70 mg per day in pregnancy and 90 to 95 mg per day in lactation is rated "Likely Safe" by the Natural Database.

Recommendations

If someone feels a cold coming on, taking 1 to 2 grams vitamin C per day for a few days may help him or her get over the cold a little quicker. Since this is a generally safe and inexpensive vitamin, it may not hurt to try, especially for people who usually have very little vitamin C in their diet. However, there is no evidence that taking the vitamin for long periods of time will prevent colds or cancer and may lead to other long-term side effects.

Dosage

The recommended dietary allowance is 75 mg per day for women and 90 mg per day for men. Smokers should take an additional 35 mg per day. The RDA for children increases gradually from 15 mg per day for one- to three-year-olds to 45 mg per day for nine- to thirteen-year-olds, up to adult levels by eighteen years of age. Those who recommend vitamin C to treat the common cold usually take 1 to 3 grams a day.

Treatment Categories

Conventional Therapy
Twice-a-day supplement in doses of 75 mg to 200 mg per day
As an antioxidant

To prevent scurvy ☺☺☺☺

To increase iron absorption from the GI tract ☺☺☺☺

When ingested in food sources containing 200 mg
or more per day to prevent cancers of the mouth,
esophagus, stomach, lung, and colon ☺☺☺

Complementary Therapy

Twice-a-day supplement in doses of up to 200 mg
per day as an antioxidant to prevent cancers of
the mouth, esophagus, stomach, lung, and colon ☺

In doses of 200 to 500 mg per day as an antioxidant ☺☺

In doses of 500 mg to 2000 mg per day as an antioxidant ☹

In doses of 2000 mg per day or more as an antioxidant ☹☹

In high doses (1000 mg to 2000 mg per day) for short
periods of time to prevent common cold ☹

In high doses (1000 mg to 2000 mg per day) for short
periods of time to treat common cold ☺☺

Prevent sunburn ☺

Scientifically Unproven

Megadoses (greater than 2 grams per day)
for any indication ☹☹☹☹

Other indications

Further Reading

Gorton, H. Clay, and Kelly Jarvis, "The Effectiveness of Vitamin C in Preventing and Relieving the Symptoms of Virus-Induced Respiratory Infections," *Journal of Manipulative and Physiological Therapeutics* 22, no. 8 (October 1999): 530–33.

Hemilä, Harri, "Vitamin C and the Common Cold," *British Journal of Nutrition* 67 (1992): 3–16.

Jellin, Jeff M., Forrest Batz, and Kathy Hichens, *Pharmacist's Letter/Prescriber's Letter: Natural Medicines Comprehensive Database* (Stockton, Calif.: Therapeutic Research Facility, 1999), 939–41.

Levine, Mark, Steven C. Rumsey, Rushad Daruwala, Jae B. Park, and Yaohui Wang, "Criteria and Recommendations for Vitamin C Intake," *Journal of the American Medical Association* 281, no. 15 (April 1999): 1415–23.

VITAMIN E

What It Is

Vitamin E is a mixture of eight different, but very similar, compounds called "tocopherols." They make up the fat-soluble vitamin that is found in vegetable oils, nuts, whole grains, and greens. Wheat-germ oil is the single richest source of the vitamin. However, the amount present naturally in foods is much lower than what is needed to get the health benefits reported from those who take a supplement of at least 100 IU per day (IU stands for International Units; 100 IU of vitamin E = 67 mg). Much of the absorbed vitamin ends up in low-density lipoprotein particles (LDL), which play a central role in transporting cholesterol around the body. The rest forms part of the cell membranes throughout the body.

Claims

Vitamin E is an antioxidant (see Antioxidants, page 298). The oxidation of LDL is an important step in the development of atherosclerosis, or hardening of the arteries. Vitamin E is said to prevent this chemical reaction, and thus to play a role in the prevention of heart disease. The vitamin is also said to help the user resist infections, to treat hepatitis B, to reverse early memory loss problems due to dementia, and to prevent some cancers. There have also been anecdotal stories of vitamin E used to restore sexual drive in former psychiatric patients believed to have temporary drug-damaged libido.

Study Findings

Laboratory studies have shown that vitamin E prevents the oxidation of LDL. Based on questionnaires (✔✔) given to tens of thousands of people, those who took the largest amount of vitamin E had lower levels of heart disease; those who took the least vitamin E had the most heart problems. However, results from more controlled studies have not been completely positive, leading to some hesitation about vitamin E's benefits. In the area of resistance to infections, one controlled study (✔✔✔) found that elderly patients taking 200 mg vitamin E per day had about one-third of the infections compared to those taking a placebo. The study on libido (✔) did not have a control group to show whether the sex drive would have recovered naturally even without taking vitamin E.

In early 2000, the Institute of Medicine (IOM) released a report on vitamins E and C and other antioxidants. This report, and the research upon which it is based, is a good example of how confusing medical research can be. It also demonstrates the importance of patience before making broad recommendations about dietary supplements. The report concluded that it remains too early to make firm statements about the ability of vitamin E, or any of the other dietary antioxidants, to prevent or treat any disease.

The effects of vitamin E on heart disease have received most of the research in this area. A 1993 study in China (✔✔✔) found that healthy volunteers who took a combination of vitamin E (30 mg), beta-carotene, and selenium for five years had 9 percent fewer deaths from heart disease compared to those taking placebo. However, a 1994 study in Finland (✗✗✗) found no effect on coronary heart disease for smokers given 50 mg vitamin E daily for five to eight years. Then the 1996 British CHAOS study (✔✔✔) found an impressive 77 percent drop in nonfatal heart attacks for those taking 400 or 800 IU vitamin E daily for a little over a year. However, deaths from all cardiovascular causes remained unchanged. And in a 1999 Italian study (✗✗✗), there was no cardiac benefit for patients given 300 mg vitamin E for three to five years.

The first major United States study (✗✗✗) was published in January 2000 in *The New England Journal of Medicine*. Almost 10,000 people at high risk for cardiovascular events were randomly assigned to one of four groups. After four to six years, no significant differences were found between those taking 400 IU (267 mg) vitamin E or placebo when a variety of cardiovascular events were measured, such as heart attacks, strokes, or death from cardiovascular causes. Other groups in the study were receiving an angiotensin-converting enzyme (ACE) inhibitor (ramipril). Their results were so much better (20 to 25 percent improvement in all areas), the journal took the unusual step of prepublishing the results on its Website so physicians could make changes in their recommendations as soon as possible.

The evidence supporting the use of vitamin E supplements for any other chronic disease is even more sparse and conflicting. Some studies (✔✔✔) suggest that vitamin E might protect the retina from the damaging effects of free radicals, and that vitamin E therapy may be a cost-effective strategy for promoting heart health.

Some studies (✔✔✔✔) also show vitamin E improves blood circulation in the extremities. This improved blood circulation may improve the body's ability to heal muscle tissue, skin wounds, and reduce formation of scar tissue. Deficiencies of vitamin E have been linked with cataracts and weakened cells in the lungs, heart, and liver as well as to infertility. High concentrations of Vitamin E are found in male testes, but its role in fertility is not fully understood, and there is little support for vitamin E as a sexual potency enhancer.

According to the IOM, the vitamin E consumed should be "alpha-tocopherol," the only type that human blood can maintain and transfer to cells when needed. Other experts contend that it is preferable to take supplements that offer "mixed tocopherols," including *d*-beta, *d*-gamma, *d*-delta-tocopherols, tocotrienols, and others. They maintain that each form of vitamin E offers different antioxidant properties, and vitamin E occurs in foods as mixed tocopherols. There is no clear evidence to make a definite recommendation.

The Tolerable Upper Intake Level of vitamin E, based only on intake from vitamin supplements, was set at 1000 mg of alpha-tocopherol per day for adults. This amount is equivalent to roughly 1500 IU of "*d*-alpha-tocopherol," sometimes labeled as "natural source" vitamin E, or 1100 IU of "*dl*-alpha-tocopherol," a synthetic version of vitamin E. People consuming more than the upper limit face a greater risk of stroke and uncontrolled bleeding because the vitamin can prevent blood clotting.

Cautions

Adverse effects from vitamin E are rare. However, it may interfere with the blood's clotting mechanisms, so it should not be taken by those already taking blood thinners (like aspirin or warfarin). In March 2001, ConsumerLab.com released the results of tests on the quality of Vitamin E products in the U.S. All but three of the twenty-eight products tested passed their standards.

Recommendations

The evidence that vitamin E is able to protect people from heart disease is conflicting. However, more studies are under way which should help determine exactly whether or not it is beneficial, whether it benefits some people and not others, and how much is needed to have an effect. There is some evidence that vitamin E may be beneficial for more than just the heart, especially given its demonstrated antioxidant and immunostimulant properties. Given its ready availability as a supplement and in many vegetable foods, it seems good advice to add more vitamin E to your diet.

Dosage

The new IOM recommended intake level of vitamin E for both women and men is 15 mg (22 IU). The old level was 8 mg for men and 6.4 mg for women. Food sources include nuts, seeds, liver, and leafy green vegetables. Another national group, the Alliance for Aging Research (a nonprofit research organization) recommends 100 to 400 IU for adults. The RDA, they contend, is designed only to prevent deficiencies, and a normal diet will not allow for consumption levels beyond approximately 20 to 30 IU. While studies show 22 IU will prevent deficiencies, many of the antioxidant benefits will not be achieved at levels this low. Therefore, recommendations for levels of 100 IU to 800 IU do occur in the medical literature. These doses remain under the Tolerable Upper Intake Levels.

Treatment Categories

Conventional Therapy

As antioxidant up to 22 IU per day	☺☺☺☺
Up to 400 to 800 IU per day for fibrocystic breast disease	☺☺
Up to 400 IU per day to promote heart health	☺☺
Eye health	☺☺

Complementary Therapy
    Preventing Alzheimer's disease   ☺☺
    Preventing cognitive decline in Alzheimer's patients   ☺
    400 to 800 IU as an antioxidant (up to 1500 IU of *d*-alpha-
        tocopherol or 1100 IU of dl-alpha-tocopherol) per day to prevent
        heart disease, atherosclerosis, prostate cancer (in smokers)   ☺

Scientifically Unproven
    Preventing lung cancer in male smokers   ☹☹
    Any other indication

Further Reading

Heart Outcomes Prevention Evaluation Study Investigators, "Vitamin E Supplementation and Cardiovascular Events in High-Risk Patients," *The New England Journal of Medicine* 342, no. 3 (January 2000): 154–60.

Institute of Medicine, *Dietary Reference Intakes for Vitamin C, Vitamin E, Selenium, and Carotenoids* (Washington, D.C.: National Academy Press, 2000).

Jellin, Jeff M., Forrest Batz, and Kathy Hichens, *Pharmacist's Letter/Prescriber's Letter: Natural Medicines Comprehensive Database* (Stockton, Calif.: Therapeutic Research Facility, 1999), 944–47.

VITAMIN O

What It Is

If the advertising in newspapers and magazines were held to the same standards as the articles the newspapers and magazines print, we would not be writing about this product. Unfortunately, product advertising that is misleading may run for days, weeks, or months before any action is taken to stop the fraudulent claims being made.

Vitamin O® is such a product. Available from mail-order nutritional supplement producers, Vitamin O was advertised as "an easy, inexpensive way to give your body the extra oxygen it needs." In March 1999, *USA Today* and other newspapers carried full-page advertisements for Vitamin O. A flyer containing thirty pages of testimonials from satisfied customers was distributed about the same time through the mail. The company's Website called Vitamin O the latest in "oxygen-based therapies." Vitamin O was said to have been developed by its inventor, William F. Koch, M.D., Ph.D., for use in the U.S. space program to ensure that astronauts receive enough oxygen to maintain their health while in space. The price tag was $20 to $25 for a 2 oz. bottle. At the recommended dose of 15 to 20 drops by mouth two to three times a day, a 2 oz. bottle would last about a month.

What did buyers get? The Website explained that the product contains highly stabilized molecules of oxygen that somehow allow a much higher concentration of oxygen than is usually possible. Just how this is accomplished is "a carefully guarded secret" created by a "NASA process control engineer." The chemical components of Vitamin O were listed on the Website as "distilled water, sodium chloride, dissolved oxygen and trace minerals." In other words: salt water! At $25 for 2 oz.!

Another product, BiOxygen™, claimed its version of Vitamin O contains water, sodium chloride (common table salt), and "activated oxygen molecules." The latter are said to be "O_4 or two O_2 molecules joined together in a very stable bond" using "breakthrough quantum physics technology."

Claims

The claims made regarding Vitamin O are nothing short of staggering. The *USA Today* advertisement warned that without the proper amount of oxygen, your body "can suffer serious health consequences." The Vitamin O is absorbed by the bloodstream, which "carries the pure oxygen straight to your cells and tissues. There, it maximizes your nutrients, purifies your bloodstream and eliminates toxins and poisons."

The testimonials in the mailed advertisement claimed people had been cured of asthma, hemorrhoids, arthritis, lupus, allergies, chronic obstructive pulmonary disease (COPD), bronchitis, fatigue, headaches, emphysema, back pain, atherosclerosis, and many other diseases. Even one man's lung cancer started to decrease in size after he started taking Vitamin O, the Website reported.

Study Findings

The producers of Vitamin O claim to have lots of research to back up their claims, but none of it has been made available for independent evaluation. After publication of the advertisement in *USA Today*, the Federal Trade Commission (FTC), an independent agency of the federal government responsible for enforcing legislation related to unfair, deceptive, or false advertisements for food, drugs, dietary supplements, or cosmetics, charged the makers of Vitamin O with false and misleading advertising.

The FTC had alleged that "Vitamin O" advertising was false on five counts:

1. Oxygen taken orally could not work as claimed because no matter what form the oxygen molecules are in, they cannot be absorbed from the intestinal tract.
2. Vitamin O does not prevent or treat any disease or physical ailment.
3. Vitamin O does not have any beneficial effect on human health.
4. Medical or scientific research has not established that Vitamin O works.
5. Vitamin O was not developed by a Dr. William F. Koch and was never used by NASA astronauts during any space mission.

In May 2000, the manufacturer agreed to a settlement with the FTC and was fined $375,000. As part of the settlement, the manufacturer was prohibited from claiming that

Vitamin O or any similar product is an effective treatment for any disease like cancer, cardiovascular disease, or lung diseases. They were also prohibited from claiming that any medical or scientific research or studies support the effectiveness of Vitamin O.

A month after the FTC settlement, Vitamin O was still for sale on the same manufacturer's Website, along with all the same testimonials (though not with the "research" claims that got them into trouble with the FTC). The company continues to advertise Vitamin O by mail, along with other companies marketing similar products, providing only anecdotal evidence to support their claims.

Cautions

Vitamin O demonstrates the importance of examining the claims made for alternative therapies. Even the power of the federal government could not stop its sale. All the FTC could do was keep the manufacturer from making false claims. The FTC cannot stop the anecdotal evidence the company provided in its thirty-page brochure.

How can consumers spot this type of worthless product before losing their money? We give a number of general guidelines on fraud and quackery in chapter 8. But let's look at Vitamin O as a specific example.

- When evaluating any medical claim, common sense is important. In medicine, as in all other areas of life, if something sounds too good to be true, it probably *is* too good to be true.
- Any product that claims to cure people of literally everything and anything is most likely a fraud.
- Advertisements with anecdotal overkill—one testimony after another (for thirty pages!)—should alert you to steer clear.
- Always read the fine print. Manufacturers put enough red flags in their own materials to warn you of the risks. Vitamin O, in its disclaimer, even warned that there was "no competent or reliable scientific evidence to suggest that the testimonialist's experience is due to the use of our products." The disclaimer also went on to warn that the company was making "no medical claims as to the benefits of any of our products to improve medical conditions."
- Find out what research has been done. Studies done on Vitamin O were said to be "on file with author." Articles listed were from obscure publications. The Website even referenced the writings of Joseph Priestley, who discovered oxygen in 1774, though these clearly had nothing to do with how Vitamin O is supposed to work.
- Don't let some explanation that sounds scientific fool you. Vitamin O ads referred to their new form of oxygen as "mono-atomic oxygen molecules" comprised of two oxygen atoms. A "mono-atomic" substance contains only a single atom and cannot be a "molecule," which has at least two atoms bonded together. Some of the Vitamin O explanations sounded highly technical but could have been seen to be false by anyone who checked them against the content of any elementary science course.

- Unnecessary use of technical language should alert you to be cautious. With fraudulent medical schemes, technical language is used to impress customers, not to inform them.

Recommendations

If you want to get more oxygen into your body, breathe it in. "Vitamin O" and its related products will give you no extra oxygen. Don't get taken in by this sort of "quick-fix remedy" for the many difficult and often painful illnesses of life. This product and its promotional materials demonstrate how important it is to critically evaluate any product before you spend money on it.

Treatment Categories

Quackery and Fraud

Further Reading

BIO2 International, Inc. Technical White Paper: "Vitamin O® Fact Sheet," at *www.rgar-den.com/vitamino.htm* (accessed March 23, 2001).

Federal Trade Commission press release (May 1, 2000) at *www.ftc.gov/opa/2000/05/rose-creek2.htm* (accessed March 23, 2001).

Jellin, Jeff M., Forrest Batz, and Kathy Hichens, *Pharmacist's Letter/Prescriber's Letter: Natural Medicines Comprehensive Database* (Stockton, Calif.: Therapeutic Research Facility, 1999), 950.

"Vitamin O and False Advertisment," [*sic*] *FDA Dietary Supplements* 1, no. 2 (March 1999): 5–8.

WILD YAM

What It Is

Wild yam *(Dioscorea villosa)* is a climbing vine that grows in the wet woodlands of North and Central America. Historically, it was very important as the sole source of steroids used to make contraceptive hormones, cortisone, and anabolic hormones. These pharmaceutical drugs are now made from other starting materials, but wild yam remains of interest as a natural source of steroids. Other species of wild yam are also used, including *Dioscorea floribunda, Dioscorea composita, Dioscorea mexicana* (also called *Dioscorea macrostachya*).

Claims

Hundreds of yam species exist worldwide and a number of cultures have discovered medicinal applications. The Chinese, for example, have long used a yam species as a liver tonic, digestive aid, and muscle relaxant. Ayurvedic practitioners in India have used a yam species as a remedy for impotence and infertility. Wild yam is also known as colic root because of its antispasmodic action. In some cultures it is a folk remedy for diverticulitis, nausea during pregnancy, and flatulence.

Modern uses include reduction of the symptoms of PMS and to alleviate discomforts associated with menopause. It is often taken to relieve menstrual or uterine cramps. Wild yam is said to promote the secretion of bile and may help to alleviate liver ailments. The herb is believed by some to have anti-inflammatory properties that make it useful against rheumatoid arthritis and other conditions. Others use it to prevent or treat indigestion.

Wild yam contains DHEA, which is the source of much publicity and controversy in its own right (see DHEA, page 338). Wild yam is recommended for many of the same conditions as DHEA, such as AIDS, cancer, chronic fatigue syndrome, fibromyalgia syndrome, multiple sclerosis, and various psychological disorders.

Study Findings

Studies of pure DHEA are starting to produce interesting results that may lead to it having a role in the treatment of some conditions. Another constituent of wild yam is dioscin, which has been shown to have anti-inflammatory activity.

The existence of DHEA and dioscin in wild yam is not the same as using either of these constituents alone. Taking either of these pure compounds is quite different from consuming wild yam, and we cannot expect the same results. For example, it is possible that long-term testing will show one form to be valuable and the other not of value.

Scientists recently tested a wild yam extract to see whether it increased blood levels of DHEA. After three weeks of *Dioscorea* supplementation, researchers found (✘✘) no effect on levels of DHEA. The researchers did find (✔✔), however, that *Dioscorea* has significant antioxidant activity and was associated with increased levels of the "good" HDL cholesterol and reduced levels of certain blood fats.

Scientists in Texas studied (✔✔) fifty patients diagnosed with fibromyalgia and/or chronic fatigue syndrome who had received some form of medical treatment without experiencing enduring success. Subjects who consumed nutritional supplements including a *Dioscorea* complex experienced, according to the researchers, "a remarkable reduction in initial symptom severity, with continued improvement in the period between initial assessment and the follow-up." However, there is no way to know if the effect was from *Dioscorea* or the other supplements.

While these products contain active steroids, how they interact with one another and impact the body as a whole is not clear.

Cautions

Preparations made from wild yam show all the natural variability of any herbal remedy and have the same lack of standardization as other dietary supplements. Given that steroids are very active in the body, often at very low concentrations, taking them in herbal remedies is risky due to the variability in dosages. These products have produced numerous side effects, all typical of steroids: acne, hair loss, headache, menstrual irregularities, and (in women) development of male voice and hair patterns.

A number of cancers have been shown to be stimulated by steroid hormones, so wild yam should be completely avoided by anyone with a family history of breast, ovarian, uterine, or prostate cancer. Wild yam should not be taken orally during pregnancy as the steroids may adversely affect fetal development.

There is insufficient information to determine if wild yam is safe when applied topically during pregnancy or lactation, therefore it should be avoided by these women.

Recommendations

Wild yam has played an important role in the development of steroid pharmaceuticals. Steroids are powerful drugs, actively involved in many different bodily functions. They are also active in very small quantities. There is much uncertainty about how much of any particular steroid may be in any particular wild yam product. Given that these wild yam products have not been shown to be effective for any particular disease, their potential side effects do not warrant their use.

When appropriate and necessary, standardized pharmaceutical steroid products should be used since they are readily available and not overly expensive.

Dosage

Some products recommend 2 to 4 grams three times a day, although recommendations vary widely.

Treatment Categories

Complementary Therapy
    Chronic fatigue syndrome   ☹
    Fibromyalgia   ☹

Scientifically Unproven
    Other indications   ☹☹

Further Reading

Fetrow, Charles W., and Juan R. Avila, *Professional's Handbook of Complementary and Alternative Medicine* (Springhouse, Penn.: Springhouse, 1999), 666–68.

Jellin, Jeff M., Forrest Batz, and Kathy Hichens, *Pharmacist's Letter/Prescriber's Letter: Natural Medicines Comprehensive Database* (Stockton, Calif.: Therapeutic Research Facility, 1999), 979–80.

WILLOW BARK

What It Is

Willow bark tea was the drink of choice of those who overindulged on the early wines and beer, as well as those suffering from arthritis. Although the ancients didn't know they were getting salicylic acid from the tea, that ingredient probably was the reason for the early popularity of willow bark tea. We now know it was the forerunner of aspirin (acetyl-salicylic acid).

Willow bark has been used as an anti-inflammatory at least since the time of ancient Egypt. Both the white willow *(Salix alba),* native to Europe but now growing widely in the United States, and the black willow *(Salix nigra),* native to North America, have bark used in powdered form or extracted with alcohol to make a tincture. A number of other *Salix* species are also used.

Claims

Various cultures around the world have been known to use willow bark medicinally, not only for its pain-relieving and fever-reducing properties but also as a digestive tonic. The ancient Chinese, Hippocrates and other Greek physicians, and the Romans all recommended willow bark remedies. Native American tribes were using willow species for pain and fever by the seventeenth century and probably knew of these medicinal effects before the arrival of Europeans.

Willow bark was a popular remedy among Colonial Americans to reduce inflammation and fever and to treat ailments ranging from gout to food poisoning. Willow leaves were also sometimes used in remedies for colic and other conditions. Ointments with willow bark were used topically for cuts and burns.

Modern uses for willow bark still rely on its aspirin-like effects, though it is considered milder and slower acting than aspirin. As a pain reliever, willow bark is said to alleviate muscle aches, tension headache, and arthritis.

Because studies have found that aspirin works as a thermogenic (heat-creating and calorie-burning) agent synergistically with caffeine and ephedrine, willow bark is sometimes included in weight-loss formulas. Willow bark is also believed to help prevent or treat bursitis, rheumatism, nerve pain, and many other diseases involving tissue inflammation.

Study Findings

Swedish scientists investigated more than fifty plants that are used in traditional Swedish medicine to treat inflammatory diseases and wounds. The goat willow *(Salix caprea)* was among the half-dozen plants that prevented a number of biochemical reactions that are involved in causing inflammation. Willow bark contains a compound called "salicin" in low levels (1 to 2 percent). The liver and intestines convert salicin into salicylic acid. This group compound is called the salicylates. Salicin, salicylic acid, and aspirin have all been shown to reduce inflammation, lower fever, and relieve pain.

We are aware of no controlled studies of the use of willow bark products in humans. This probably reflects the widespread use of aspirin, which was developed from extracts of willow bark. Early in the nineteenth century, pure samples of salicylic acid, salicin, and other salicylates were isolated from willow bark. In 1852, salicylic acid was chemically manufactured from other, readily available compounds, thus eliminating the need to use plant material. In 1899, the German company Bayer chemically modified salicylic acid to make a form less irritating to the stomach: aspirin. This represented one of the first successes for pharmacognosy, the science of taking an herbal remedy, identifying the active ingredient, and chemically producing a form that was better tolerated and more readily available. Aspirin has been extensively studied in human trials, with the results in many ways validating the traditional uses of willow bark.

Cautions

Aspirin, and all salicylates, can have some adverse effects and drug interactions. These also apply to willow bark. They can be irritating to the stomach, and a condition known as salicylate toxicity can develop (nausea, vomiting, diarrhea, dizziness, and lethargy). Some people are hypersensitive to salicylates, and people with a history of allergies or asthma should avoid using willow bark products.

Willow bark shouldn't be given to children who have a fever that may be due to certain viral illnesses, including chicken pox or influenza, because of the risk of Reye's syndrome. Willow bark should also be avoided by pregnant women and anyone with ulcers. Side effects are infrequent but may include nausea, diarrhea, and digestive upset. Excessive long-term use could cause stomach ulcers.

Aspirin slows blood clotting, and it is now recommended for some people at risk of strokes (caused by blood clots). However, if someone is already taking anticoagulant medication, using willow bark products may increase the risk of bleeding.

The Natural Database rates willow bark "Possibly Unsafe" in lactation. It is rated "Possibly Unsafe" during childhood because it theoretically could cause Reye's syndrome (as does aspirin in children under seventeen years of age who take aspirin during viral infections, such as influenza or chicken pox). It is recommended that willow bark not be taken during lactation due to inadequate information to establish its safety.

Recommendations

While modern research has validated the traditional uses of willow bark, this doesn't mean that taking willow bark instead of aspirin is the best thing to do. Willow bark, like all other herbs and plants, varies in the concentrations of active ingredients, depending on when and how it is harvested, stored, and processed. Since aspirin is widely available, inexpensive, and standardized, it should always be used by those taking these products for extended periods. For occasional use in relieving headaches or other aches and pains, willow bark is an effective and safe alternative.

Dosage

Usually 120 to 240 mg salicin is recommended per day, although products vary considerably in their strengths.

Treatment Categories

Complementary Therapy

Pain in adults	☺☺
Soft tissue inflammation in adults	☺☺
Headaches in adults	☺☺
Fever in adults	☺☺
Warning: Do not use in children under seventeen years of age	☹☹☹☹

Further Reading

Fetrow, Charles W., and Juan R. Avila, *Professional's Handbook of Complementary and Alternative Medicine* (Springhouse, Penn.: Springhouse, 1999), 669–71.

Jellin, Jeff M., Forrest Batz, and Kathy Hichens, *Pharmacist's Letter/Prescriber's Letter: Natural Medicines Comprehensive Database* (Stockton, Calif.: Therapeutic Research Facility, 1999), 981–82.

WITCH HAZEL

What It Is

Witch hazel, or *Hamamelis virginiana*, is a small tree, native to North America. It forms distinctive yellow treadlike flowers in the fall while other trees are losing their leaves. Hamamelis water, a witch hazel extract used medicinally, is made by passing steam through the plant parts and adding alcohol to keep the cooled material soluble.

Claims

An extract of witch hazel was used by Native Americans to reduce inflammation and as an astringent for the treatment of diarrhea, hemorrhoids, and a variety of skin conditions. All astringents contract tissues and thus reduce fluid secretions. In Europe, an alcohol witch hazel extract is recommended for the treatment of varicose veins.

The Iroquois, Cherokee, Chippewa, and other Native Americans had multiple uses for witch hazel, employing it as a chew stick, in steam baths, as a gargle, and to make teas and poultices. The tea would be drunk or gargled for relief of colds, flu, and sore throat. Witch hazel was also taken internally for diarrhea, internal bleeding, and menstrual pain. Topical remedies were used to stop minor bleeding or soothe insect bites, sunburn, and poison ivy. Witch hazel also helped relieve the pain and inflammation of sore backs and muscle pain.

Another traditional topical use is to add witch hazel extract to cold water to cool a victim of heatstroke. Witch hazel was used to make eyewashes. The herb became a common ingredient in patent medicines of the nineteenth century and was the active ingredient in the popular Pond's Extract.

Many of witch hazel's topical uses remain popular today. Astringent compounds in witch hazel are believed to stem bleeding, whether from abrasions or from minor cuts like shaving nicks. Witch hazel is said to reduce the pain and swelling of hemorrhoids and bruises. Many people use witch hazel pads, small pieces of thin cloth packaged in a witch hazel solution, to cool sunburn and other minor burns, to help relieve the itching of insect bites and poison ivy, and to dry out cold sores. Witch hazel is used as a remedy for varicose veins and other venous conditions. Hospital personnel use witch hazel pads to soothe the itching and burning of rectal or vaginal surgical stitches.

Some companies sell witch hazel in teething preparations. Witch hazel is also said to help to prevent or treat inflammations of the mouth, eczema, skin ulcers, and bedsores.

Study Findings

Some studies have been done on the compounds extracted from witch hazel. The astringent compounds are called "tannins." Alcohol extracts of witch hazel leaves contain the highest concentration of tannins. However, the most commonly available preparations are made by steam distillation to which alcohol is later added. These contain no tannins. Since alcohol is an astringent, this may account for any observed astringent activity of these preparations.

German scientists determined that a witch hazel bark extract exhibited significant antiviral activity against herpes simplex type 1. Witch hazel was also shown to have antioxidant and anti-inflammatory properties. Japanese researchers tested sixty-five plant extracts (✔) for antioxidant activity. Witch hazel was one of two herbs (the other being horse chestnut) found to have strong free-radical scavenging activity. The researchers concluded that these herbs were likely candidates for use in antiaging or antiwrinkle products for protecting the skin—although no clinical trials have been completed. An extract of horse chestnut seeds (*Aesculus hippocastanum*) is quickly becoming popular in topical preparations to improve blood flow in the veins. Some studies (✔✔✔) support this.

In one of the few controlled human trials (✔✔✔) of witch hazel's anti-inflammatory properties, an after-sun lotion containing witch hazel was shown to protect the skin from ultraviolet-induced inflammation and redness.

Cautions

Topical use of witch hazel is very safe, although it may on rare occasions cause minor skin irritations. "Witch hazel water" and other commercial products are often for external use only. Drinking witch hazel tea is thought to be relatively safe, with one drawback being the possibility that when taken internally, the high level of tannins may cause nausea, vomiting, or constipation (✘✘). There is some concern they may also cause liver damage. Since there is insufficient reliable information on which to judge its safety, the Natural Database recommends that it be avoided during pregnancy and lactation.

Recommendations

Alcohol extracts of witch hazel may have some value as astringents, but this is not a readily available form of the remedy. Varro Tyler quotes from a 1947 pharmacy manual: "Hamamelis [witch hazel] is so nearly destitute of medicinal virtues that it scarcely deserves official recognition." He claims it would be better to use red wine as an astringent since it does contain tannins, and about as much alcohol as witch hazel extract. Witch hazel preparations appear to bring relief for different skin injuries, though we question whether this is due to witch hazel or the other ingredients in the preparations—or even the pad itself. Regardless, when used externally, these are safe. Conventional therapies should be pursued if the irritation persists or worsens in any way.

Dosage

A tea made from 2 grams of dried leaves is taken three times a day. The extract is used to make creams and various preparations and pads for topical application.

Treatment Categories

Conventional Therapy
Itching and burning of anorectal disorders
and external hemorrhoids ☺☺
As an antiseptic for mild skin injury ☺☺

Complementary Therapy
Fever blisters, sunburn, varicose veins ☺

Scientifically Unproven
    Any internal use   ☺
    Other indications

Further Reading

Foster, Steven, and Varro E. Tyler, *Tyler's Honest Herbal: A Sensible Guide to the Use of Herbs and Related Remedies*, 4th ed. (New York: Haworth Herbal Press, 1999), 383–85.

Jellin, Jeff M., Forrest Batz, and Kathy Hichens, *Pharmacist's Letter/Prescriber's Letter: Natural Medicines Comprehensive Database* (Stockton, Calif.: Therapeutic Research Facility, 1999), 988–90.

ZINC

What It Is

Zinc is a naturally occurring mineral that is required in the diet. In the body, it is incorporated into a number of enzymes that are involved in a variety of reactions throughout the body. Zinc deficiencies are rare and occur primarily when other problems prevent the absorption of zinc from the intestines. Deficiencies lead to skin problems, diarrhea, problems with the immune system, and failure to thrive among babies. Zinc is present in legumes, grains, peanuts, and many meats. Both meat eaters and vegetarians generally get enough of the mineral in their diet.

Claims

Zinc supplements have been recommended for acne, diabetes, high blood pressure, ulcers, enlarged prostates, and to fight off infections. The most recent interest in zinc has been as lozenges to cure the common cold, but prior to that, zinc supplements were widely taken by people who were HIV positive.

Study Findings

Zinc lozenges have been popularly advertised as an effective way to treat the common cold. However, numerous clinical trials (✗✗✗✗) have failed to back up these claims, at least when lozenges with lower doses (less than 5 mg) are used. Meta-analyses in 1997 and again in 2000 concluded that while there had been at least eight randomized, controlled trials in this area, the results were very weak. Given the side effects discussed below, both reviews concluded that zinc lozenges should not be recommended for the common cold.

However, a small number of studies continue to report positive results for zinc lozenges, including the most recent one (✔✔✔) we examined at the end of 2000. Positive effects seem most clear for reducing cough symptoms. In those studies with positive effects, the zinc lozenges contained 13.3 to 23 mg of zinc, whereas some of the negative studies used lozenges containing about 5 mg each. Although the evidence is still unclear, the higher-dose lozenges do appear to somewhat reduce the duration of cold symptoms.

There is much more clear evidence that zinc is beneficial for enhancing wound healing. Taken before and after surgery, zinc supplements have been shown in numerous studies (✔✔✔✔) to speed recovery time and reduce the incidence of postoperative complications, such as wound infections. In some studies (✔✔✔✔), the hospital stay has been reduced by more than half. Zinc may be helpful in speeding healing after burns or injury. The results seem to be particularly pronounced when there is zinc deficiency prior to the treatment. In many of the wound-healing studies, zinc dosages of 150 mg per day were used. It is possible that lower amounts, even 30 to 60 mg per day, would produce these effects.

Zinc has been said to be useful in treating such skin problems as boils, bedsores, general dermatitis, and acne; however, research (✔✔✔) on zinc and acne shows variable results. Leg ulcers have healed more rapidly with zinc treatment in a dose of 150 mg per day. Gastric ulcers have responded favorably to zinc in a similar dosage. Psoriasis (✔✔) is even occasionally responsive to zinc supplementation. White spots on the fingernails, which can be a result of zinc deficiency, may respond also to zinc treatment. Cataracts have been associated with zinc deficiency in some individuals and have been helped by treatment.

For male prostate problems, there is no compelling scientific evidence (✘✘) that zinc works. There is some suggestion that the prostate enlargement that comes with age, termed benign prostatic hyperplasia (BPH), is related to low zinc (and cadmium toxicity), and that regular zinc supplementation may prevent this common problem. More research is needed to clearly evaluate zinc's relationship to prostate health.

Zinc may also be beneficial in rheumatoid arthritis, for which it has been shown (✔✔) to reduce symptoms in some patients. Zinc treatment may help (✔) with the loss of taste sensation that comes from zinc deficiency.

Use of zinc by people infected with HIV became popular after it was noticed that many infected people had lower than normal zinc levels. Since zinc deficiency is known to adversely affect the immune system, it was logical to conclude that supplements might help those with HIV. However, studies have now shown (✘✘✘) that HIV patients taking zinc supplements were twice as likely to develop AIDS and more likely to die sooner. The reasons for these connections are not known.

Cautions

Zinc lozenges have a really bad taste, yet they are to be taken every two hours or so. The taste is so bad that about one-third of the research subjects had nausea, and about 10 percent had diarrhea.

High doses of zinc have been found to negatively impact the immune system and to lower HDL levels (which can lead to higher blood cholesterol levels), and hinder the absorption of copper (another essential element). The Tolerable Upper Intake Limit is 40 mg per day for adults, which would quickly be exceeded taking high dose lozenges every two hours. The upper limit for children ranges from 4 mg per day during the first six months to 23 mg for nine- to thirteen-year-olds and 34 mg for adolescents.

Zinc, when used at the recommended dietary allowances (RDA) during pregnancy and lactation, has been rated "Likely Safe" by the Natural Database. It is "Unsafe" when taken in large doses during pregnancy

Recommendations

There is no evidence to suggest that low-dose (less than 10 mg) zinc supplements help relieve or shorten cold symptoms. High zinc intake can also have adverse effects, especially in HIV-infected patients. Taking more zinc than is present in a healthy diet is presently unwarranted. However, zinc supplementation can help a variety of disorders in people deficient in this trace element.

Dosage

Most lozenges contain 9 to 24 mg zinc, with one being recommended every two hours. The new RDA recommended by the Institute of Medicine in 2001 is 11 mg per day for men and 8 mg per day for women. Vegetarians require an additional 50 percent because chemicals commonly found in plants hinder the absorption of zinc. Pregnant and breast-feeding women should increase their consumption of zinc by a few milligrams per day, but should discuss dosage with a physician.

Treatment Categories

Conventional Therapy
    Zinc deficiency ☺☺☺☺

Complementary Therapy
    Zinc lozenges in doses of greater than 13.3 mg to reduce
        the duration of symptoms for the common cold in adults ☺
    Oral supplements for the prevention or treatment of BPH ☺
    Enhance wound healing ☺☺
    Topically with the antibiotic erythromycin for acne ☺
    Rheumatoid arthritis symptoms ☺
    Zinc lozenges in doses of less than 5 mg to treat
        the common cold in adults ☹☹
    Zinc lozenges should not be given to children or adolescents
        in any dose to treat the common cold ☹☹

Scientifically Unproven
    Other indications

Further Reading

Jackson, Jeffrey L., Cecily Peterson, and Emil Lesho, "A Meta-Analysis of Zinc Salts Lozenges and the Common Cold," *Archives of Internal Medicine* 157 (1997): 2373–76.

Jellin, Jeff M., Forrest Batz, and Kathy Hichens, *Pharmacist's Letter/Prescriber's Letter: Natural Medicines Comprehensive Database* (Stockton, Calif.: Therapeutic Research Facility, 1999), 1012–14.

Marshall, I., "Zinc for the Common Cold (Cochrane Review)," in *The Cochrane Library* (Oxford: Update Software, 2000), Issue 4.

14

Effectiveness of Therapies: Listed by Disease or Symptom

This table shows the authors' rating for the effectiveness of each therapy, herb, vitamin, or supplement, listed alphabetically by disease, condition, or symptom.

For more information on any of the author-rated therapies, see the listing for that therapy. Therapies or remedies for which insufficient evidence exists for a reliable recommendation are not included in this section. Before acting on these recommendations, please read the complete entry. This chapter is intended to guide you to the evidence discussed in each entry.

The Key: Reader Guide

Since the evidence for any particular therapy can include evidence that not only supports its benefits but also shows its potential for harm, we have compiled a single guide that we hope will be useful. This rating is our "best estimate" of the benefit or harm of any particular therapy for any particular indication. Others could (and often do) look at the same evidence and derive different conclusions:

☺☺☺☺ 75%–100% confidence that the therapy is potentially beneficial

☺☺☺ 50%–74% confidence that the therapy is potentially beneficial

☺☺ 25%–49% confidence that the therapy is potentially beneficial

☺ 0%–24% confidence that the therapy is potentially beneficial

☹ 0%–24% confidence that the therapy is of no benefit or potentially harmful

☹☹ 25%–49% confidence that the therapy is of no benefit or potentially harmful

☹☹☹ 50%–74% confidence that the therapy is of no benefit or potentially harmful

☹☹☹☹ 75%–100% confidence that the therapy is of no benefit or potentially harmful

Disease, Condition, or Symptom

AIDS

☹☹☹ St. John's wort, Therapeutic Touch
☹☹☹☹ chaparral

ACNE

☺ tea tree oil (topical), witch hazel, zinc
☹☹☹☹ aloe

ALLERGIES

☹☹ megavitamin therapy
☹☹☹ applied kinesiology, colonics, homeopathy
☹☹☹☹ iridology, Qigong, Reiki, shamanism

ALTITUDE SICKNESS (SEE MOUNTAIN SICKNESS)

ALZHEIMER'S DISEASE

☺☺☺ ginkgo biloba
☺☺ milk thistle, vitamin E (prevention)
☺ evening primrose oil

ANGINA

☺☺ Coenzyme Q_{10}
☹☹ bilberry, megavitamin therapy
☹☹☹ homeopathy
☹☹☹☹ chelation, comfrey, iridology, Qigong, Reiki, shamanism

ANXIETY

☺☺☺☺ aromatherapy, biofeedback, massage therapy, meditation, Shiatsu massage, visualization
☺☺☺ kava, reflexology, Tai Chi, yoga
☺☺ chamomile, St. John's wort
☺ valerian
☹☹ megavitamin therapy
☹☹☹ colonics, homeopathy
☹☹☹☹ iridology, Qigong, Reiki, shamanism

ARTHRITIS

☺☺☺☺ capsaicin (topically), chondroitin sulfate
☺☺☺ evening primrose oil, glucosamine
☺☺ willow bark
☺ ginger, honeybee venom, selenium
☹ magnet therapy
☹☹ bilberry, black cohosh, craniosacral therapy, megavitamin therapy
☹☹☹ colonics, homeopathy
☹☹☹☹ aloe, chaparral, iridology, Qigong, Reiki, shamanism

ATHLETE'S FOOT

    ☺☺ tea tree oil

ATHLETIC PERFORMANCE ENHANCEMENT

    ☺☺☺ creatine (during brief high-intensity anaerobic exercise)
    ☺ creatine (possibly increasing muscle mass)
    ☹ pyruvate
    ☹☹ Coenzyme Q_{10}, DHEA, ginseng
    ☹☹☹ androstenedine, chromium, creatine (for recreational or aerobic exercise or for increasing endurance or improving performance in most highly trained athletes)
    ☹☹☹☹ ephedra

ASTHMA

    ☺☺ yoga
    ☺ ginkgo biloba
    ☹☹ acupuncture, megavitamin therapy
    ☹☹☹ aromatherapy, colonics, evening primrose oil, homeopathy
    ☹☹☹☹ aloe, iridology, Qigong, reflexology, Reiki, shamanism

BACK PAIN

    ☺☺☺☺ chiropractic, massage therapy, Shiatsu massage
    ☺☺ biofeedback, meditation
    ☺ reflexology
    ☹☹ acupuncture, craniosacral therapy, magnet therapy, megavitamin therapy
    ☹☹☹ colonics, homeopathy
    ☹☹☹☹ iridology, Qigong, Reiki, shamanism

BENIGN PROSTATIC HYPERPLASIA (BPH)

    ☺☺☺☺ saw palmetto
    ☺ zinc
    ☹ magnet therapy
    ☹☹ megavitamin therapy
    ☹☹☹☹ Reiki, shamanism

BREAST PAIN (MASTALGIA)

    ☺☺☺ evening primrose oil

BRUISES

    ☺ St. John's wort (topical)
    ☹ comfrey (topical)

BURNS (MILD)

    ☺☺☺ aloe
    ☺ St. John's wort (topical), witch hazel

CANCER

- ☺☺☺☺ diet and nutrition (for prevention)
- ☺☺☺ selenium (for prevention), vitamin C (in food sources, as a cancer preventive)
- ☺ vitamin C (supplement, as a cancer preventive), vitamin E
- ☹ magnet therapy
- ☹☹ megavitamin therapy
- ☹☹☹ Gerson diet therapy, homeopathy, macrobiotic diet
- ☹☹☹☹ chaparral, comfrey, iridology, Qigong, Reiki, shamanism, shark cartilage

CATARACTS

- ☹☹ bilberry

CHEMOTHERAPY–INDUCED NAUSEA

- ☺ ginger

CHOLESTEROL, HIGH

- ☺☺☺☺ diet and nutrition, red yeast rice
- ☺ chromium, evening primrose oil, garlic
- ☹ ginseng, pyruvate
- ☹☹ Tai Chi

CHRONIC FATIGUE SYNDROME (CFS OR CFIDS)

- ☹ wild yam

CLAUDICATION

- ☺☺ ginkgo biloba

COLDS

- ☺☺☺ echinacea (to alleviate symptoms)
- ☺ vitamin C (to alleviate symptoms), zinc (high-dose lozenges in adults)
- ☹ vitamin C (for prevention)
- ☹☹ black cohosh, echinacea (for prevention), megavitamin therapy
- ☹☹☹ goldenseal, homeopathy
- ☹☹☹☹ chaparral, comfrey, iridology, reflexology, Reiki, shamanism

COLIC

- ☺ chamomile
- ☹☹☹☹ aloe

COLITIS

- ☺ evening primrose oil (ulcerative colitis)
- ☹☹ megavitamin therapy
- ☹☹☹ colonics, homeopathy
- ☹☹☹☹ iridology, Qigong, reflexology, Reiki, shamanism

CONSTIPATION

- ☺☺☺☺ aloe, colonics, diet and nutrition, senna

CORONARY ARTERY DISEASE

☺☺☺☺   diet and nutrition
☺☺   Coenzyme Q$_{10,}$ hawthorn
☹☹   megavitamin therapy
☹☹☹   homeopathy
☹☹☹☹   chelation, iridology, Qigong, reflexology, Reiki, shamanism

DENTAL PAIN

☺☺☺☺   acupuncture
☺☺   willow bark

DEPRESSION

☺☺☺☺   light therapy, St. John's wort
☺   evening primrose oil
☹   DHEA, magnet therapy
☹☹   craniosacral therapy, megavitamin therapy
☹☹☹   colonics, homeopathy, Therapeutic Touch
☹☹☹☹   aloe, iridology, Qigong, reflexology, Reiki, shamanism

DIABETES

☺☺☺☺   diet and nutrition
☺☺☺   chromium
☺☺   ginseng
☺   bilberry, burdock, evening primrose oil
☹   Coenzyme Q$_{10}$
☹☹   megavitamin therapy
☹☹☹   homeopathy
☹☹☹☹   aloe, iridology, Qigong, reflexology, Reiki, shamanism

DIARRHEA

☺☺   bilberry
☹☹☹   goldenseal, homeopathy
☹☹☹☹   comfrey

DIZZINESS ASSOCIATED WITH VASCULAR DISEASE

☺☺   ginkgo biloba

ECZEMA

☺☺   evening primrose oil
☹☹☹☹   aloe

ENERGY IMPROVEMENT

☺☺☺☺   diet and nutrition
☺   ginseng
☹☹   chromium
☹☹☹   androstenedione

ERECTILE DYSFUNCTION

☹ DHEA
☹☹☹☹ reflexology, Reiki, shamanism

FEVER

☺☺ willow bark (in adults)
☹☹☹ colonics, homeopathy, Therapeutic Touch
☹☹☹☹ willow bark (in children with viral infections)

FIBROMYALGIA SYNDROME

☺☺ willow bark (for pain)
☺ honeybee venom
☹ wild yam

FLU

☺☺ echinacea
☺ elderberry (European)
☹☹ megavitamin therapy
☹☹☹ goldenseal, homeopathy
☹☹☹☹ reflexology, Reiki, shamanism, willow bark (for children)

GOUT (SEE ARTHRITIS)

HEADACHE (VARIOUS)

☺☺☺ acupressure, biofeedback, hypnosis, massage therapy, meditation, Shiatsu massage
☺☺ acupuncture, gingko biloba, willow bark
☺ reflexology
☹ magnet therapy
☹☹ megavitamin therapy
☹☹☹ colonics, homeopathy
☹☹☹☹ iridology, Qigong, Reiki, shamanism

HEART DISEASE

☺☺☺☺ diet and nutrition
☺☺ hawthorn
☺ evening primrose oil, ginseng, grape seed extract, vitamin E
☹☹ bilberry, megavitamin therapy
☹☹☹ chelation, colonics, homeopathy
☹☹☹☹ iridology, Qigong, reflexology, Reiki, shamanism

HEART FAILURE (CONGESTIVE HEART FAILURE)

☺☺ Coenzyme Q_{10}
☺ ginseng

HEAVY METAL POISONING

☺☺☺☺ chelation

HEMORRHOIDS

☺☺☺☺ senna (for constipation)

☺☺ witch hazel (for burning and itching)

HEPATITIS

☺☺ milk thistle

☺ licorice

HIGH BLOOD PRESSURE

☺☺☺☺ biofeedback, meditation

☺☺☺ diet and nutrition, Tai Chi

☺ Coenzyme Q_{10}, garlic

☹☹ chromium, megavitamin therapy

☹☹☹ colonics, homeopathy, Therapeutic Touch

☹☹☹☹ chelation, iridology, Qigong, reflexology, Reiki, shamanism

HOT FLASHES

☺☺☺ black cohosh

☹ DHEA

HUNTINGTON'S DISEASE

☹ Coenzyme Q_{10}

INCONTINENCE

☺☺ biofeedback

INSECT BITES

☺☺☺ aloe, marigold

IRRITABLE BOWEL SYNDROME (IBS)

☺☺ evening primrose oil (IBS exacerbated by PMS)

☹☹☹☹ aloe

LABOR PAIN

☺☺☺ hypnosis

LEARNING DISABILITIES

☹☹ craniosacral therapy, megavitamin therapy

☹☹☹ colonics, homeopathy

☹☹☹☹ chelation, iridology, Qigong, reflexology, Reiki, shamanism

MACULAR DEGENERATION

☺☺ bilberry

MEMORY LOSS, AGE-RELATED

☺☺☺ ginkgo biloba

☺ ginseng

MENOPAUSE SYMPTOMS

☺☺☺ black cohosh
☹ DHEA

MENSTRUAL PROBLEMS

☺☺ black cohosh
☹☹☹ aloe, comfrey

MERCURY POISONING

☺☺☺☺ chelation

MIGRAINE HEADACHE

☺☺☺ biofeedback, feverfew (for prevention), hypnosis, meditation, Shiatsu massage
☺☺ willow bark
☺ reflexology
☹ feverfew (for treatment), magnet therapy
☹☹ megavitamin therapy
☹☹☹ colonics, homeopathy
☹☹☹☹ Reiki, shamanism

MORNING SICKNESS

☺☺☺☺ acupressure
☹ ginger
☹☹ megavitamin therapy
☹☹☹ homeopathy

MOTION SICKNESS

☺ ginger

MOUNTAIN SICKNESS PREVENTION

☺☺ ginkgo biloba

MULTIPLE SCLEROSIS

☹ honeybee venom
☹☹☹☹ aloe

MUSCLE ACHES

☺☺ willow bark
☺ St. John's wort (topical)

MUSCLE STRENGTHENING OR GROWTH

☺ creatine
☹☹ DHEA
☹☹☹ androstenedione

MUSCULAR DYSTROPHY

    ☺   Coenzyme Q$_{10}$

NAIL INFECTIONS (FUNGAL)

    ☺☺   tea tree oil (topical)

NAUSEA

    ☺☺☺☺   acupuncture
    ☺☺☺   acupressure
    ☺   ginger
    ☹☹   megavitamin therapy
    ☹☹☹   homeopathy, Therapeutic Touch
    ☹☹☹☹   iridology, Qigong, reflexology, Reiki, shamanism

NEUROPATHY

    ☺☺☺☺   capsaicin (topically)
    ☺   evening primrose oil (diabetic neuropathy)

OSTEOARTHRITIS (SEE ARTHRITIS)

OSTEOPOROSIS

    ☹   DHEA

PAIN (ACUTE OR CHRONIC)

    ☺☺☺   hypnosis, massage therapy, meditation
    ☺☺   aromatherapy, biofeedback, massage therapy, Shiatsu massage, willow bark, yoga
    ☺   reflexology, senna
    ☹   magnet therapy
    ☹☹   craniosacral therapy, megavitamin therapy
    ☹☹☹   homeopathy
    ☹☹☹☹   iridology, Qigong, Reiki, shamanism

PERIPHERAL ARTERIAL DISEASE

    ☺☺☺   ginkgo biloba
    ☹☹   megavitamin therapy
    ☹☹☹☹   chelation, iridology, Qigong, Reiki, shamanism

POSTOPERATIVE NAUSEA

    ☺   ginger

PREMENSTRUAL SYNDROME

    ☺☺   black cohosh
    ☹☹☹   evening primrose oil
    ☹☹☹   Therapeutic Touch

PROSTATE PROBLEMS (SEE BENIGN PROSTATIC HYPERPLASIA, BPH)

PSORIASIS

- ☺☺☺☺ light therapy
- ☺ capsaicin, zinc
- ☹☹☹ evening primrose oil
- ☹☹☹☹ aloe

RESPIRATORY PROBLEMS

- ☺☺ licorice, massage therapy
- ☹☹ megavitamin therapy
- ☹☹☹☹ comfrey

RHEUMATOID ARTHRITIS (SEE ARTHRITIS)

- ☺☺☺ evening primrose oil
- ☺☺ willow bark
- ☺ ginger, glucosamine, honeybee venom, zinc
- ☹☹ feverfew

RINGWORM

- ☺ tea tree oil (topical)

SEASICKNESS

- ☺☺ ginger

SEIZURES

- ☹☹ megavitamin therapy
- ☹☹☹ colonics, homeopathy
- ☹☹☹☹ aloe, iridology, Qigong, Reiki, shamanism

SEXUAL DYSFUNCTION ASSOCIATED WITH SSRI (SELECTIVE SEROTONIN REUPTAKE INHIBITOR) ANTIDEPRESSENTS

- ☺☺ ginkgo biloba

SJOGREN'S SYNDROME

- ☺ evening primrose oil

SKIN DISORDERS

- ☺☺☺☺ light therapy (in selected disorders, especially psoriasis)
- ☺☺☺ aloe
- ☺☺ chamomile, tea tree oil, witch hazel
- ☹☹ megavitamin therapy
- ☹☹☹ colonics, homeopathy
- ☹☹☹☹ iridology, Qigong, reflexology, Reiki, shamanism

SLEEP

☺☺☺ valerian (for chronic insomnia)
☺☺ chamomile
☺ ginseng
☹☹☹ valerian (for occasional sleep problems)

SMOKING CESSATION

☹☹☹ acupuncture, homeopathy, hypnosis
☹☹☹☹ Reiki, shamanism

SORE THROAT

☺☺ bilberry
☺ slippery elm
☹☹☹ comfey

STRESS, IMPROVED RESPONSE TO

☺☺☺☺ aromatherapy
☺☺ kava
☺ ginseng

STROKE

☹☹ craniosacral therapy, megavitamin therapy
☹☹☹☹ iridology, Qigong, reflexology, Reiki, shamanism

SUNBURN (SEE BURNS, MILD)

TENSION (MUSCLE CONTRACTION)

☺☺☺☺ aromatherapy, biofeedback, massage therapy, meditation
☺☺☺ reflexology, Shiatsu massage, Tai Chi
☺☺ kava, valerian
☹☹ megavitamin therapy
☹☹☹ colonics, homeopathy
☹☹☹☹ iridology, Qigong, Reiki, shamanism

TINNITUS ASSOCIATED WITH VASCULAR DISEASE

☺☺ ginkgo biloba

ULCERS (INTESTINAL)

☺ chamomile, evening primrose oil, licorice, slippery elm, zinc
☹☹☹☹ comfrey, goldenseal, willow bark

URINARY TRACT INFECTION

☺☺ cranberry

VISION PROBLEMS

☺☺ chondroitin, vitamin E
☺ vitamin C
☹☹ bilberry

VOMITING

- ☺☺☺☺ acupuncture
- ☺☺☺ acupressure
- ☹☹☹ homeopathy
- ☹☹☹☹ iridology, Reiki, shamanism

WEIGHT LOSS, DESIRED

- ☺☺☺☺ diet and nutrition, exercise, social support
- ☹☹ hypnosis, megavitamin therapy, pyruvate
- ☹☹☹ colonics, homeopathy
- ☹☹☹☹ acupuncture, chromium, ephedra, iridology, Qigong, reflexology, Reiki, shamanism

WOUNDS, MINOR SKIN

- ☺☺☺ aloe, echinacea (topical), marigold
- ☺☺ chamomile, witch hazel, zinc
- ☺ slippery elm, St. John's wort (topical)
- ☹☹ comfrey

Scripture Index
According to Topics

Subject Index

A

AA. *See* Arachidonic acid

Abortion, caused by: goldenseal, 379; juniper oil, 154; licorice, 392; marigold, 394; parsley seed oil, 154; pennyroyal, 33, 154, 411; slippery elm, 430

ACE inhibitor, 327, 385, 449

Acetylsalicylic acid. *See* Aspirin

Achillea lanulosa. See Yarrow

Achillea millefolium. See Yarrow

Acne: aloe, 293; burdock, 311; chromium, 323; megavitamin therapy, 404; reflexology, 264; tea tree oil, 437; zinc, 462

Acupoint, 145, 146, 147, 272, 281

Acupressure, 144–47, 271, 281

Acupuncture, 76, 139, 147–50, 193, 279, 281

Adam and Eve, 47, 108, 205, 209

Adaptogen, 372

Addiction, treatment of: acupuncture, 147; hypnosis, 226; Reiki, 266

ADD. *See* ADHD

ADHD: martial arts, 82; megavitamin therapy, 404; valerian, 439

Adjustment disorder: kava, 389

Aesculus hippocastanum. See Horse chestnut

Agitated nerves: chamomile, 315; kava, 389

Agoraphobia: kava, 389

Ahaziah, King, 73

AIDS: chaparral, 318; Coenzyme Q_{10}, 326; echinacea, 341; marijuana, 396; prayer, 252; selenium, 422; St. John's wort, 432; Therapeutic Touch, 275; wild yam, 454; zinc, 462

Alcoholism: colonics, 167; milk thistle, 408

Alexander the Great, 293

Alkaloid, 120, 330–31, 347–48, 352

Allantoin, 330

Allergies: acupuncture, 147; applied kinesiology, 150; chiropractic, 163; colonics, 167; echinacea, 341; ephedra, 346; evening primrose, 350; grape seed extract, 381; homeopathy, 222; magnet therapy, 240; megavitamin therapy, 404

Allicin, 358–61

Alliin, 358, 361

Alliinase, 358, 361

Allium sativum. See Garlic

Aloe, 293–95

Aloe barbadensis. See Aloe

Aloe vera. See Aloe

Alpha blockers, 419

Alpha-tocopherol. *See* Vitamin E

Alpine cranberry, 333

Altered states of consciousness (ASC), 77–79, 139, 156, 226, 247, 248, 282, 429, 479

Alternative medicine, definition, 17–18

Altitude sickness: valerian, 439

Alzheimer's disease: antioxidants, 298; chelation therapy, 161; DHEA, 338; ginkgo biloba, 368; milk thistle, 408; vitamin E, 448

Ama, 156

Amanita phalloides, 408

American dwarf palm tree. *See* Saw palmetto

American elder. *See* Elderberry

American ephedra. *See* Ephedra

American ginseng. *See* Ginseng

Amotivation syndrome, 402

Anabolic steroid, 296, 454

Anabolic Steroids Control Act, 295

Analgesic: aromatherapy, 152; evening primrose, 350; kava, 389; marijuana, 396; senna, 425; willow bark, 457

Analgesic cream: capsaicin, 313

Anandamide, 399

Andro. *See* Androstenedione

Androgenic steroid, 296

Androstenedione, 295–98

Stay in Touch and Find Out What Is New!

Thank you for your interest in *Alternative Medicine: The Christian Handbook.* Since the field of alternative medicine is a rapidly growing field, we want you to be informed about the most recent alternative practices and available therapies.

Subscribe to our Email list to:

- Receive current updates on new treatments and remedies
- Gather information about articles and newsletters pertaining to alternative treatments
- Learn more about other Zondervan health related books

Visit *www.zondervan.com/alternativemedicine* to sign up today!

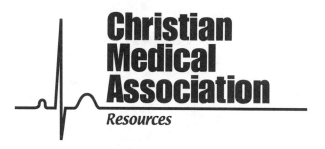

Christian Medical Association Resources

Medically reliable ... biblically sound. That's the rock-solid promise of this dynamic new series offered by Zondervan and the Christian Medical Association. Because when your health is at stake, you can't settle for anything less than the whole truth.

Finally, people of faith can draw from both the knowledge of science and the wisdom of God's Word in addressing health care and medical ethics issues. This series allows you to benefit from cutting-edge knowledge of experienced, trusted, and respected medical scientists and practitioners. Now you can gain their insights into the vital interconnection of health and spirituality—a critical unity largely overlooked by secular science.

While integrating your faith and health can actually improve your physical well-being and even extend your life, it can also help you make health care decisions consistent with your beliefs. A sound biblical analysis of emerging treatments and technologies is essential to protecting yourself from seemingly harmless—yet spiritually, ethically, or medically unsound—options.

Founded in 1931, the Christian Medical Association helps thousands of doctors minister to their patients by imitating the Great Physician, Jesus Christ. Christian Medical Association members provide a Christian voice on medical ethics to policy makers and the media ... minister to needy patients on medical missions around the world ... evangelize and disciple students on more than 90 percent of the nation's medical school campuses ... and provide educational and inspirational resources to the church.

To learn more about Christian Medical Association ministries and resources on health care and ethical issues, browse the Web site at www.christianmedicalassociation.org or call Christian Medical Association Life & Health Resources toll free at 888-231-2637.

> "Dear friend, I pray that you may enjoy good health and that all may go well with you, even as your soul is getting along well."
>
> (3 John 2 NIV)

Jesus, M.D.

A Doctor Examines the Great Physician

David Stevens, M.D.,
with Gregg Lewis

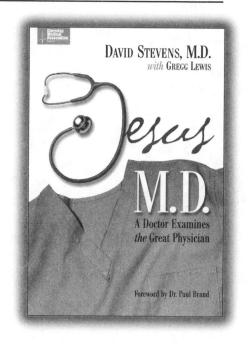

Jesus—the ultimate doctor. His touch extended grace to the sick and sinful of ancient Palestine and left a miracle in its wake. And his ministry hasn't ceased. Today, he looks for willing hearts and hands through which he can heal a needy world.

Dr. David Stevens knows. His eleven years at Tenwek Hospital in Kenya have shown him more than the drama and sacrifice of missionary medicine. In *Jesus, M.D.* Dr. Stevens shares the insights he has gained into the character, power, and purposes of the Great Physician and what it means for *you* to follow in his footsteps.

This is more than a book of dramatic, true-life stories. It is an inspiring and challenging invitation to partner with Jesus in his "practice," accompanying him on his rounds to people whose lives he wants to make whole. Discover how to participate with him in bringing his healing touch to your corner of the world. You don't need a medical education—just determination to trust God as your "attending physician," your mentor, and your source of guidance, discipline, and encouragement.

Dr. Stevens takes you inside stories from the Bible to obtain challenging perspectives and life-changing truths. You'll also get an inside look at life-or-death surgeries; the tense, powerful relationship between resident and attending physicians; the overcrowded patient quarters of a missionary hospital; what it's like to improvise an emergency facial reconstruction; and much more. Best of all, you'll gain surprising insights from the life and methods of Jesus, the ultimate doctor, in his ministry to desperately needy people two thousand years ago . . . and today.

Electrifying, moving, and thought-provoking, *Jesus, M.D.* will help you see your relationship with God and your world in a brand-new light. Your life is filled with incredible possibilities waiting to unfold one by one as you walk in the presence and provision of Dr. Jesus.

Some books address the health of our bodies. Others nurture the mind. A few of them have a story to tell. Still others touch the soul. This one brings all of these strengths with profound and practical wisdom.

Ravi Zacharias
President, Ravi Zacharias
International Ministries

Hardcover 0-310-23433-6

Pick up a copy at your favorite bookstore today!

We want to hear from you. Please send your comments about this book
to us in care of the address below. Thank you.

ZondervanPublishingHouse
Grand Rapids, Michigan 49530
http://www.zondervan.com